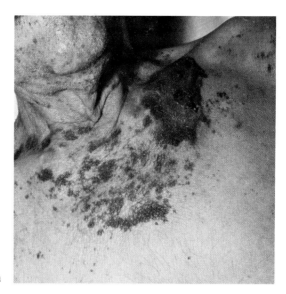

A Purpura

B Scale (psoriasis)

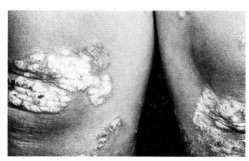

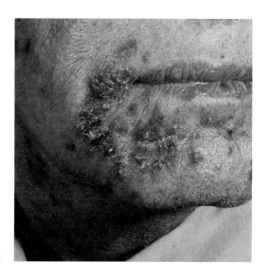

C Crust (impetigo)

dermatology and skin care

dermatology and skin care

John A. Parrish, M.D.

Assistant Professor of Dermatology, Harvard Medical School
Clinical Assistant in Dermatology, Massachusetts General Hospital

McGraw-Hill Book Company

A Blakiston Publication

New York
St. Louis
San Francisco
Aukland
Düsseldorf
Johannesburg
Kuala Lumpur
London
Mexico
Montreal
New Delhi
Panama
Paris
São Paulo
Singapore
Sydney
Tokyo
Toronto

Library of Congress Cataloging in Publication Data

Parrish, John Albert, date
    Dermatology and skin care.

    "A Blakiston publication."
    Includes index.
    1. Dermatology. I. Title. [DNLM: 1. Dermatology—Popular works. WR100 P261d]
RL71.P27   616.5   74-20984
ISBN 0-07-048508-9

NOTICE

Medicine is an ever-changing science. As new research and clinical experience broaden our knowledge, changes in treatment and drug therapy are required. The editors and the publisher of this work have made every effort to ensure that the drug dosage schedules herein are accurate and in accord with the standards accepted at the time for publication. The reader is advised, however, to check the product information sheet included in the package of each drug he plans to administer to be certain that changes have not been made in the recommended dose or in the contraindications for administration. This recommendation is of particular importance in regard to new or infrequently used drugs.

Dermatology and Skin Care

1 2 3 4 5 6 7 8 9 0 D O D O 7 9 8 7 6 5

This book was set in Times Roman by Bi-Comp, Incorporated.
The editors were Cathy Dilworth and Michael Weber;
the cover was designed by Anne Canevari Green;
the production supervisor was Leroy A. Young.
The drawings were done by Gale Cooper, M.D.
R. R. Donnelley & Sons Company was printer and binder.

Contents

	Preface	vii
Chapter 1	Introduction	1
Chapter 2	The Integument	4
Chapter 3	Variations of Normal Skin and Common Incidental Disorders	33
Chapter 4	General Pathologic Descriptions and Mechanisms	51
Chapter 5	Normal and Abnormal Reactions of Skin	70
Chapter 6	Tools and Laboratory Tests Used in Evaluating and Treating the Skin	99
Chapter 7	Common Dermatoses of Otherwise Well People	111
Chapter 8	Infection and Infestation	146
Chapter 9	Disorders of Mucous Membranes	184
Chapter 10	Skin Cancer	201
Chapter 11	Cutaneous Signs of Systemic Disease	214
Chapter 12	Blisters, Ulcers, and Bedsores	238
Chapter 13	The Psychological Importance of Skin	257
Chapter 14	Principles of Dermatologic Therapy	276
	Index	289

COLOR PLATES   Front Endpapers

Color Plate I
   A Hives
   B Telangiectasia
   C Petechiae

Color Plate II
   A Purpura
   B Scale (psoriasis)
   C Crust (impetigo)

Back Endpapers

Color Plate III   Malignant Tumors of the Skin
   A Basal cell carcinoma
   B Squamous cell carcinoma
   C Lentigo maligna
   D Malignant melanoma type I
   E Malignant melanoma type II
   F Malignant melanoma type III

Color Plate IV   Cutaneous Manifestations of
Systemic Disease
   A Drug eruption
   B Scarlet fever
   C Measles
   D Necrobiosis lipoidica diabeticorum

Preface

This is a book about skin. It is written primarily for student members of the health-care team. More specifically, it is a textbook of cutaneous anatomy and physiology and of dermatology for nursing students. It may also serve as a survey of dermatology for the medical student, as a guide for the practicing nurse, nurse practitioner, or physician's assistant, or as a review or overview for the nondermatologist physician.

In the past decade, much progress has been made in dermatology. For example, knowledge of many of the causative factors and anatomic sequences of acne has led to effective, logical treatments of this common disfiguring disorder. Determination of the factors causing or worsening eczema has made preventive medicine an important part of eczema treatment. Certain skin signs have been found to be characteristic of specific systemic diseases and therefore can provide useful diagnostic information. Determination of the early signs of malignant melanoma allows life-saving early recognition of these tumors. This type of information should be presented to all persons who deliver health care.

The emphasis in this book is on normal skin, on the frequently occurring normal variants, and on the common skin diseases. The goal is to provide concepts, mechanisms of disease, and examples of disorders, instead of specific, detailed lists of information. The attempt is to provide the framework or hooks for further accumulation and placement of meaningful data. For example, the discussion of treatments furnishes reasons, goals, concepts, and general methodology, instead of specific brand names, cookbook treatment regimens, and artful dressings.

The language of the book is simple. Beginning chapters use minimal medical terminology. General concepts of inflammation, immunology, allergy, and infection are introduced, and the skin is used to give examples of their normal and abnormal functioning. New terms are explained throughout the book as the dermatological vocabulary is gradually expanded. Some general medical orientation is assumed in the later chapters, which deal with cutaneous manifestations of systemic disease. The language is also honest. When different terms mean the same thing, or when one disorder has many names, there is no attempt to add to existing confusion by insisting on one definition or by adding new names.

Pictures are essential to a dermatology book. Skin disorders are obvious and noticeable. The photograph is the permanent record, the example, the means of communication, and the teaching tool of the dermatologist. It carries more information than does an EKG for the cardiologist. This text presents 135 black-and-white and 16 color photographs. Basic examples of the microscopic appearance of normal and disordered skin are presented with photomicrographs and simple diagrams. It is unnecessary for the nondermatologist to be able to interpret skin histology, but some appreciation of vascular and cellular responses increases one's understanding of disease. It is helpful to correlate clinical reaction patterns with microscopic happenings.

Making things simple while preserving accuracy maximally stresses one's understanding of a topic and one's ability to conceptualize. Prejudices about skin, unwillingness to question the old, and reluctance to admit our collective and individual ignorance compound the difficulties. The author, however, has attempted to make dermatology simple and interesting and to relay accurate information useful to the health-care team. He has been greatly aided by the fact that the skin is a fascinating organ.

John A. Parrish

Acknowledgments

I am grateful to Anne Dubin for typing the manuscript and to Diane Patry for typing and clerical organization. All the black-and-white prints were prepared by John Charles. The graphs were prepared by Rox Anderson.

Drs. Kenneth A. Arndt, Maurice Tolman, S. M. Moschella, and Martin C. Mihm, Jr., provided some of the clinical photographs. Drs. Harley A. Haynes, Irvin H. Blank, Lewis Z. Tanenbaum, Robert S. Stern, Kenneth A. Arndt, and David S. Feingold reviewed and criticized the text. I am especially grateful to Rob Stern, who assisted in organizing the photographs and the preparation of Chapter 13, and to Lew Tanenbaum, who assisted in selecting appropriate references. Dr. Thomas B. Fitzpatrick criticized the text and provided the author with much of his approach to dermatology and skin care.

All drawings are by Gale Cooper, M.D.

John A. Parrish

Acknowledgments

dermatology and skin care

Chapter 1

Introduction

The skin is visible, viable, and vital. It is one of the largest organs of the human body and is the most easily observed. The purpose of the skin is to protect man from his noxious environment and to maintain a homeostatic internal milieu. The skin shields us from chemicals, sunlight, and bacteria and absorbs most of the mechanical stresses of our world. Acting as an insulator and a membrane, the skin keeps the environment within the body at a relatively constant temperature and saltwater content. The skin has a vast network of nerve endings which mediate the sense of touch and many other essential messages about our world. When the skin performs these life-supporting functions normally, we notice it only for its aesthetic, cosmetic, racial, and nonverbal communications. But if any of the cutaneous protective mechanisms malfunction or become overwhelmed, we suffer discomfort, disfigurement, and possible death.

The skin is alive. The outer layer of skin is continuously growing throughout life. Cells are constantly dividing and moving outward to replace dead cells which fall off the surface. Any interference with this unending process leads to the problems we recognize as skin diseases.

Skin diseases range from an unnoticed wart to ego-destroying teenage acne to skin cancer and fatal spontaneous blistering diseases. Although less than 5 percent of inpatients are hospitalized because of skin diseases, dermatology clinics account for a large proportion of outpatient clinic visits in many medical centers. In a large-city children's hospital, as many as one of every six patients brought to the emergency ward had a rash. Dermatologists' figures underestimate the real frequency of skin disorders, because most are treated by general practitioners, pediatricians, pharmacists, and concerned mothers.

The skin can be an important indicator of general health. Patients may be pale, sweaty, jaundiced, red, or cyanotic, and skin temperature may be elevated or decreased. The increase or decrease of certain pigments from blood products or skin pigment cells can give clues to the cause of certain illnesses.

Since the skin is an organ which is exposed, and can be seen and felt, its importance in both health and sickness extends beyond its ability to perform the life-supporting function of protection. The molding and modeling of our skin and its fatty layers give us much of our individual identity, and the skin, its glands, and hair provide a major aspect of sexual attraction. The skin is an important means by which people communicate. We judge people immediately upon seeing the 4 to 5 percent of the skin which covers the face. We communicate our emotions by blushing, sweating, wrinkling our brows, or frowning. At all stages of our lives, the most intimate messages we as humans are able to communicate to one another are those mediated by touching skin surfaces.

Psychic disturbances are both a result and a cause of skin diseases. Chronic skin disorders often result in marked emotional derangements. Infantile eczema can distort mother-child relationships and severe skin disease in children may make them unable to relate normally to the world around them. Uncontrolled cystic acne can be socially and psychologically damaging during the critical teenage years. Skin disorders which cause severe itching can lead to markedly altered behavior and even to suicide. On the other hand, emotionally disturbed people sometimes purposely damage their skin in a conscious or subconscious attempt to manipulate their families, doctors, or caretakers.

Informed concern about the function, care, and treatment of the skin in sickness and health is necessary for any person planning to provide medical care. This text will briefly examine the anatomy, physiology, and function of the skin as an organ system and outline basic normal cutaneous reaction patterns by which the skin maintains or alters its integrity and function. By examining some of the ways in which normal skin reacts to stress we can better understand the altered physiology, anatomy, and function seen with many skin disorders. Simple tools and easily understood rapid microscopic tests aid greatly in diagnosing such disorders.

In order to relay accurate information about the skin consistently, it is necessary to learn certain descriptive words and concepts which allow medical personnel to communicate, not only with each other, but also with hospital records and literature of the past and future. Using this vocabulary, one can examine some of the common disorders of the skin and the mucous membranes, as well as some of the more serious diseases of the skin which lead to hospitalization and special treatments. In addition, there are certain cutaneous signs of potentially fatal disorders that, if recognized early enough, can lead to prompt diagnosis and life-saving treatment. Ideally, all medical personnel should be able to recognize such lesions.

Finally, knowledge of the physiology and function of normal skin and of malfunction and the mechanism of disease permits a logical approach to treatment, skin care, and cutaneous preventive medicine. Here, as in all medicine, we must be sensitive to the patients' emotional needs. Supportive concern and touching the skin may often do what medicines alone cannot.

REFERENCES

Clinical Dermatology, Demis, D. J., R. G. Crounse, R. L. Dobson, and J. McGuire, eds., Harper & Row, Publishers, Incorporated, New York, 1972.

Dermatology in General Medicine, Fitzpatrick, T. B., K. A. Arndt, W. H. Clark, et al., eds., McGraw-Hill Book Company, New York, 1971.

Textbook of Dermatology, Rook, A., D. S. Wilkinson, and F. J. G. Ebling, eds., F. A. Davis Company, Philadelphia, 1968.

Wilkinson, D. S.: *The Nursing and Management of Skin Diseases: A Guide to Practical Dermatology for Doctors and Nurses,* Faber and Faber, Ltd., London, 1969.

The Integument

Function of skin
Anatomy and physiology of skin
  Epidermis
  Dermis
  Subcutaneous tissue
Epidermal appendages
  Hair
  Glands of the skin
    Sebaceous glands
    Apocrine glands
    Pilosebaceous apocrine unit
  Eccrine sweat glands
  Nails
Melanocytes

FUNCTION OF SKIN

The skin is the integument, or covering, of the body. When animal and plant life became multicellular and complex, certain groups of cells became specialized and developed into organ systems. Each of these organ systems performed functions previously carried out within the cell itself. The skin is a large organ which has assumed the protective role once performed by cell walls. It is the limiting membrane or outer envelope which defines the boundaries of the organism.

Mammals have developed a complex outer covering. Extensive hair growth forms a protective coat that provides warmth in frigid regions and blocks the sun's rays in tropical areas. Mammals have claws, hooves, horns, nails, and scales to provide protection and to assist in locomotion and food gathering. Mammals also have a large number and variety of skin glands which secrete substances that lubricate the skin and hair or emit odors for sexual attraction.

Human beings are relatively naked; they are distinguished from the other mammals by their lack of insulating fur. Instead, they have developed a unique combination of features: thick outer layers of skin with a well-developed dead horny layer, a widespread system of thermal-sensitive sweat glands, and an extensive layer of fatty tissue at the undersurface of the skin. This complex arrangement allows humans to survive in a wide range of temperatures and humidities.

Since humans are exposed to heat, cold, water, trauma, friction, and pressure, the integument must be durable. Because humans are active and mobile and use many delicate and gross motions, the skin must be pliable. The skin must be strong enough to be protective, yet sensitive enough to give us many important messages about our environment. Our covering must be tough enough to save us from a hostile world, yet soft enough to relay our earliest, most meaningful and most intimate human message, that of touch.

Healthy, normal skin behaves primarily as a barrier, preventing or limiting passage of fluids or chemicals into or out of the body, thereby permitting the body to maintain a relatively constant internal environment. Aside from sweat, there is very little transfer of water across the skin. Since we live in a world of air and our cells are bathed in salt water, the skin's barrier properties keep the internal tissues from drying out. It is a two-way barrier, for we can also immerse ourselves in water for hours without the body becoming waterlogged by absorbing water.

Blood flow to the skin is under neural control and is adjustable to help regulate the body temperature. The skin can also absorb frictional forces, cushion against physical trauma, and protect against certain electromagnetic or radiational energy emitted by the sun or from artificial sources. The dry external surface inhibits the growth of microorganisms. The skin also acts as a sophisticated neuroreceptor with a vast, complex network of nerves that give information to us about our surroundings. Many of the cells within the skin are specialized to perform one or more of these functions.

In keeping foreign chemicals out, resisting mechanical stress, absorbing ultraviolet radiation, and preventing water loss, the skin acts, in part, as a passive physical structure. It is a complicated shell with specific physical and chemical characteristics that provide protection. Skin is a well-structured, thin, pliable material made of components that absorb, reflect, cushion, and restrict various substances and forces that might otherwise enter or alter the body. Yet each of these protective properties results from the activities of the cells of the skin. Metabolic processes actively create the protective substances of the skin. Maintenance and repair of the layers of protection and physical barriers depend upon continual replacement and repair by living cells.

ANATOMY AND PHYSIOLOGY OF SKIN

The skin is a living organ. Since it makes up about 15 percent of the total body weight, it may be considered one of the largest organs of the body. In an adult, it is as if it were a living tissue system 6 feet long and 3 feet wide (2 square yards or 1.8 square meters). The thickness of whole skin ranges from $\frac{1}{2}$ millimeter ($\frac{1}{50}$ inch) over the eardrum or eyelids to well over ten times that thickness (up to $\frac{1}{4}$ inch) over the soles or upper back. In most areas, fatty tissue on the inner layer of the skin adds to the thickness of the integument, while in some areas the skin closely approximates the underlying bone (as on the shin), cartilage (as on the outer ear), joint capsules, or deep fascia (as on the palms).

Figure 2-1 is a diagrammatic cross section of the skin showing three major tissue levels or tissue layers. Figure 2-2 is an actual photograph of a cross section of skin magnified about 300 times. The thin, outermost layer, or *epidermis,* is composed of closely packed skin cells. It is that part of the skin which is normally visible, and it is only as thick as a piece of paper or a very thin coat of paint. The middle layer, or *dermis,* is much thicker, has proportionately fewer cells, and is mostly connective tissue containing blood vessels, lymphatics, nerves, and special supportive and structural fibers. The dermis provides substance to the skin. The lowest layer, or *subcutaneous tissue,* consists mostly of fatty tissue and acts as an insulator and shock absorber or cushion.

The thickness of the skin varies from one region of the body to an-

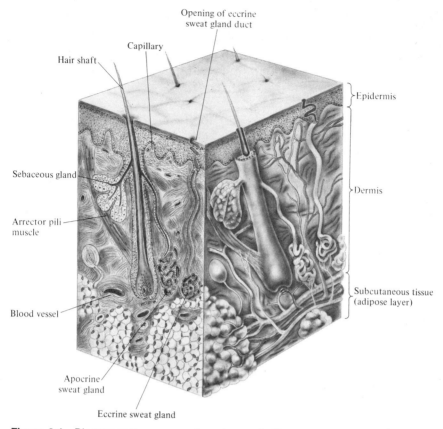

Figure 2-1 Diagrammatic cross section of normal skin.

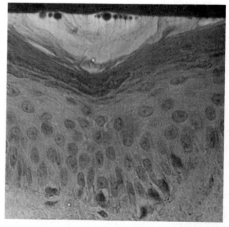

Figure 2-2 Cross section of normal skin.

other. It is thickest over the back and thinnest over the scalp or wrist. Most of this variation in thickness is accounted for by the differences in thickness of the dermis. The epidermis is of relatively uniform thickness over the entire body, except on palms and soles, where it is much thicker (Figure 2-3).

Epidermis

The epidermis is a stratified squamous epithelium which grows from within outward. It is the actively regenerating part of the skin. As it grows outward it differentiates to make a special protein outer membrane. All the glands of the skin, as well as the hair and nails, are derived from the epidermis.

The skin cells which make up most of the epidermis are called the keratinocytes because they produce keratin, the special protective proteins of skin. The keratinocytes are all derived from the lowermost cell layer of the epidermis which is adjacent to the dermis. They constantly change size and shape as they move outward toward the surface, and are sometimes called by different names in different layers of the epidermis (Figure 2-4). The lowest or innermost layer consists of evenly distributed, tall, columnar keratinocytes called *basal cells*. As these basal cells divide to produce two cells, some daughter cells are gradually pushed upward to

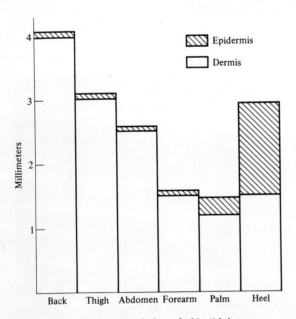

Figure 2-3   Regional variation of skin thickness.

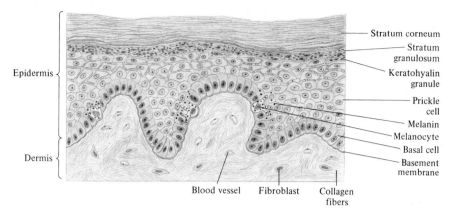

Epidermis

Dermis

Stratum corneum

Stratum granulosum

Keratohyalin granule

Prickle cell

Melanin

Melanocyte

Basal cell

Basement membrane

Blood vessel Fibroblast Collagen fibers

Figure 2-1 Diagrammatic cross section of epidermis. This drawing is a magnification of part of Fig. 2-1.

form the next layer, which is composed of close-fitting, many-sided *prickle cells*. The chemical processing and fixation techniques used to prepare the skin for microscopic examination cause a change in the appearance of these cells. The cells shrink and, as they are pulled apart from one another, the intercellular bridges (sites where the cells are normally closely joined) seem to protrude. Such protrusions have been termed "prickles" and the cells distorted by the many protrusions pulled out from their cell walls are referred to as spinous cells or prickle cells. Above this layer, granules appear within the cells; the keratinocytes are simply called *granular cells*. In the outermost layers of the epidermis, above the granular layers, the keratinocytes lose their nuclei and flatten out to become the *stratum corneum*. This layer consists mostly of the protein (keratin), cell walls, and lipid residue of the dead keratinocytes (Figure 2-5).

New keratinocytes are constantly being produced by the division of the basal cells into daughter cells. Each basal cell forms two daughter cells. These same cells are actually pushed outward or upward by new

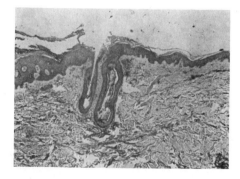

Figure 2-5 Cross section of normal epidermis.

cells being formed beneath them. The keratinocytes flatten and become dehydrated into thin, flat plates as they move outward, and eventually die, leaving their proteins and cell walls as a protective layer in the outermost part of the epidermis. The pancake-like keratinocyte layered out and blending into the stratum corneum has a surface area 25 times that of its top surface when it was a basal cell (Figure 2-6). Although the various layers of the epidermis look quite different, they are really composed of the same cell, the keratinocyte, which has different characteristics as it matures, dehydrates, and manufactures its special proteins on its way to the outer surface of the skin.

Another way to view the cell layers of the epidermis is not only to consider what the keratinocytes look like (their morphology), but also to focus on their activities. When considering the reproduction, function, and physiology of the skin, we can divide the epidermis into three compartments.

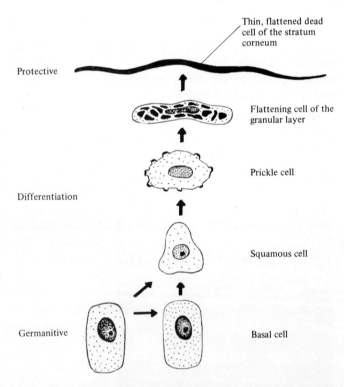

Figure 2-6 Cell kinetics. Basal cells divide and provide new basal cells as well as cells which differentiate to become the flattened cells of the stratum corneum.

The *germinative,* or reproductive, compartment is the bottom, or innermost, row, the basal row. Morphologically, it is composed of a single layer of the tall basal cells which divide constantly to repopulate the skin with cells. Each time a basal cell divides, on the average, one daughter cell stays behind as another basal cell which can later divide again. The process provides a continuous source of cells, with the basal cell layer remaining as a single row of cells. A daughter cell moves upward into the next compartment, the differentiated cell layer.

The *differentiation* compartment consists of the spinous (prickly) layer and the granular layer. It is made up of cells which are becoming different in appearance and activity from the parent cells and are specializing in making proteins, fibers, and adherent cell walls. It may be several rows thick. The cells are alive. Enzymes are present, cell respiration and metabolism are active, food substances are being used, and complex proteins and fats are being produced. The specialized cells lose their ability to reproduce. As they are pushed toward the skin surface, they gradually become more dehydrated, flatter, less metabolically active, and more closely compact, and they eventually form the third and final compartment, the lifeless stratum corneum or protective compartment.

The horny layer, or stratum corneum, is the dead, outer *protective* compartment. Its cells are incapable of any metabolic activities. All of the materials synthesized in the busy differentiation compartment are passively pushed outward. There may be as many as 20 to 25 or more layers of keratinocytes packed into this compartment even though it is the thinnest compartment in most sites. The keratinocytes are almost unrecognizable as individual cells. It is their tightly packed corpses and layered end products which protect us, keep our body fluids within, and keep us alive. Normally, it takes about two weeks for a daughter cell to make its migration from basal layer to stratum corneum. It usually takes about two more weeks for the remnants of that cell to fall off the outer surfaces of the skin.

It is the outermost layer of the epidermis, the stratum corneum, with its tightly packed layers of cell products, cell walls, and protein that constitutes the important semipermeable membrane that keeps the fluids within the body and noxious substances outside the body. Most of the barrier function of the skin is a result of this important thin outer layer. Besides holding in water and electrolytes and keeping the body from becoming dehydrated, the stratum corneum also is fairly resistant to corrosive chemicals, and its high electrical impedance resists passage of electric current. The dry external surface discourages the growth of microorganisms which need moisture for their growth.

Stratum corneum is hard and brittle when it is dry, pliable and strong when it is wet. It is normally thicker on palms and soles, and may thicken at any site as a response to repeated friction or pressure. When the skin is submerged, the stratum corneum absorbs much water. Absorption of water may make the palms appear white, wrinkled, and waterlogged. If the stratum corneum becomes overdried, it becomes brittle and cracks may occur (chapping). In winter the ambient humidity may be sufficiently low to cause excessive dryness of the skin.

The outer surface of the stratum corneum is constantly scaling, breaking up, or sloughing off. Although we constantly shed dead cells, under normal circumstances this process does not provide enough scales to become noticeable. In order for the skin to maintain appropriate thickness and important barrier functions, there must be a constant balance between the formation of new keratinocytes by division of the basal cells and the rate of falling off of the dead keratinocytes from the outermost stratum corneum. The balanced process of division or creation of new cells and sloughing off of cells at the surface continues throughout life. If dead skin cells fall off faster than new cells are formed, then the skin becomes thin, eroded, or atrophic. If new cells are formed faster than dead cells are sloughed off, then the stratum corneum piles up and appears as scales or thickened skin. The skin must be constantly viable or its barrier functions deteriorate and alterations and erosions occur.

The tough, hard protein made by the live cells of the differentiated compartment of the epidermis, which makes up a major part of the stratum corneum, is called *keratin*. Keratin is actually a mixture of fibrous and amorphous proteins whose exact chemical structure has not been discovered. It is the relatively insoluble material which makes up much of the stratum corneum, hair, and nails. It is hard and brittle when dry, pliable and strong when adequately hydrated. Other examples of keratin, besides stratum corneum, hair, and nails, are the scales of fish, the feathers of birds, and the hooves, claws, and horns of certain animals. The process by which epidermal cells synthesize protein fibers, dehydrate, lose their nuclei, and become compact layers of protein is called keratinization.

In most parts of the body, the whole epidermis, including all of its cell layers, is only as thick as a page of this book. Although thin, the epidermis is the part of the skin which is visible. It does, however, transmit light, and we can partially see through it. Part of what we view as skin color resides in the epidermis, and part is color which we see through the epidermis.

Dermis

The dermis (Figure 2-1) is the thicker layer beneath the epidermis that gives skin much of its substance, mass, or feel. The dermis varies from

1 to 4 millimeters in thickness in different anatomic sites (Figure 2-3). The dermis has far fewer cells than does the epidermis. Whereas the epidermis is almost a solid sheet of cells, the dermis is mostly a semisolid mixture of fibers, water, and a gel called *ground substance*. There are three types of fibers made by the scattered cells of the dermis: collagen, reticulum, and elastin. *Collagen,* which makes up a large part of the dermis (70 percent of the dry weight), is a long molecule woven together in fibrils in such a manner that it allows stretching and contraction, but still maintains striking tensile strength. Collagen is the major source of the mechanical strength of the skin. Its bundles of fibers course through the dermis, providing structure and substantiveness. The pattern of the larger bundles can be seen with the light microscope. Laying down new collagen is an important part of wound healing. Vitamin C is essential to normal collagen synthesis, and its absence causes poor wound healing and an easily damaged dermis.

Reticulum fibers are present in a fine branching pattern in all normal connective tissue, and may help to link bundles of collagen fibers together. *Elastin* fibers are also scattered throughout the dermis and, since these protein fibers appear to be reversibly extensible, may add to the elastic quality of the dermis. The ground substance in which all of these fibers rest is a gelatinous, viscous, compressible, and elastic mixture of water, mucopolysaccharides, and colloidal elements.

Blood vessels, nerves, and lymphatics course through the dermis. Scattered cells called fibroblasts produce the fibers, proteins, and viscous materials of the dermis and, therefore, maintain its integrity as well as take part in the healing process. Scattered throughout the dermis there are also cells which take part in other aspects of wound healing, in removal of foreign bodies from the skin, in combatting infection, and in mediating certain reactions of the skin.

The dermis provides the structural support for the epidermis, for the skin glands and hair, and for the blood vessels, nerves, and lymphatics. It envelopes the whole body in a protective viscous gel and, since it can be compressed and stretched, it can absorb and reduce environmental stress and strain on the body. The dermis is also a storage place for a significant amount of the body's water.

In the outermost part of the dermis the collagen bundles are smaller, fewer, and loosely arranged in a haphazard fashion. This part of the dermis is called the *papillary dermis.* The extensive plexus of capillaries, lymphatics, and nerves, and scattered lymphocytes, or histiocytes, which leave the blood vessels to enter the dermis give this upper part of the dermis a slightly more cellular appearance. Beneath the papillary dermis, the protein fibers become thicker and more regular, and are oriented longitudinally.

This lower, more densely fibered area is called the *reticular dermis*. There are fewer cells and less ground substance in the reticular dermis.

The junction between epidermis and dermis is far from flat or smooth. The outer dermis has many tiny projections (as many as 100 per square millimeter) up into the epidermis. These projections from which the papillary dermis gets its name, are called *papillae,* and fit into corresponding sockets in the underside of the epidermis (Figure 2-7). Because of this arrangement, when the skin is cut in cross section and viewed under the microscope, the dermoepidermal junction appears as waves. The cut section of the ridges of epidermis appear as pegs projecting into the dermis and are referred to as rete pegs, rete ridges, or epidermal pegs. The nutrients and oxygen for the cells of the epidermis are brought by the capillaries of the papillary dermis and must diffuse across the dermoepidermal junction and among and into the keratinocytes. Epidermal cell metabolites, waste products, and cell products to be resorbed and conserved by the body must make their way back to the dermal capillaries. The skin appendages (hair, nails, glands) are epidermal structures which grow down into the dermis (Figure 2-1), and also obtain nutrient supply by diffusion from the dermal vessels.

Fluid freely bathes the fibers and cells of the dermis, and can cross the dermoepidermal junction to pass between the cells of the epidermis. It is the stratum corneum which acts as the retainer or barrier to keep body fluids from leaking out. This arrangement allows the epidermal cells to obtain nutrients and metabolites from and return waste products to the

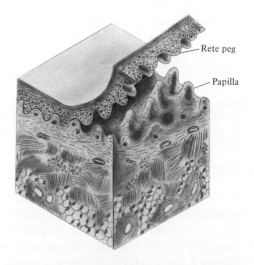

Rete peg

Papilla

Figure 2-7 The dermoepidermal junction. The projections of the dermis fit into depressions of the epidermis.

blood vessels of the dermis. It is only logical that the water and nutrient barrier must be outside of the last living cell layer.

The dermis is tough and strong. The complex nature of the dermis and its fibers creates a tissue with very high tensile strength which can resist compression but, at the same time, remains pliable and movable. Leather is animal dermis which has been modified by dehydration and certain chemical treatments and processes (tanning) which render it stable and resistant to decomposition or bacterial decay.

Subcutaneous Tissue

Beneath the dermis, the fibrous proteins become loosely textured and widely spaced and, in most areas of the body, separated by collections of fat cells (Figure 2-1). This fatty tissue is sometimes called the *subcutaneous tissue,* because it is beneath the true skin (dermis and epidermis). Because of the fat content, it is sometimes called the adipose layer or panniculus adiposus. The subcutaneous layer varies in different parts of the body. In most areas, it is thicker than the dermis, but in some regions such as eyelids, penis and scrotum, nipple and areola, and tibia, it is absent. The different distribution of fatty tissue in males and females makes up one of the secondary sex characteristics. The thickness and the fat content of the subcutaneous layer in various parts of the body are influenced by heredity, sex hormones, age, and eating habits.

The subcutaneous tissue layer can be viewed as a specialized layer of connective tissue in which the fat cell is the primary cell. It is like the dermis except for the enormous quantities of fat stored between the protein strands, blood vessels, nerves, and lymphatics. The fat is stored within cells. Subcutaneous tissue serves as an insulator to conserve body heat. It is also an excellent mechanical shock absorber to reduce the effects of trauma on deeper structures. In some areas, such as the orbit of the eye, the fatty tissue can be viewed as the perfect packing material, in this case, cushioning the eyeball. Finally, fatty tissue can serve as a source of fuel. When adequate calories are not available by mouth, the fat cell can be broken down to provide energy.

EPIDERMAL APPENDAGES

Early in fetal life some of the epidermal cells change or differentiate into cells that set them apart from the normal keratinocytes. The cells specialize to make specific added structures or appendages of the epidermis. Some cells become specialized in making unique kinds of keratin structures: the hair and nails. Other epidermal cells become specialized to produce the glands of the skin (sebaceous glands, eccrine sweat glands).

These appendages begin as a small collection of epidermal cells, which protrude down into the dermis (Figure 2-8). As these cells multiply, they migrate or extend down further into the dermis from which they receive their nutrients, electrolytes, fluids, and innervation. The appendages maintain their connection with the epidermis. The hair, nails, and glands are therefore epidermal in origin and character. The cells lining the ducts or walls of the tubular appendages may be similar to keratinocytes, and, indeed, these cells maintain the potential ability to make stratum corneum. If the epidermis is removed by disease or trauma and the hair follicles

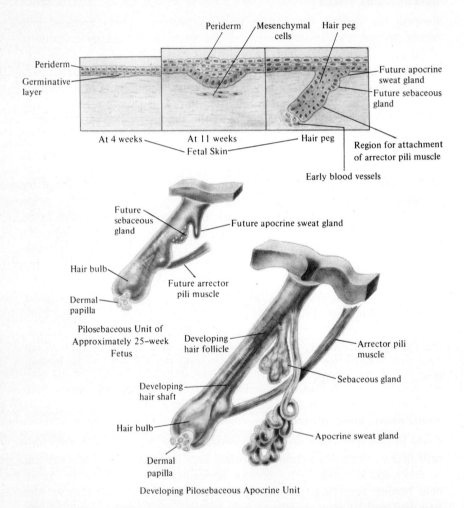

Figure 2-8 The origin of the epidermal appendages: the primary epithelial germ of the embryo gives rise to the hair, sebaceous gland, and apocrine gland.

are left behind, the cells of the hair follicle walls can move up to repopulate or reepithelize the injured area with normally functioning keratinocytes.

Embryologically, the formation of the epidermal appendages occurs during the third fetal month. At this time, thousands of small buds of epidermal cells begin to push into the dermis. A clump of cells, called the primary epithelial germ (PEG), elongates, becomes hollow, and forms many of the important skin appendages. The bottom of the column of cells is influenced by collections of cells and blood vessels gathering in the dermis to become a hair bulb. The epidermal cells at the base of the tube formed by the PEG become capable of making the special hard keratin of hair and the tube of the invaginating epidermis (PEG) becomes the *hair follicle.* As the column of cells from the PEG grows deeper into the dermis to form the hair follicle, three bulges become apparent in the lateral wall of the column of cells. The epidermal cells of the uppermost bulge form another column of cells which differentiate to form the *apocrine gland* and its duct. The middle bulge further differentiates to become the *sebaceous gland,* while the lower one becomes the attachment for the small muscle (the *arrector pili*) which makes hairs stand straight.

Hair

By the fourth intrauterine month, hair is being formed on the face and scalp. Throughout the remainder of fetal life, hairs continue to form from the original epidermal downgrowths. After birth, however, the epidermis loses its capacity to generate new hair follicles. Epidermis no longer can be influenced to invaginate into the dermis and form a new hair-producing structure. As noted above, the inverse is not true. The epidermal cells which line the wall of the hair follicle maintain their ability to behave as keratinocytes. They can reproduce as normal basal cells, form a covering layer over the dermis, and manufacture normal stratum corneum. Once hair follicles are destroyed, no new hairs will be formed to replace the missing hairs. This is the basis of electrolysis. If hair is plucked or cut, but the hair follicle remains, a new hair may grow in the follicle. If, on the other hand, the epidermis between hair follicles is destroyed but the follicle remains, then the keratinocytes lining the follicle can reform the epidermis (see section on wound healing in Chapter 5).

Hair, like stratum corneum, may be regarded as a protein product of specialized epithelial cells. Just as epidermal cells (keratinocytes) manufacture protein, dehydrate, die, and become packed together to make stratum corneum, so also the cells of the hair follicle make protein, dehydrate, die, and become packed together. As they are pushed upward by the division of the basal cells of the hair follicle, their nonviable end products become hair.

Some type of hair is found on all skin surfaces except palms and soles, which have no hair follicles. Two main types of hair are found on human skin. *Terminal hairs* are long, coarse, thick, easily visible, and usually more important clinically. The hair we easily see on the scalp, beard, arms, and legs is all terminal hair. The other type of hair, which is tiny and almost unnoticeable, is called *vellus hair*. Vellus hairs are analogous to the underfur on animals, and are shorter, finer, and only visible on close inspection. (The word *lanugo* is sometimes used interchangeably with vellus, but it more commonly refers to fetal hair.) It is important to remember that terminal hairs vary considerably in size in different areas of the body and on the normal female face they are not readily distinguishable from vellus hairs.

Hair growth is continuous in some animals (merino sheep, some dogs). Each follicle produces hair continuously from fetal life until the death of the animal. In most hairy animals, however, hair growth is cyclic. Hair grows in all the follicles for a time. Then growth stops. The old hair rests in place for a while before it is pushed out as a new hair begins to grow beneath it in the same follicle. The animal sheds its old hairs and a new cycle begins.

In humans, although all hairs are growing at birth, within the first few weeks of life all hairs are converted into a resting state. Cell multiplication at the base of the hair follicle ceases, and no new cells are pushed upward and outward to keratinize, dehydrate, form more protein, and die. The hair gets no longer. Thereafter, human hairs demonstrate a relatively unique property. As new hairs begin to grow beneath the old ones, there is a random distribution of growth cycles of each follicle, independent of its neighbors, yet a relatively constant total number of hairs is maintained. Throughout life, each hair follicle continues to go through its growth or *anagen* phase followed by a nongrowing phase (*telogen* or resting phase) after which the hair falls out, being pushed out by the new hair beginning to grow in the same hair follicle. The new hair then proceeds through the same phases. In humans, hair growth, therefore, is cyclic but the hair follicles are not all in the same phase of growth. There is no synchrony of growth cycles. One hair may be growing while another is in the resting state and a third is being pushed out by a brand new hair. This cyclic growth pattern for each hair, without synchrony with neighboring follicles but with overall constant numbers of hairs, is called *mosaic* pattern of growth.

On the normal adult scalp, about 85 to 90 percent of hairs are in anagen phase and 10 percent in telogen phase. The telogen hairs (also called club hairs) rest in place for a time (often several months) before they are pushed up and out of the follicle when the growth cycle begins again within that follicle, and a new (anagen) hair is formed. The old club hair is shed. We normally lose about 75 to 100 scalp hairs per day through this process of shedding old hairs as the growth of new ones pushes them out of their follicles.

Anagen phase varies from months to years on various parts of the body, accounting for different hair lengths. The duration of the growing phase obviously dictates how long a hair will be. Scalp hairs, which remain in anagen phase for years, become very long, while hairs of the pubic area or limbs, which only grow for months before stopping growth and entering resting (telogen) phase, are much shorter.

During anagen phase, the rate of mitosis (cell division) is the same in large and small hairs, and all scalp hair bulbs reproduce their population of cells approximately every twenty-four hours. Therefore, a large hair (having a larger population of cells) will produce a greater bulk and length of hair shaft each day than a small hair. Mitotic activity of hair matrix ranks among the highest of any of the body tissues. Scalp hair grows about ⅓ millimeter each day (1 centimeter per month, 1 inch in two to three months). Since there are about 100,000 scalp hairs, this growth produces about 100 feet of practically solid protein each day (7 miles per year). In considering physiology and pathologic conditions of hair, it is important to emphasize three primary means through which hair growth expresses itself and by which it can be measured, namely: cycle (anagen vs. telogen), rate of growth, and size. Changes in any one of the parameters in a sufficient number of hairs may lead to clinically noticeable abnormalities.

A change in the hair *cycle* is a break in the regular pattern of growth. The cycle of growing (anagen), resting (telogen), falling out, and being replaced is interrupted. The change may be caused by hairs prematurely stopping growth and becoming resting hairs before their usual length has been reached. As a result, a greater proportion of hairs enter the telogen state. (In extreme cases, all anagen hairs make this conversion.) Many severe stresses can cause this sudden cessation of growth and subsequent premature conversion to resting phase. As new hairs begin to grow in these follicles, the old hairs are displaced at nearly the same time and thinning or near balding may occur temporarily before the new hairs become long and obvious. Examples of this phenomenon, called *telogen effluvium,* are seen after pregnancy, severe illness, high fever, and heparin therapy.

In considering changes in *rate* of hair growth, one must consider environmental temperature and general state of health. Warm weather stimulates growth and antarctic environments reduce growth of hair and nails. These changes are not clinically noticeable unless the environmental changes are extreme and prolonged. Starvation reduces mitotic activity of hair matrix. Chemotherapeutic drugs used to treat malignancies may decrease the intrabulbar expansion forces by inhibiting mitosis. This reduces the volume of the hair bulb and thereby reduces the caliber of the hair shaft. Although the bulb will reexpand when the inhibitory agent is withdrawn, the segment of constriction remains. This narrow segment is pushed outward as hair growth continues and the hair shaft lengthens. The hair may be easily broken off at the point of constriction. *Alopecia* (loss of hair) due to such breakage should be separated from alopecia due to change in cycle.

Hair loss following irradiation with x-rays is not due as much to suppression of mitosis as it is to conversion to telogen state. This is made worse by the fact that x-ray-induced atrophy of perifollicular structures compromises anchorage of the hairs.

Changes in *size* of hair are of fundamental importance when studying hypertrichosis (excessive amount of hair). The clinical impression of increased hairiness is actually the result of an increase in length and caliber of existing hairs and not an increase in the absolute numbers of hairs present. Unnoticed vellus hairs may become obvious terminal hairs or previously existing terminal hairs may enlarge. Hypertrichosis may be localized or generalized. Hypertrichosis secondary to Dilantin may be caused by enlargement of connective tissue supporting a hair bulb similar to that seen in gingival (gum) hyperplasia, another side effect of the drug.

In the male, large terminal hairs normally develop in the face, chest, and body in response to the higher levels of male hormone (*androgens*). In women and children, such a male distribution of hair represents an excess number of visible terminal hairs, referred to as *hirsutism*. While the appearance of marked hirsutism suggests abnormalities of gonads or adrenal glands, modest excess hair in male distribution may occur in women as a normal variant, e.g., a familial trait.

Hair follicles in different regions of the body respond differently to the presence of male hormones. The same androgenic (male hormone) stimuli which cause facial hirsutism in women by increasing the size of normally inconspicuous hairs can cause scalp hairs to become progressively smaller and fewer as seen in male pattern baldness.

Alopecia simply means "baldness" or a noticeable decrease in number of hairs. Alopecia may be focal or diffuse, scarring or nonscarring (Figure 2-9). Most nonscarring alopecia is hereditary. The most common hereditary alopecia is "male pattern baldness" with its typical distribution: frontal recession, followed by loss of hair on the vertex (tip) of the head, with relative sparing of the temporal (lateral) regions. Seen commonly in adult males, this pattern of hair loss also may occur in women, especially in later life. It may be considered a normal part of the aging process.

Alopecia areata is an asymptomatic circumscribed patch of hair loss

---

Scarring
   Healed congenital ectodermal defects
   Severe infection (bacterial, fungal, viral, spirochetal)
   Chemical agents (acid, alkali)
   Physical agents (burns, frostbite, x-ray)
   Skin diseases (lupus erythematosis, lichen planus, morphea, sarcoidosis)
   Neoplasms
   Nevi

Nonscarring
   Congenital defects
   Physiologic (post partum, neonatal)
   Hereditary ("male pattern baldness")
   Drugs, toxins, chemicals (thallium, heparin, methotrexate)
   Infection (fungus, secondary syphilis)
   Skin diseases (severe eczema, exfoliative erythroderma)
   Endocrine (hypopituitary, hypothyroid, hyperthyroid)
   Acute and chronic illness (high fever, systemic lupus erythematosus)
   Alopecia areata
   Friction, physical trauma, x-ray

Figure 2-9   Causes of alopecia.

of unknown etiology. All of the hair falls out of a slowly growing round or oval area. Any hairy region of the body may be affected, but it is most common, or at least most noticeable, on the scalp. Alopecia areata is more common in young persons, and has frequently been seen to follow several weeks after a severe emotional trauma, such as the real or threatened loss of a loved one. The direct relationship of emotional stress has not been explained. The hairless scalp skin is usually otherwise normal in appearance.

Alopecia areata may remain as a small localized patch, or may become extensive, leaving the whole head (alopecia totalis) or whole body (alopecia universalis) completely hairless. Hair often regrows spontaneously. Repeated episodes of hair loss may occur. The prognosis for return of hair is worse if age of onset is low and also if the first episode is extensive. Systemic steroids may temporarily stimulate regrowth of hair but the hair falls out when such treatment is discontinued. Long-term systemic steroid therapy of this cosmetic and chronic problem is therefore usually not justified, because of the potential side effects of such therapy. Intralesional steroid injections sometimes lead to regrowth of hair; topical steroids are much less effective. No safe therapy is consistently effective in stimulating regrowth of hair.

Nonscarring alopecia may also be caused by repeated friction, rubbing, traction on hairs such as that caused by tight curlers, changes in hair cycle, x-irradiation, and antimetabolites. Hair loss may actually be the result of a person pulling, twisting, or removing his own hair in an act of nervous tension, or in order to manipulate his family or doctor. Children may pull out their hairs when they think they are not being observed. Such an act is referred to as *trichotillomania.* The resulting areas of hair loss may be round, as in alopecia areata, but are usually not completely bald. Short hairs and stubs of varying length remain.

Scarring alopecia occurs after any infection, inflammation, or trauma sufficient to destroy hair follicles. Healed ectodermal defects are hairless. Thermal and chemical burns may destroy hair follicles. Scars on the scalp may be caused by *lupus erythematosis, lichen planus, sarcoidosis,* or *neoplasms.* Since destroyed hair follicles do not regenerate, scarring alopecia is irreversible.

Hair that is oval in cross section has a tendency to curve on itself as it grows out of the follicle and produces curly hair. The bonds that help hold the protein bundles of hair together can be broken with chemicals. The hair can then be curled or straightened or waved and the bonds then chemically rejoined (setting or permanent).

Hair served many functions in man's predecessors. It not only protected from cold, sun, wind, and physical trauma, but also served as sensory receptors. By conducting motion of touch or wind to the many nerve endings that surround the base of the follicle, hairs could serve to communicate, warn of danger, or provide sensual pleasure. In some animals, hair, like feathers, serves as ornament for sexual attraction. Manes, tails, and tufts of hair provide the same attraction for some animals as hair styles and beards for modern men and women.

Although the hair seen above the layer of the skin is dead and can be painlessly cut or altered chemically without affecting the growth of the hair, it is constantly being replaced by a living, growing group of specialized epidermal cells. Any sickness, drug, or trauma which interferes with the metabolism of these cells results in damage or loss of hair.

Glands of the Skin

Just as keratinocytes of the epidermis multiply and make the keratin of stratum corneum, and some epidermal cells specialize to make the keratin of hair and nails, still other epidermal cells specialize to become the various glands of the skin. During embryonic development, these cells also push down as downgrowths of epidermis into the dermis from which they receive their nutrition.

Sebaceous Glands   The sebaceous glands, or "oil glands," actually develop during fetal life as outgrowths from the newly forming hair follicles (Figure 2-8). Sebaceous glands are found on all areas of skin except for palms, soles, and the dorsa of the feet. Their distribution varies from place to place on the body. They are most numerous and largest on the face, scalp, upper chest, and back (face and "cape areas"). The sebaceous glands of the skin are not grossly visible, but when they appear on mucous membranes, they can be seen as tiny white to yellow papules.

The sebaceous glands produce a large amount of a very complex lipid mixture called *sebum*. Sebum is the end product of sebaceous gland cells in the same way that keratin is the end product of keratinocytes. The sebaceous gland is a *holocrine* gland. This means that the entire gland cell ends up in the excretory stream. The cells of the gland divide, and as the daughter cells move outward and into the lumen (opening or duct), they themselves become the basic part of the secretion. The dead cell products disintegrate, decompose, and change as they are moved outward to become sebum. In this sense, the hair and nails and, in fact, the entire stratum corneum–producing epidermis, may also be considered as holocrine organs.

Sebaceous glands are hormone dependent. The male hormones (androgens), cause them to enlarge and function. Once the glands are functioning, the formation of sebum is continuous, and seems to be based on the constant cellular proliferation of the glands, and not on any stimulation by nerves.

Infants have functioning sebaceous glands because of the androgens they have received from maternal blood. In fact, the *vernix caseosa*—the cheesy, unctuous substance which covers the newborn—is largely a mixture of sebum and desquamated cells from the skin of the fetus. The sebaceous glands become inactive shortly after birth and remain relatively non-functional throughout childhood. At puberty they become large and active because of the presence of male hormone. Postpubertal males and females have enough male hormone to keep the glands stimulated.

It is not certain to what degree, if at all, sebum provides lubrication, antibacterial action, antifungal properties, or suppleness to the skin. Some of the fatty acids present in sebum may inhibit the growth of some bacteria and fungi, and water loss from hair may be retarded when hair is coated with sebum. Still, the sebaceous glands may not have a significant useful function in modern man. However, their role in acne makes them important objects of study. Acne results from plugging and rupture of the sebaceous gland ducts and, therefore, occurs in areas of high concentration of large sebaceous glands. Another common dermatologic entity, *seborrheic dermatitis,* is a red, scaly, greasy eruption which also occurs in these areas, but its relationship to sebum production is unclear.

Apocrine Glands   The Apocrine gland arises from the same bud of epidermal cells (PEG) that moves down into the dermis to create the hair follicle and the sebaceous gland. In most areas of the body, the attempts to form apocrine glands are abortive and only represent ontogeny (embryological development of the individual organism), faithfully recapitulating phylogeny (the evolutionary development of the race or group of animals), but in a few body areas, the apocrine sweat gland develops into a recognizable organ which is capable of secreting a milky fluid. The usual locations of apocrine glands in the adult are the axillae, areolae (nipples), periumbilical region, and perianal and genital areas. These glands contribute significantly to the secretions and odors of the armpit. The apocrine sweat gland is large enough to be visible under direct observation during dissection of the subcutaneous tissue of the axillae, and is seen as a 1-millimeter red or yellow-brown sphere which is actually a highly coiled gland whose duct joins the hair follicle just above the duct of the sebaceous gland. Comparative anatomy and physiology studies show that the cerumen (earwax) glands of the ear canal and certain glands of the eyelids are modified apocrine glands, and that the mammary gland represents a highly specialized group of apocrine glands.

Apocrine secretions are continuous. The lumen of the gland acts as a reservoir, its contents being discharged under appropriate nerve stimuli. The total quantity of secretion of all apocrine glands is so small that no physiologic alterations result from their overactivity or underactivity. The apocrine sweat glands in man are not important for fluid regulation or for temperature control, but only as a source of odor and a site of dermatologic disease.

The maturation of apocrine glands depends upon hormonal factors; they become active at puberty and atrophic in later life. *Secretion* by each cell of the gland is actually a growth process beyond direct pharmacological or chemical control. *Excretion* of glandular contents to the surface of the skin is achieved by contraction of a myoepithelial sheath surrounding the gland and results from neural (adrenergic) stimulation, usually influenced by emotional stress. The gland is indifferent to heat stimuli.

Apocrine glands present personal problems to some because of the odor produced when bacteria grow and degrade its secretions. Apocrine secretions are odorless, but when certain bacteria grow and decompose the secretions, the resulting odor can be offensive and is sometimes called "body odor." That odor occurring in the axillae where moisture and occlusion promote bacterial growth may be quite noticeable. Antiperspirants are designed to reduce moisture so that it is difficult for bacteria to grow; deodorants kill bacteria and provide counter smells. Some antiperspirants work by helping to occlude the ducts of the apocrine glands. Rarely, the milky sweat from the axillary apocrine glands is colored and stains clothing.

Apocrine glands may produce clinical problems. Duct occlusion, cysts, infections, and sweat retention may occur. Apocrine gland tumors are rare.

The Function of the Pilosebaceous Apocrine Unit   The pilosebaceous apocrine unit develops *in utero,* as a bud from the epidermis (PEG). The complicated structure begins its development over the entire skin surface, except for palms and soles. The various offshoots begin to form hair, sebaceous glands, apocrine gland, and the attachment for the arrector pili muscle. The prominence of any one of these epidermal appendages varies from one region of the body to another. The hair bulb becomes more prominent on the scalp, while the sebaceous gland is the most prominent part of the pilosebaceous apocrine unit on the nose. By the time of birth, the apocrine gland disappears completely from most of the body areas.

The pilosebaceous apocrine unit is largely a vestigial or rudimentary structure in human beings. Its appendages may once have served the ancestors of humanity well, but any essential role in survival of modern men and women is unclear. We no longer have enough hair to provide protection against cold, sun, or trauma. Now, hair has mostly cosmetic significance. People are quite concerned about too much or too little hair, and about hair styles for social, sexual, and psychological, but not medical, reasons.

The sebaceous glands serve no clear function. They may have once been essential to coat the hairs with sebum and make the fur coats of our ancestors more pliable and water resistant. The persistent prominence of these glands on the face, chest, and back plays a role in causing acne, a severe cosmetic problem.

The apocrine glands may have once been scent glands for sexual attraction. Odors from sexually aroused animals or from frightened animals can attract or warn other animals from great distances, even in thick brush that prevents visualization. In modern men and women, apocrine glands serve as a source of body odor. They are present in greatest quantity in the axillae, but are also found in the anogenital region and around the nipples. They have largely disappeared from the rest of the body except in areas where they have become further specialized to serve special functions (earwax glands, mammary glands).

The sebaceous glands and apocrine glands are both responsive to androgens. Both postpubertal males and females have enough androgen to support growth and function of these glands. Hairs in certain parts of the body are also influenced by androgens to change from almost unrecognized vellus hairs to long, thick, obvious terminal hairs. The hairs in the pubic area and the axillae are so sensitive to androgens that the smaller amount of male hormone present in normal females causes hair to grow after puberty. Growth of the hair of the beard, chest, and lower abdomen requires the higher levels of androgens seen in males. Strangely enough, some regions of scalp hair may be genetically predisposed to stop growth in the presence of the higher androgen levels (male pattern baldness).

Eccrine Sweat Glands

Eccrine sweat glands are part of the skin's sophisticated heat regulatory system. They deliver water to the skin so that heat may be lost by evaporation. Most mammals have no eccrine glands. Those who do, have them on palms and soles, paw pads, or friction surfaces, where they provide moisture to improve grip and tactile sensitivity. In the human being, the naked mammal which lost its fur coat, millions of eccrine sweat glands are found all over the body and they are used for heat control.

Eccrine sweat glands are also appendages of the epidermis but they arise independently of the pilosebaceous apocrine apparatus (Figure 2-1). During the fifth and sixth fetal months, the body becomes covered with eccrine sweat glands derived from tiny germinal buds growing down from primitive epidermal cells. The epidermal downgrowth and its supporting dermal blood vessels and nerves grow down to the deeper dermis, where they form a coiled secretory tube maintaining communication with the surface via the sweat duct, a tube lined with cells which are continuous with the epidermis. Although the entire body is covered by the 2 to 3 million glands, the distribution varies considerably, being greatest on palms, soles, and forehead.

Many investigators believe that no true anatomically open pore is present in the epidermis where the sweat duct exits, but that the eccrine duct ends in an opening which is actually a loose mesh of stratum corneum. Using a hand lens, one can see these openings on the palm. They appear as tiny depressions spaced along the epidermal ridges. No significant intralumenal storage of eccrine sweat takes place.

Although all the eccrine glands are morphologically the same, there are functionally two different groups of glands. Those on the palms and soles function continuously and markedly increase their output in response to mental or emotional stimuli. Sweaty palms are a common problem during emotional stress. These glands develop earlier in the embryo and may be analogous to similar glands on the gripping surfaces of lower animals. The remainder of the eccrine sweat glands over the rest of the body function in response to heat stress. In addition, there are morphologically normal glands which do not function at all. The axillae contain both emotion-sensitive and heat-sensitive clusters of eccrine sweat glands.

Although the epidermis functions essentially as a poikilothermic organ (assumes the temperature of its environment), man is basically homeothermic (maintains a fairly constant internal temperature), and the skin and its appendages play a role, not only as a protective interface but also as an active heat-regulating organ. Secretion by eccrine sweat glands (to provide water for evaporation) and regulation of cutaneous blood flow (to conserve or dissipate heat) are the major specializations for this function.

Metabolism, burning of food stuffs, muscular activity, and respiratory activities constantly create heat deep within the body. Increase in blood flow to the skin carries more of this body heat toward the surface of the body where it can be dissipated. Conversely, when body heat needs to be conserved, the blood vessels of the skin constrict, and keep the warm blood within the deeper layers of the body. Therefore, the skin appears red when we are overheated (vessels are dilated to deliver the heat to the surface) and white when we are cold (vessels of the skin are constricted to conserve heat).

Excess internal heat can be lost to the environment by radiation or convection from the skin surfaces. If body heat production is not increased or if the ambient temperature is low, this method of heat loss may be sufficient. But if large amounts of internal heat are created (as with exercise), or if the external environmental temperature is high, an additional method of heat loss is necessary. The excess heat is lost by evaporation of water from the skin surface.

When the body is overheated, the increase in blood temperature causes a thermoregulatory center in the hypothalamus to send impulses to sweat glands to begin to function. The eccrine sweat glands secrete dilute salt water onto the surface of the skin. The glands are supplied by the sympathetic nervous system, but the effective mediator is acetylcholine, not epinephrine. Local increases in skin temperature may also cause local sweating by a reflex arc mechanism, and local or systemic cholinergic agents can induce sweating. Atropine, a cholinergic blocker often used to decrease oral secretions in surgical patients, interferes with the sweating mechanism.

The exact composition of sweat varies depending upon the rate of sweating. Sweat contains sodium and chloride in concentrations less than that of serum, and also contains potassium, lactate, and urea in concentrations greater than that of serum. Sweat is always hypotonic. The mechanism of sweat formation has been likened to that of the action of the nephron of the kidney in that a two-step process occurs: filtration by the coiled segment and active resorption of sodium and chloride in the tube section. Aldosterone can increase the sodium resorption both by the tubules of the kidney and by the sweat duct. However, unlike the kidney, the original solution in the coiled segment does not appear to be a simple passive filtrate of plasma and probably represents an active transport of solutes from interstitial fluid. In any case, it should be remembered that the sweat gland is not involved in regulating body fluids or eliminating body wastes. Its job is to deliver water to the surface of the skin for evaporation and heat loss. Any solutes or metabolites carried out in such a process represent a compulsory or obligatory drain on the body necessary to the formation and delivery of sweat.

Fever results when a readjustment of the hypothalamus thermostat maintains body temperature at a higher setting, bringing the blood vessels and sweat glands into action to maintain an abnormally high body temperature. When the hypothalamic setting returns to normal, profuse sweating is often the mechanism by which heat is rapidly lost in the return to normal body temperature. Under maximum stimulation, up to 2 liters of sweat may be lost in an hour.

The pathologic conditions caused by eccrine sweat glands include hyperhidrosis (excessive sweating), anhidrosis (abnormal decrease or absence of sweating), and blockage of sweat ducts, with its resulting eruptions, called heat rash (*miliaria*). Primary infection and tumors of eccrine sweat glands are uncommon.

Nails

Nails are epidermal specializations which are homologous with the claws of lower animals. Their formation begins in the middle of the third intrauterine month, when a thickened plaque of epidermal cells begins to sink down into the dorsal tip of the digit, and the *invaginated* group of cells begins to make the modified keratin of the nails. Growth forward from this base is slow and takes until the final month of gestation to reach the tip of the digit. From this time on, growth is continuous, and the nail would extend indefinitely if the free edge were not worn away or deliberately cut.

The nail-forming tissue is metabolically highly active and, therefore, very sensitive to physiologic alterations, whether they arise locally or as the result of systemic disease. Nails are 0.5 to 0.75 millimeters thick and grow at a rate of about 0.1 millimeter per day, with some variations. Nails of the right hand grow faster than corresponding nails of the left hand; middle fingernails grow faster than the rest; toenails grow one-third to one-half as fast as fingernails.

There are three varieties of nail disorders: (1) congenital developmental disorders of the nail-forming structures, (2) interference with the process of nail formation during postembryonic life, as in psoriasis, and (3) changes effected in the finished product after the nail has been formed, as in fungal infections.

The source of specialized epidermal cells which dry out, keratinize, stack up, and die to make the special protein of the nail is called the nail matrix. The white quarter-moon seen through the proximal part of the thumbnail of most people is the distal part of the matrix. The matrix in the other fingers is usually hidden by the skin covering the proximal part of the nail plate. The nail plate keratin is usually clear, and the pink color of the vascular nail bed can be seen through the nails.

Any skin disease that can affect epidermis can affect the matrix and alter the nails. Fungi which can live in the keratin of stratum corneum can also live in the keratin of nails.

MELANOCYTES

Scattered throughout the basal layer of the epidermis between some of the basal cells are special cells called *melanocytes* which produce pigment granules. These granules are actually passed on to the keratinocytes to give skin most of its color. The pigment granules are called melanosomes because they contain a complex protein called melanin. Melanin is a brown-black pigment. In Greek, *melas* means brown or black.

The melanocytes could actually be viewed as a tiny, one-celled gland. The melanocytes are actually derived from nerve tissue, not from the epidermis itself. In fetal life, melanocytes migrate into the epidermis and reside scattered among the basal layer of the keratinocytes (Figure 2-10). Each melanocyte has long projections or dendrites which reach many surrounding keratinocytes and act to pass the pigment particles (melanosomes) into the keratinocytes. As the keratinocytes migrate upward, they carry the pigment particles with them. Pigment is constantly being made by the melanocytes and passed on to the keratinocytes. The keratinocytes are constantly carrying the pigment upward and outward, until they finally degrade and dump it on the surface of the skin as they die. Melanocytes are also present in the lowest layers of the hair bulb cells and pass pigment granules on to color the hair itself.

Melanin acts as a screen or filter to prevent the damaging ultraviolet rays of the sun from entering the deeper parts of the skin where they might affect blood vessels, damage cells, and cause wrinkling and aging or skin cancer. Melanin pigmentation of the skin is the most efficient sunscreen known. This is why black people have less sunburn, wrinkling, and skin cancer.

When solar ultraviolet light in large quantities strikes the skin, not all of it is absorbed by the melanin sunscreen. The ultraviolet light which does get through to strike blood vessels, melanocytes, and lower keratinocytes causes sunburn. Such radiation also causes the melanocytes to begin working harder to provide more melanin as sunscreen. The increased pigmentation results in an acquired darkening we popularly refer to as "tan." Since this tan provides more pigment-sunscreen, it serves to protect us from

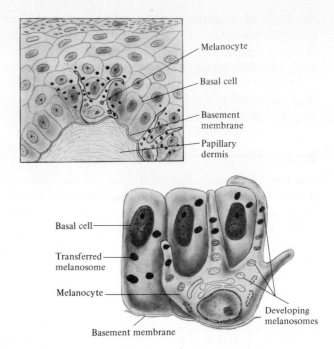

Figure 2-10 Melanocytes. The long dendrites serve to transfer pigment to the keratinocytes.

further sunburn. Ability to tan is inherited and is generally less efficient in lighter individuals.

The various races have roughly the same number of melanocytes. The melanocytes of the darker races are simply much more active in producing melanosomes, and they produce more and larger pigment particles. Caucasians have less active, or at least less productive, melanocyte pigment cells, while blacks have very active pigment cells. The fair Irishman ends up with the least melanin in his skin; the darkest black has the most. Our base-line color is inherited.

Anthropologists usually divide mankind into groups, such as Caucasoid; Asiatic, which includes Chinese and Japanese; American Indian; and Negroid, in which color is one of the most obvious identifying features. The term "race" as applied by biologists refers to groups of animals that have physical characteristics in common. Race is a taxonomic subclassification of a biologic species.

Since *Homo sapiens* is the one species of humankind, race is the major distinguishing subgrouping. A race is a group of peoples who are distinct by virtue of genetic isolation and natural selection. It has nothing to do with persons arbitrarily selected from a population, or with religion or nationality. Racial differences, including body size and shape, density and configuration of various bones, number of cusps on teeth, form and distribution of body hair, blood grouping, fingerprint differences, amount of pigmentation, and susceptibility to certain diseases are hereditary as groups of gene dominances which tend to occur together.

The present populations of the world are hybrid. Blood groups are so widely scattered geographically that miscegenation must always have taken place. Skin color as a precise guideline to racial differentiation is also futile because of the wide spectrum and subtle variations of hues and intensities. Some East Indians are darker in color than many American Negroes. Yet centuries of prejudice have left their mark; the "aristocracy of the skin" which has been called the "most stupid of nobilities" continues to be a common persuasion. Skin color variability provides modern man with convenient but inappropriate markers for segregation and prejudice.

Many people are dissatisfied with their skin color. Some light-skinned individuals spend hours of time and millions of dollars to acquire the sun-tanned hues that have become hallmarks of wealth and leisure. Conversely, "black" is not always equated with "beauty," for many darkly pigmented people give high priority to artificial lightening of their complexions. The social implications and psychological ramifications of skin color are deeply rooted and far-reaching.

Certain systemic diseases and skin diseases cause the pigment cells either to become overactive, resulting in darkening, or to become underactive, causing lightening of the skin. In some disorders, the pigment cells are destroyed completely and the result is a totally white area of skin.

The color of skin is actually made up of several components. The epidermis contains the brown-black of melanin. The skin also contains small amounts of yellow from carotenoids, exogenous substances obtained by ingestion of fruits and vegetables. Since the epidermis permits some transmission of light, we are also able to see the bright red of oxygenated hemoglobin and the bluish-red of reduced hemoglobin in the superficial blood vessels in the dermis of the skin.

REFERENCES

Advances in Biology of Skin, Vol. 6, Aging, Proceedings of Symposium Held at the University of Oregon Medical School, 1964, Montagna, W., ed., Pergamon Press, New York, 1965.

Advances in Biology of Skin, Vol. 3, Eccrine Sweat Glands and Eccrine Sweating. Proceeding of Brown University Symposium on Biology of Skin, 1961, Montagna, W., R. A. Ellis, and A. F. Silver, eds., Pergamon Press, New York, 1962.

Biology of Normal and Abnormal Melanocytes. Seminar on the Biology of Normal and Abnormal Melanocytes, Tokyo, 1969, Kawamura, T., T. B. Fitzpatrick, and M. Seiji, eds., University Park Press, Baltimore, 1971.

Cage, G. W., and R. L. Dobson: "Sodium Secretion and Reabsorption in the Human Eccrine Sweat Gland," *J. Clin. Invest.* **44:**1270–1276, July 1965.

Church, R.: "Drugs and the Hair," *Practitioner* **202:**109–116, January 1969.

DeFeo, C. P., Jr.: "Dysfunction of Hair Growth," *Med. Clin. Am.* **49:**603–620, May 1965.

Hair Growth, Proceedings of Symposium on the Biology of Skin, University of Oregon Medical School, 1967, Montagna, W., and R. Dobson, eds., Pergamon Press, 1969.

Hurley, H. J., and W. B. Shelley: *The Human Apocrine Sweat Gland in Health and Disease,* Charles C Thomas, Publisher, Springfield, Ill., 1960.

Kligman, A. M.: "Pathologic Dynamics of Human Hair Loss: Telogen Effluvium," *Arch. Derm.* **83:**175–198, February 1961.

Kuno, Y.: *Human Perspiration,* Charles C Thomas, Publisher, Springfield, Ill., 1956.

Lewin, K.: "The Finger Nail in General Disease," *Brit. J. Derm.* **77:**431–438, August–September 1965.

Maguire, H., and A. M. Kligman: "Hair Plucking as a Diagnostic Tool," *J. Int. Coll. Surg.* **42:**77–79, July 1964.

Montagna, W.: *The Structure and Function of Skin,* Academic Press, Inc., New York, 1962.

Muller, S., and R. K. Winkelmann: "Alopecia Areata," *Arch. Derm.* **88:**290–297, September 1963.

Orentreich, N.: "Hair Transplants—Long-Term Results and New Advances," *Arch. Otolaryng.* **92:**576–582, December 1970.

Pardo-Castello, V., and O. Pardo: *Disease of the Nails,* Charles C Thomas, Publisher, Springfield, Ill., 1960.

Saitoh, M., U. Makoto, and M. Sakamoto: "Human Hair Cycle," *J. Invest. Derm.* **54:**65–81, January 1970.

Samman, P. D.: *The Nails in Disease,* William Hienemann Ltd., London, 1965.

Sims, R.: "Beau's Lines in Hair: Reduction of Hair Shaft Diameter Associated with Illness," *Brit. J. Derm.* **79:**43–49, January 1967.

Sneddon, I. B.: "Nail Changes in Systemic Disease," *Current Med. Drugs* **4:**17–23, July 1964.

Stroud, J.: "Hair Shaft Defects," *Cutis,* **5:**1375–1382, November 1969.

Van Scott, E. J.: "Physiology of Hair Growth," *Clin. Obstet. Gynec.* **7:**1062–1074, December 1964.

Chapter 3

Variations of Normal Skin and Common Incidental Disorders

Skin of the newborn
Diaper dermatitis
Common benign malformations of the skin
  Nevus
  Hemangioma
  Mole
  Dermal melanocytosis
  Lentigo
  Freckles
Skin of the adolescent
Dry skin
Common benign tumors of the skin
  Seborrheic keratosis
  Skin tags
  Dermatofibroma
  Lipoma
  Wen
Skin of the aged

SKIN OF THE NEWBORN

At birth, the skin is frequently covered with a greasy or cheesy film, the vernix caseosa. This film is largely a product of the sebaceous glands of the infant's skin mixed with sloughed skin and dried amniotic fluids.

Since sebaceous glands are sensitive to maternal androgens, the glands are developed and functioning before birth. The vernix is usually washed off or wears off in a few days or weeks. It can, however, partially dry up and harden and can persist in the scalp area as so-called cradle cap.

The infant's skin usually becomes a red-blue during delivery but appears increasingly pink to red over the next several hours. This redness normally fades over two to three days and is often followed by a fine scaling. This generalized desquamation (scaling) may be impressive in some infants, especially on hands and feet.

Differentiation of the epidermal appendages may not be complete at birth. Tiny white cysts called *milia* commonly appear scattered over the face. These represent aberrant, faulty, or partially occluded pilosebaceous follicles. The formation of milia may be related to hormone stimulus of sebaceous glands in a pilosebaceous unit not yet mature or fully patent. The sebaceous glands gradually become smaller and inactive after birth, and remain quiescent until adolescence. The amount of scalp hair present at birth is quite variable. Frequently only fine vellus hairs (often called lanugo hair) are present, but most infants have some terminal hairs on their scalps. More than 75 percent of scalp hairs are in resting (telogen) phase at birth. The child may become more bald as these hairs fall out over the ensuing weeks, as they are displaced by new hairs beginning to grow in the follicle. It may take as long as six to twelve months before the asynchronized adult growth cycles become established to provide constant scalp hair. The friction of rubbing often accelerates the normal shedding at the occipital and temporal areas.

Eccrine sweat glands may not function for several days after birth and even then they are often not fully effective at delivering large quantities of sweat. Inadequate or immature sweat ducts or duct orifices may result in sweat retention and subsequent inflammation. As a result, tiny red inflammatory papules occur at the site of such occluded glands. Such a "heat rash" is called *miliaria*.

Maternal or placental hormones have other influences on the fetus. The newborn may have swollen, slightly enlarged, and edematous sex organs or hyperplastic vaginal mucosa with a white discharge. The breast tissue of male and female infants may be engorged, and may secrete small amounts of milk. These changes are all reversed within several weeks as the maternal sex hormones are metabolized.

The blood vessel tone and the vascular distribution of the infant is not fully functional at birth. Blood tends to pool centrally, and the skin may have poor or intermittent circulation. Blotchy red, white, or cyanotic areas may appear after crying or if the room temperature is lowered. At times, when a child is lying on his side, the half of his body which is uppermost may suddenly become pale, while the dependent side flushes red. The colors of the two sides may be reversed by turning the child to the opposite side. This nonpathologic and temporary event is sometimes referred to as the *harlequin color change.* Another reversible sign of poor vascular tone is localized pitting edema.

Relatively obese infants have many skin folds in which friction and occlusion cause intertriginous irritation and redness. If room temperature and humidity are elevated, *intertrigo* (dermatitis of opposed surfaces of skin) is more likely to occur. In the absence of any complicating factors, the process is usually self-limiting and lasts only days to weeks. These areas may become superinfected with yeast or bacteria and may require definitive therapy.

Colonization by bacteria begins immediately after birth and within a few weeks the normal flora of the adult is present on the infant's skin. Infants obtain bacteria from the vaginas of their mothers, from nursery objects and personnel, and from the air. The establishment of harmless bacteria which reside on the skin is important because their presence helps prevent invasion by pathogenic organisms. Occasionally, certain staphylococci carried by hospital staff cause nursery epidemics of *impetigo,* a superficial bacterial skin infection. Periodic checks for asymptomatic nose and throat carriers of pathogenic staphylococci among doctors and nurses is advisable. Proper observation of nursery and ward cleaning techniques and isolation procedures is essential.

Erythema neonatorum is a common, benign, blotchy redness of the skin of the newborn which begins at birth or within the first few days of life. The lesions are usually flat, but occasionally there may be small raised areas or pustules. The pustules contain numerous eosinophils. The infant may appear slightly restless but is otherwise normal. The condition is temporary, nonserious, and requires no treatment. The fact that no cause is known is reflected by the confusing list of names for this eruption (*toxic erythema* of the newborn, *erythema neonatorum, urticaria neonatorum, erythema neonatorum allergicum*).

DIAPER DERMATITIS

Diaper dermatitis (napkin rash) is an inflammatory reaction in areas normally occluded by pads or diapers. It is induced by prolonged contact with urine or feces, or other irritants. It is very common in infancy, but is also seen in incontinent children and adults. Confluent redness is confined to the lower abdomen, anogenital region, and upper thighs (Figure 3-1). The areas of maximum occlusion at the apex of the body creases may be less involved than the surrounding skin, because urine and feces and soiled diapers do not reach into these areas. The opposite is true of simple intertrigo in which maximally occluded skin folds are maximally involved. Scattered small pustules, erosions or papules may be superimposed on the redness.

Most diaper dermatitis is caused by a combination of factors. Prolonged contact with urine macerates the skin. Totally occlusive dressings, rubber pants, and diapers with outer plastic lining prevent any evaporation, and increase the maceration. Bacteria normally present in feces break down the urinary urea to produce ammonia, which causes irritation. Other enzymes in skin or feces, or bacteria, may cause inflammation from additional irritants created from body wastes.

Local superimposed miliaria caused by occlusion of immature eccrine sweat ducts adds to the disorder. Contactants, contaminants, and primary irritants in the diaper itself may further complicate the dermatitis. Once skin is irritated and the stratum corneum is not intact, it is far more suscep-

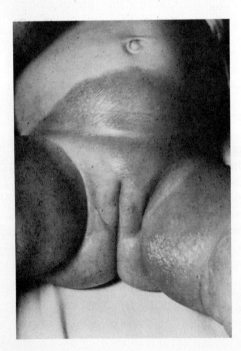

Figure 3-1 Diaper dermatitis. Erythema is confined to the areas of diaper occlusion. There is relative sparing of the normally occluded region of the inguinal crease.

tible to such irritants. Finally, bacteria or yeast may take advantage of the moisture and of the organic food supply of feces and macerated skin, and cause superinfections.

Treatment is aimed at removing the causes of occlusion, maceration, and irritation. Thorough cleansing after soiling is essential. Since the skin appears clean after a urine saturation, all too often it is just wiped with a dry area of the diaper or a dry cloth, and a new diaper applied. Instead, the area should be rinsed before drying and recovering. Removal of rubber or plastic, frequent diaper changes, air drying, and proper cleansing are frequently all that is needed to treat diaper dermatitis. Diaper material should be washed in mild soap, and rinsed thoroughly. Quarternary ammonium compounds may be used for laundering. More severe irritations may require protective creams such as zinc oxide or petrolatum or may require treatment with topical steroids. Absorption through scrotal skin and macerated skin is greater than normal, and so it is critical that irritating medicines or sensitizers not be used topically and that diapers be rinsed thoroughly. Marking inks used by laundries may cause aniline poisoning. Diapers stored in mothballs may cause hemolytic anemia because of naphthalene poisoning.

COMMON BENIGN MALFORMATIONS OF THE SKIN

Minor abnormalities in development are probably present in the skin of every person. In an organ that covers 2 square yards and contains millions of hairs and glands, it is to be expected that aberrant growth and local malformations will occur frequently. Probably most of these are microscopic and unnoticed. Some, like the *milia* of the newborn, are transient and unimportant. Other malformations are large enough to cause more serious functional or cosmetic difficulties.

Malformations in the skin may result from an excess of a certain cell or constituent of the skin, or from too few cells or too little of one of the skin substances. Malformations can be generalized or local. The popular term "birthmark" is often nonspecific, referring to any kind of localized malformation of the skin which is visible at or shortly after birth. The term is most often used to describe vascular malformations in the skin, more correctly called *hemangiomas*.

Nevus

The word nevus is an ancient medical term often used to describe circumscribed developmental abnormalities in the skin. In its broadest sense, "nevus" is even less specific than "birthmark," as it includes those lesions which are evident at or shortly after birth and also lesions which may not become apparent for years but which are suspected as being developmental in origin.

Using this broad definition, nevi may be made up of epidermal components, glands or parts of glands, dermal components, or melanocytes. Usually, one tissue or cell type predominates. In any case, it is a benign overgrowth (rarely a deficiency), or aggregation, or relatively stable proliferation of a normal skin component. It is localized, usually ovoid or linear in shape, and may occur as single or multiple lesions. Such nevi of primarily *epithelial* (epidermal) components would include sebaceous nevi (nevus sebaceous), apocrine nevi and hair-follicle nevi. Nevi made up of a *dermal* skin constituent would include vascular nevi (hemangiomas), lymphangiomas, and connective tissue nevi. Nevus lipomatosus is a local excess of fat-laden cells in the *subcutaneous* tissue. A nevus can also be made of *melanocyte-like* cells. Such collections of melanocytes may be in the epidermis or dermis, or may extend into both.

Some pigmented lesions are present at birth and are large. They may contain hair and are often found on the lower trunk (bathing suit nevus), but can be found anywhere. Large congenital pigmented hairy nevi may be associated with neurologic disorders. A significant number of these large congenital lesions develop malignant change within them, so that it is best to remove them early in life.

Of the localized proliferation or aggregation of melanocytes, those which are smaller than 1 centimeter appear well after birth and are made up of nests of normal cells, have been referred to as *moles*. Some dermatologists and pathologists confine the use of the word nevus only to this very common group of pigmented lesions and, in fact, refer to the nesting deviated or malformed melanocyte cells which make up the mole as "nevus cells." Most textbooks use the term nevus in both the broad sense listed above (any circumscribed excess of normal tissue leading to a benign, stable malformation of skin), and in the more specific sense, describing the nesting "nevus" cells (moles) derived from melanocytes. The confusion is magnified because moles (nevus cell nevi) are not always obviously pigmented. Both uses of the word are so entrenched that change is not likely. Therefore, it is best to be as specific as possible when using the term nevus—describing epithelial nevus, sebaceous nevus, nevus cell nevus (mole), comedo nevus, etc. Hemangioma is another name for vascular nevus.

The reason for the occurrence of these local circumscribed malformations is not known. Intrauterine pressure, trauma, and externally applied pressures play no role in their location. Hereditary etiology for most of the nevi has not been documented, but some genetic syndromes do have increased incidence of certain nevi, and the number and location of moles is sometimes familial.

Nevi of all types, including moles, are very common, being present in over 95 percent of all adults, with an average of more than 10 per person. Few are present at birth, and incidence increases with age. While prominent hemangiomas occur in 1 percent of newborns, some transient neonatal malformation, caused by an excess of capillaries or fixed vasodilatation, occurs in more than half of all males and females. The most common nevus is the mole. Most appear in childhood, increase in number over the first three decades, and diminish thereafter. The skin is not unique in its tendency to form stable benign developmental defects. Clinically, unimportant malformations can be found in the internal organs of most people carefully examined at autopsy.

Hemangioma

Nevus flammeus (diffuse capillary hemangioma, plane nevus, telangiectatic nevus) is a red, partially blanchable, flat lesion present at birth, which is caused by fixed dilatation of mature capillaries in otherwise normal skin (Figure 3-2). The mildest form is a flat pink area (salmon patch, "stork bite") as the nape of the neck or on the forehead, at the base of the nose, or over the upper eyelid, which fades away over the first months or years of life. The more impressive but less frequent presentation is the port wine stain, which is purple, is present at birth, may enlarge for a few months, and then remain stable throughout life. Lesions may be small or may cover a large proportion of the face, cape area, or extremity, but usually do not cross the midline. Mucous membranes, including conjunctiva, may also be involved.

Port wine stain usually occurs as a purely cosmetic defect in otherwise normal people, but if present in the trigeminal nerve area may signal Sturge-Weber syndrome (venous angioma of the leptomeninges over the cerebral cortex resulting in central nervous system symptoms). Rarely, hypertrophy of a limb or a communicating arteriovenous fistula may be associated findings. Treatments are usually unsatisfactory. Since port wine stains are flat and have little tendency to fade, the best therapy is reassurance and an opaque cosmetic covering cream, such as Covermark®.

Capillary hemangioma of infancy (strawberry mark, nevus vasculosus, hypertrophic hemangioma, circumscribed capillary hemangioma) has a predilection for the head and neck region. It is usually not present at birth, but begins to be noticeable in the first month of extrauterine life. It is bright red, lobulated, elevated, soft, and blanchable, and frequently grows very rapidly for nine to twelve months. Progressive involution then occurs over several years, with eventual complete remission in the majority

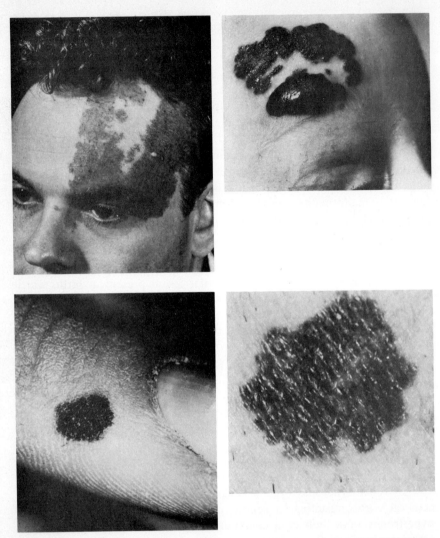

Figure 3-2 (*a*) Nevus flammeus (port wine stain); (*b*) capillary hemangiomas (strawberry); (*c*) mole (compound nevus); (*d*) lentigo.

of cases. Histologically, dilated vessels and immature proliferative endothelial cells are mixed with connective tissue.

Careful observation but intelligent neglect is often the best management because many of the treatment modalities leave scarring and distortion. The hemangioma left alone may disappear without a trace. If growth rate is alarming and if no involution occurs after six or seven years, or if clotting and thrombocytopenia develop, then such things as surgical intervention, systemic steroids, x-ray, or cryotherapy may be considered.

Cavernous hemangiomas are deeper and have larger vascular spaces. They appear as irregular, soft, blue-red palpable lesions. The boggy mass consists of thin-walled vascular spaces resembling venous sinuses, which may extend down to and into the subcutaneous tissue, and may protrude from the skin, distorting some other areas. They may also involve internal organs, but usually do not cause symptoms. Some have a tendency to persistent and continual growth, but most resolve. Many hemangiomas are mixed, having components of both capillary and cavernous hemangioma.

Mole ("Nevus Cell" Nevus)

Moles are very common lesions that usually appear after birth. They are clumps of normal cells derived from melanocyte-like precursor cells. They usually begin as flat spots, but often become raised over several years. They are usually pigmented, and may be determined by heredity (Figure 3-2c).

The excess cells may be present only in the epidermis, where they appear as normal mature melanocytes. The lesion differs from normal skin only in the fact that melanocyte-like cells are present in large numbers, may aggregate into clumps, and usually make more pigment. When the excess cells are present deep in the dermis, they lose their pigment and dendrites and begin to look like neural elments. Those cells which may occur high in the dermis or near the dermoepidermal junction have histologic features midway between these two types of cells.

The mole may be flat, slightly elevated, dome-shaped, polypoid, pedunculated, or papillomatous. Skin lines or markings are usually preserved over the lesions. The pathologists classify these moles as junctional (intraepidermal), dermal, or compound (in both epidermis and dermis), depending upon the location of the collection of cells. The individual cells within these lesions are probably no more prone to malignant change than are other melanocytes in the skin. Malignant lesions of melanocytes arise more often from moles simply because there is a much greater density of melanocyte-like cells present in moles than in normal skin and this increases the chances of such change within a mole. Also, malignant melanomas may begin as small pigmented lesions thought to be moles. This misapprehension creates the illusion of a transformation from mole to malignant lesion. Unless a mole is frequently traumatized, secondarily inflamed, rapidly growing, or has features suggestive of malignant melanoma (see Chapter 10), there is no reason to remove it, except for cosmetic reasons.

Dermal Melanocytosis

Melanocyte precursor cells or clumps of melanocyte-like cells en route to the epidermis may collect in the dermis. Because the cells are deeper within the skin, the brown-black melanin which they produce may appear blue through the skin. There are several types of collections of functioning melanocytes in the dermis.

The *Mongolian spot* is a poorly circumscribed, flat lesion, usually present at birth, and most often seen on the lower back or over the buttocks. It is found predominantly in Mongoloids, Negroids, Polynesians, and American Indians, but may occur in Caucasians. Elongated melanocyte precursor cells in the lower dermis cause the blue-black color. These spots often disappear over many years, but may remain noticeable for life.

A *dermal melanocytoma* (blue nevus) is a benign neoplasia of fibroblast-like melanocyte precursor cells, which is often removed for cosmetic reasons or to differentiate it from malignant melanoma.

A *compound melanocytoma* (Spitz juvenile melanoma) is a rapidly growing, dome-shaped, pink, or pigmented lesion, which usually occurs on the faces of children. Although the clinical and histologic features often suggest melanoma, there is little evidence to support such a relationship. Therefore, the lesions may be only of cosmetic importance, but they are often removed surgically because of the rapid growth and histologic findings, which are similar to those of malignant melanoma.

Lentigo

Lentigines are common pigmented lesions of the skin which are small, flat, and usually of an uniform brown to black color (Figure 3-2*d*). They arise at any age and may appear anywhere. Those that appear in early or middle life do not seem to be related to sun. They occur in covered sites, and show little seasonal variation in color. The lentigines which appear late in life (senile lentigo, "liver spots") appear on the dorsum of the hand and on the face and may be related to aging and sun (see section on aging skin).

Histologic examination simply shows an increased number of normal melanocytes in the basal layer of the epidermis. Lentigines, therefore, fit into the broad definition of nevus and also into the definition of mole. They differ from the junctional or intraepidermal mole in that the increased numbers of melanocytes remain in the basal layer, whereas in the junctional mole they may clump into nests. Lentigines are simply localized increased numbers of melanocytes. The melanocytes are of usual morphology, and remain located in their normal site in the basal layer.

Freckles

Freckles (ephelides) are flat, well-circumscribed brown lesions scattered over sun-exposed areas. Freckles are caused by local groups of melanocytes, which are genetically determined to be more sensitive to solar stimulation than those of the surrounding skin. After ultraviolet radiation, these melanocytes become large, very active cells which make increased pigment.

Freckles are inherited and do not occur without sun exposure. They are harmless. The number of melanocytes in freckles may be normal or reduced. The production of pigment granules is increased in these areas and is responsible for the hyperpigmentation.

SKIN OF THE ADOLESCENT

At puberty, the gonads begin to secrete hormones which cause the genitals to grow and secondary sexual characteristics to appear. The skin also responds. Androgens made by the adrenals, ovaries, and testes stimulate the enlargement, maturation, and secretory activity of hair follicles, sebaceous glands, and apocrine glands in certain body areas. Many of the vellus hairs of the pubic and axillary region change to coarse terminal hairs. The higher levels of androgens present in males also cause facial hair to grow. Unlike sebaceous and apocrine glands, the hair follicles in the beard area are not sensitive to the levels of androgens found in both male and female, but are stimulated only by the higher levels of androgens present in males. Females would also grow beards if given exogenous androgens to supplement their endogenous male hormone. At the time of this stimulation of hair growth, the incidence of occlusion, irritation, and infection of hair follicles increases. The resulting inflammation, called *folliculitis,* is most often seen over the thighs, buttocks, or beard areas.

Sebaceous glands of the face, chest, and upper back become large and functional. Acne and seborrheic dermatitis begin to appear. Apocrine glands begin to function in the axillae and around the genitalia. As bacteria act on the secretions from these glands, young people begin to notice odors for the first time. Increased activity of the eccrine sweat glands causes hyperhidrosis of the palms and increased axillary sweating. The skin is also affected by the menstrual cycle. Vascularity may be increased during the last half of the cycle, and premenstrual retention of salt and water may cause breast enlargement, ankle edema, or swelling of the fingers. Acne often flares four to seven days before onset of menstrual flow, and the hair may be slightly greasy due to increased sebaceous gland activity in the scalp.

With all the skin glands working fulltime, body hygiene begins to require more careful attention and more active measures. Some teenagers overreact; they use too much soap and too many cosmetics, antiperspirants, powders, and medications, all of which cause skin irritation. They pinch, squeeze, and manipulate their skin, hair, and nails excessively. Other teenagers exercise such a proud and practiced neglect of their skin that occlusion, folliculitis, untreated acne, and infection cause unnecessary skin damage and possible scarring.

Puberty is a time of identity crisis, contests of will between parent and child, sexual awakening, maximum peer group pressure, increasingly difficult school work, and a first hard look at individual responsibility. It is no wonder that those skin diseases that are precipitated or worsened by emotional tension or anxiety become very active. Eczema and psoriasis are very clearly worsened by such stress.

Warts occur most frequently in the teenage years. This is true of plantar warts and digital warts. The cause of this increased incidence is not known.

Sexual maturity and activity brings with it the risk of venereal disease. Many adolescents have unverbalized fears about V.D., based on misinformation. Medical personnel must know enough about V.D. to give advice and must be receptive and understanding enough to be asked for advice.

DRY SKIN

Relative dehydration of the stratum corneum occurs gradually with age and may occur within hours in decreased environmental humidity. Some persons may be genetically predisposed to be more susceptible to drying than others. There is a genetically determined group of disorders called *ichthyosis* in which this tendency is evident to a marked degree. The many domestic cleansers, solvents, and chemicals which touch skin remove lipids that normally help maintain the water-holding properties of the stratum corneum. Nutritional deficiencies of several types may result in dryness of the epidermis and thickening of the stratum corneum at hair follicle openings.

Fully hydrated stratum corneum swells and, when subsequentially dried, shrinks and becomes brittle and hard. Repeated wetting and drying may lead to cracks in the stratum corneum which, in turn, result in fissures.

Dry skin is rough, finely flaky, and less flexible, and it feels dry to the touch. The hair follicle openings may feel rough, because they have elevated plugs of stratum corneum. As the skin becomes drier, cracks or fissures may occur and a fine lacework of erythema or even hemorrhages can be seen. *Pruritus* (itching) is caused by the dryness and the resultant scratching and rubbing leads to thickening of the skin and to excoriations. If dryness and rubbing become extensive, generalized eczematous dermatitis (see Chapter 5) may result.

The best therapy consists simply of rehydrating the skin and providing an environment with adequate relative humidity. Minimizing contact with soap and other irritants is helpful. Occlusive ointments or greases prevent evaporation of water from the skin surface and help restore adequate water content to the skin. Oils added to bath water help somewhat, but ointments applied to the skin immediately after bathing are much more effective in holding water in the skin. Cool mist humidifiers operated in the bedroom during the dry winter months may prevent symptomatic drying of the skin.

COMMON BENIGN TUMORS OF THE SKIN

Seborrheic Keratosis

Seborrheic keratosis is a common benign epidermal tumor, which occurs with increasing frequency with advancing age. It may be an epithelial nevus of markedly delayed onset. Seborrheic keratoses usually do not appear before the fourth decade, and are seen most often on the trunk, face, or scalp. They are the most common epidermal growth on aged skin; some persons may have more than twenty. The occurrence of large numbers of seborrheic keratoses may be familial.

They appear as small, light-yellow or tan, thin, sharply circumscribed plaques which have a "stuck on" appearance but are not easily removed (Figure 3-3). As the lesion ages, it thickens, becomes more verrucous (wart-like, see Chapter 7) or papillomatous (many tiny projections), and

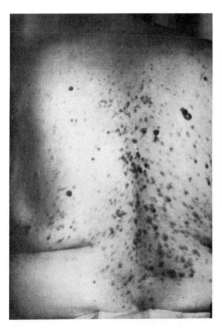
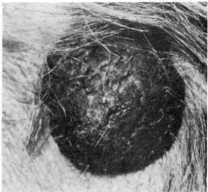

Figure 3-3 Seborrheic keratoses. (a) Multiple lesions on the trunk are frequent in the elderly; (b) close-up of single lesion; the lesion is dirty brown and appears as if it is stuck on or could be crumbled away.

may darken considerably. Some become black. Follicles within the lesion tend to become plugged. The surface may be greasy or rough and dry. Even the large lesions maintain their superficial nature.

The lesion is made by a proliferation of epidermal cells which maintain some of the features of basal cells but are somewhat differentiated and many even form keratin cysts within the lesion. Melanin pigmentation is usually present in variable amounts, accounting for some of the color of the lesion.

The lesions grow slowly, and do not disappear spontaneously. Since they do not become malignant, their presence is simply a cosmetic problem and no treatment is required. Curettage or freezing with liquid nitrogen will successfully remove the lesions.

Skin Tags

Skin tags (Figure 3-4) (acrochordon, cutaneous tag, fibroepithelial polyp) are tiny, soft, pedunculated protrusions or polyps of normal-colored skin. Eyelids, neck, axillae, and upper trunk are the usual sites. They are often found in flexural creases of obese individuals. Most common among the elderly, they sometimes cause cosmetic concern to middle-aged women. They may become irritated when traumatized but are usually asymptomatic.

The stalk contains loose connective tissue and the overlying epidermis may be thickened but has no abnormal cells. Cutaneous tags are easily removed surgically but are harmless if left in place. They are sometimes accidentally removed by minor trauma.

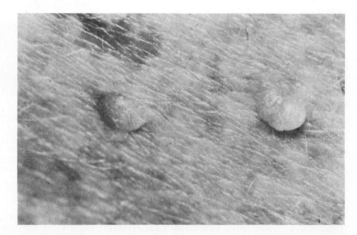

Figure 3-4 Skin tag (acrochordon). The tip of pedunculated lesion is easily movable.

Dermatofibroma

Dermatofibroma is a common, benign, firm dermal nodule which is covered with epidermis of normal or slightly hyperpigmented color. Most dermatofibroma occur during the fourth and fifth decade. The lesion is partially fixed to the deep dermis, so that it is not as movable as the surrounding skin. If the examining thumb and index finger attempt to grasp and raise the entire lesion, the nodule puckers or dimples, to allow it to remain close to its deep attachments as the surrounding skin is lifted.

It is caused by focal proliferation of fibroblasts and/or histiocytes and may represent a kind of dermal tissue reaction, not a true neoplasm. In any case, it is benign and requires no treatment. Dermatofibromas are often removed by simple excision for diagnostic or cosmetic reasons.

Lipoma

Lipoma is a benign tumor made up of an excess of normal mature fat cells encompassed in variable amounts of connective tissue. It can occur anywhere that subcutaneous fat or other fatty tissue exists. The soft, movable, rounded masses occur anytime in life and are more frequent in females. One to many lesions of almost any size may exist on one person.

Lipomas are subcutaneous structures, obviously deep within the skin. They are asymptomatic and are covered with normal dermis and epidermis. They are spongy-feeling and easily movable. They should be excised if extremely rapid growth occurs, if they are unsightly, or if they happen to press on a nerve. The vast majority require no treatment.

Wen

A wen is a benign cystic structure in the skin usually found in young and middle-aged adults. It is located in the dermis; the normal epidermis may appear tense, as it is raised over the dome-shaped protuberance. The cyst is movable, semifirm, and may be 4 millimeters to 4 centimeters in size. Most wens appear on the face, neck, shoulders, or chest.

Although such cysts are most often called sebaceous cysts, they are seldom lined with fat-filled cells or sebum. Most wens could more correctly be termed epidermal cysts because the wall of the cyst looks like normal keratinizing epidermis and the material in the cyst is keratin. Epidermal cysts may be caused by aberrant growth of cells which normally line the pilosebaceous duct. Trauma, duct obstruction, acne, and genetic influences may also be causative factors. *Milia* are small (less than 2 millimeters) epidermal cysts. Cysts may be surgically removed if they are tender or of cosmetic concern.

SKIN OF THE AGED

From birth to old age, skin gradually changes: it has less water and more mature, more insoluble, and less flexible collagen. Since many of the changes we tend to relate to age are actually the result of accumulative ultraviolet damage from years of sun exposure, the sun-exposed skin appears to age faster than the unexposed skin. Although skin aging is gradual and is influenced a great deal by sun-exposure habits, a more rapid acceleration of the cutaneous changes we normally relate to old age occurs after the level of sex hormones begins to fall and the skin and epidermal appendages begin to atrophy.

Although the most conspicuous effect of hormones is that of androgens on the hair, sebaceous glands, and apocrine glands, the sex hormones may play some poorly understood general supportive role in skin growth and function. Testosterone stimulates basal cell reproduction in some laboratory animals and stimulates human dermal fibroblasts to proliferate. Male castrates have pasty, finely wrinkled, pale, thin skin, which appears normally thick and heavy after appropriate hormone replacement.

Normally the diminution of output of the gonads that occurs with aging is more clearly announced in the female body. Although menopause, the cessation of menstruation, may precede the climacteric, the cessation of ovulation, the two events are usually related within a few years. The anovulatory ovaries gradually become atrophic and fibrotic and sex hormone output falls. At this time, vasomotor instability may cause hot flashes, headaches, and spontaneous sweating. These changes are so frequent that they have been accepted as physiologic events, although the mechanism escapes explanation. Many of the other frequent symptoms of menopause, such as insomnia, fatigue, emotional lability, and backache are probably related to the understandable emotional difficulties of a transition to the generation of the grandparent.

Other changes are observable, grossly and microscopically. The breasts lose some of their glandular tissue and firm structural support. The vagina becomes shorter and narrower. The epithelium that lines the vagina, distal urethra, and urethral meatus becomes atrophic. Intercourse may be painful, urination may become painful, and vaginal discharges may irritate the skin. Vulvitis and vaginitis and some of the genital symptoms can be reversed by the local or systemic administration of estrogens. Estrogens lead to increased basal layer cell division, faster transit time, and thickening of the vaginal mucosa. The facial hirsuitism and increasing incidence of male pattern baldness in old females may be related to falling levels of estrogens or to a cumulative androgen effect on hair follicles which were genetically predisposed to respond late in life. Male pattern baldness in males is similarly increased late in life. Hormone therapy does not reverse the baldness.

The skin of the aged is dry and wrinkled. Caucasian skin develops a pale-yellow complexion, and is covered with many lentigines and seborrheic keratoses. Purple spots occur at the sites of minor trauma because fragile and easily broken capillaries permit blood to leak into the dermis. Thinning of the epidermis may occur and the skin may appear more transparent. The cells of the epidermis show irregularity in size and shape and the dermoepidermal junction is flattened. The thin stratum corneum allows the skin to be more easily dehydrated and decreases its effectiveness as a barrier.

With aging, there is gradual reduction in the number of active eccrine sweat glands and a reduced sweat output per gland. The apocrine glands and sebaceous glands become less active because their function is hormone dependent. They do not atrophy to any great extent and their activity can be restimulated by exogenous hormones. The scalp hair becomes sparse and gray and the rate of nail growth diminishes. With increasing age, there is a progressive reduction in the number of active melanocytes, and a reduced capacity to tan. Paradoxically, senile lentigines (age spots, "liver spots") develop on the face and on the backs of the hands and represent an increased number of melanocytes in the basal layer.

The dermis displays many changes which cause some of the signs we recognize as aged skin. Collagen becomes stiffer as it "matures," with more chemical cross links, more cross bonds, and higher collagen to ground-substance ratio. The dermis may be thin and the amount of subcutaneous tissue decreased, which adds to the wrinkled or sagging appearance of the skin. These dermal changes are magnified in the sun-exposed areas where chronic actinic damage has also caused increased elastic tissue and has changed the fibers of the dermal proteins into amorphous granular material. Such skin appears wrinkled, coarse, and leathery.

Altered function of the skin, as a consequence of aging, dryness, the cumulative effects of decades of environmental hazards, and other factors, leads to increased frequency of certain dermatoses in the aged. Skin tags, seborrheic keratoses, and lentigines are common. Small 2- to 5-millimeters dome-shaped, soft, purple lesions on the trunk, called cherry angiomas, are benign hemangioma-like growths of vascular tissue. Seborrheic dermatitis, chronic localized eczema, and dry skin are frequent. Stasis dermatitis and leg ulcers are manifestations of the poor circulation seen in the lower extremities. Skin cancers are more frequent with advancing age. Pruritus is common among older patients and, at times, may become severe. Since the thin, dry skin seems to react to minor stimuli to cause itching and rubbing, bathing with soap, decreased humidity, and sudden changes in temperature may precipitate generalized pruritus. Stasis dermatitis (and chronic venous insufficiency) or insufficient arterial supply often lead to localized itching of the lower extremities. The thin atrophic skin around the genitalia is also a common site of itching.

REFERENCES

Advances in Biology of Skin, Vol. VIII. The Pigmentary System. Proceedings of Symposium on the Biology of Skin, University of Oregon Medical School, 1966, Montagna, W., and F. Hu, eds., Pergamon Press, New York, 1967.

Becker, S. W., Jr., S. W. Becker, Sr., W. R. Nickel, and W. B. Reed: "Giant Pigmented Nevi, Melanoma and Leptomeningeal Melanocytes," *Arch. Derm.* **91:**100–119, February 1965.

Bowers, R. E., E. A. Graham, and K. M. Tomlenson: "The Natural History of the Strawberry Nevus," *Arch. Derm.* **82:**667–680, November 1960.

Burgoon, C. F., Jr., F. Urbach, and W. D. Grover: "Diaper Dermatitis," *Pediatric Clin. N. Am.,* **8:**835–856, 1961.

Holt, L. E.: "Conference on Infantile Eczema," *J. Pediat.* **66:**153–262, January 1965.

Korting, G. W. T., translation of Hautkrankheiten bei Kindern und Jugendlichen: *Diseases of the Skin in Children and Adolescents,* W. B. Saunders Company, Philadelphia, 1970.

Margileth, A. M., and M. Museles: "Cutaneous Hemangiomas in Children: Diagnosis and Conservative Management," *JAMA* **194:**523–526, November 1965.

Solomon, L. A., and N. B. Esterly: *Neonatal Dermatology, Vol. IX: Major Problems in Clinical Pediatrics,* W. B. Saunders Company, Philadelphia, 1973.

Chapter 4

General Pathologic Descriptions and Mechanisms

Definitions
  Macule
  Papule
  Nodule
  Plaque
  Erythema
  Hyperpigmentation
  Hypopigmentation
  Wheal
  Vesicle
  Cyst
  Scale
  Crust
  Ulcers
  Excoriations
Pruritus

The skin does not invariably perform its functions normally. The skin is so available for inspection that we are usually very much aware when things go wrong with it. If the internal organ systems were as visible, many more diseases would probably be described for the heart, lungs, gastrointinal tract, or bones. Changes in skin not sufficient to impair physiologic function but enough to alter appearance are included as "skin diseases." When skin does not perform its function, we not only suffer the consequences, we see the pathology.

Learning to recognize certain skin disorders is not enough. In order to understand the components of skin diseases and to communicate accurately, it is necessary to learn some descriptive words and concepts about skin lesions. In order to understand the etiology of skin disorders, it is important to be able to translate what we see on the surface of the skin into the possible pathologic mechanism occurring within and beneath the skin. It should be remembered that each descriptive word is not only a shorthand account of what we see on the surface of the skin, but also relays specific information about processes going on within the skin. We must think anatomically and mechanistically when we see skin lesions.

DEFINITIONS

Every nursing student, medical student, or paramedical trainee must learn several thousand new words in preparing to care for patients. Below are listed some of the most important vocabulary words of the skin. Most of these words can be used as nouns or adjectives; various combinations of a few key words create short phrases which relay much specific information.

Macule

A macule is a circumscribed area of change of skin color, without elevation, depression, or change in consistency of the skin. A macule is a skin spot which can be seen but not felt. A macule looks different from the surrounding skin because the skin in that area contains a different amount of pigment, blood, or blood products. A macule is perfectly flat and flush with the surrounding skin (Figure 4-1a).

Papule

A papule is a small, elevated, solid lesion which not only can be seen but also can be felt to rise above the level of the surrounding skin. Papules are usually smaller than 0.5 centimeter in diameter, and may be caused by collections or proliferations of cells, by accumulation of fluid, or by metabolic deposits in the dermis or epidermis. A papule is a spot on the skin which can be felt (Figure 4-1*b*).

Nodule

A nodule is a palpable solid bump which is usually deeper and larger than a papule and which results from collections of cells or metabolic substances within the dermis or subcutaneous tissue. Nodules are usually larger than 1 centimeter (Figure 4-1*c*).

Plaque

A plaque is a relatively flat-surfaced elevation of the skin surface; it may cover large surface areas. It may result from thickening of any of the layers normally present in the skin, as well as from infiltration of substances not normally present (Figure 4-1*d*).

Erythema

Erythema simply means redness. Redness of the skin is caused by dilatation of capillaries which leads to the presence of more blood in the superficial dermis. Capillary dilatation has many causes.

Hyperpigmentation

The presence of excessive pigment causes the skin to be darker than is normal or darker than the surrounding skin. This condition is usually caused by an increased production of melanin, from either a normal or an increased number of melanocytes. If the excess melanin is present in its usual site—the epidermis—it is brown-black in appearance. If the melanin should be formed in or find its way into the dermis, the skin has a blue-gray appearance. Hyperpigmentation may result from a tiny local increase in melanin, as in freckles, or from an increase in melanin-producing cells, as in moles. Or it may be a generalized process causing darkening of all of the skin and mucous membranes as is seen in certain disorders of the adrenal or pituitary gland which lead to the production of hormones which stimulate melanocytes.

Hypopigmentation

A decrease in the amount of pigment normally present may result from genetic, endocrine, or nutritional abnormalities or may be induced by topical chemicals, which selectively destroy melanocytes. Sometimes severe trauma to the skin irreversibly damages melanocytes. Thermal burns frequently leave hypopigmented scars. Certain infections or inflammatory dis-

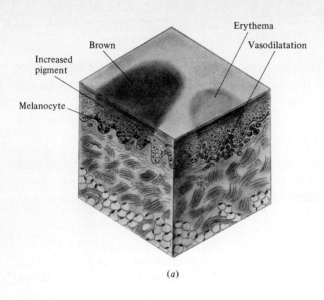

(a)

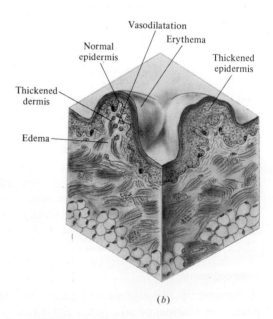

(b)

Figure 4-1 *(a)* Macule; *(b)* papule; *(c)* nodule; *(d)* plaque.

54

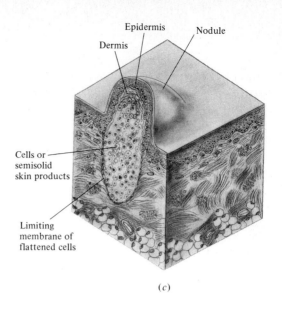

(c)

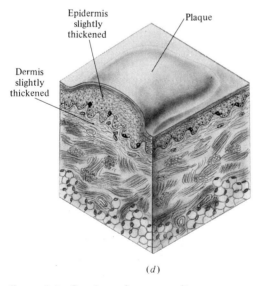

(d)

Figure 4-1 See legend on opposite page.

orders (tinea versicolor, leprosy, severe eczema) may lead to hypopigmentation. Vitiligo is a focal complete loss of pigment (amelanosis) of unknown etiology which occurs in 1 percent of the human race and varies from tiny barely noticeable lesions on the hands, face, and genitalia to extensive absence of pigment over the entire body.

Each of these nouns may also be used as adjectives. Lesions may be described as macular, papular, or nodular. Areas of skin may be hyperpigmented, hypopigmented, or erythematous. The words are usually used in combinations to paint verbal pictures, such as "hypopigmented macules," "erythematous nodules," or "hyperpigmented plaques."

A great many of the changes that take place in skin diseases can be explained by considering the patterns of reactions of blood vessels of the skin. Ultraviolet light, bacteria, toxins, foreign bodies, and many skin and systemic diseases may cause damage to the skin. The superficial blood vessels may be damaged directly or may be influenced by mediators, such as histamine, released from cells in the skin. The result is dilatation of the capillaries of the superficial dermis which is observed in the skin as erythema. There is simply more blood present in the erythematous areas of the skin. If the blood flow through the damaged area is markedly increased, the blood brings more heat from the central body core and the local skin temperature is increased. More severely damaged and swollen vessels may begin to leak fluid into the surrounding dermis, and *edema* results. If the pathologic process continues, more fluid and proteins begin to leak out and to infiltrate the dermis, causing considerable swelling of the tissue.

Inflammatory cells may proceed to the site of the insult and collect in great numbers, adding to the swelling and resulting in palpable lesions. A markedly damaged vessel may allow red blood cells to escape or whole blood to leak into the dermis or subcutaneous tissues. If the insult to the vessels is so severe that they can no longer function to carry blood and nutrients, the skin supplied by those vessels may die, and may become necrotic because its metabolic demands are not fulfilled.

During inflammatory reactions in the skin, fluids and cells collect and congregate in various ways, which results in different grossly visible patterns. When we observe such patterns, we can best understand the significance of the lesions if we mentally reconstruct the most probable microscopic mechanism of the cause.

Wheal

A wheal is a slightly rounded or plaque-like elevation in the skin which is caused by the presence of edema in the upper dermis (Figure 4-2*a*). Spontaneously occurring wheals are called *urticaria* or "hives" (Color Plate

1A, front endpaper). They are usually slightly erythematous. Although new urticarial lesions may continue to appear for several days to weeks, each individual hive usually lasts less than a day. Hives may be tiny or may cover large areas of the body. Lesions may come and go for several days to several months, and often cause itching. Urticaria usually results from some allergic phenomenon (Chapter 5).

Vesicle

If fluid accumulates in a circumscribed focal area within the skin, an elevated bubble results. If the bubble is small (less than 0.5 centimeter), it is usually called a vesicle (Figure 4-2b). A larger, elevated, fluid-filled space is called a *bulla* (plural: bullae) (Chapter 12).

Cyst

A cyst is a thick-walled lesion which contains fluid or semisolid matter. Cysts are usually formed by an aberrant or misdirected growth of epidermal cells which gradually fill the space within the cysts with products of their own making. A cyst differs from a vesicle or a bulla. Cysts form more slowly, are firmer and more fixed to the skin, and are usually found deeper in the skin than are vesicles or bullae. They are often covered with normal epidermis (Figure 4-2c).

Fluid accumulates in the skin from many different causes. Damaged or inflamed blood vessels may leak large amounts of fluid. Necrosis or destruction of epidermal cells may simply leave spaces in the epidermis; tissue fluids accumulate in these spaces. Inflammatory changes may lead to the collection of fluid between the various layers of the skin. Sometimes edema fluid collects beneath the basement membrane which separates the epidermis from the dermis and actually lifts the epidermis up off the dermis.

Knowledge of the site of fluid collection within the skin is often helpful to the dermatologist in deciding the etiology of a vesicle or bulla. Certain groups of blistering diseases occur in the upper dermis, or beneath the basement membrane, while other diseases such as certain viral infections (Chapter 8) and *pemphigus vulgaris* (Chapter 12) always occur within the epidermis.

The fluid in the vesicles and bullae is usually clear initially and simply contains serum. As time goes by, a blister may fill with white blood cells, and become turbid, white, or green-yellow. Such body fluid filled with white blood cells is called purulent fluid or pus. Vesicles filled with such material are called *pustules*. Occasionally blisters may fill with blood and become hemorrhagic vesicles or hemorrhagic bullae.

Blood and blood products may accumulate in the skin in other ways besides simply filling in blister cavities. Blood is sometimes seen in the skin because of relatively permanently dilated blood vessels. Birth marks or congenital hemangiomas represent permanently dilated overgrowths of blood vessels. Single large dilated capillary-like vessels are sometimes visible in the skin and are called *telangiectasias* (Color Plate I*B*). These relatively permanent dilatations appear as fine bright red branching lines, which

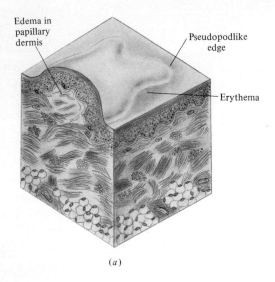

(*a*)

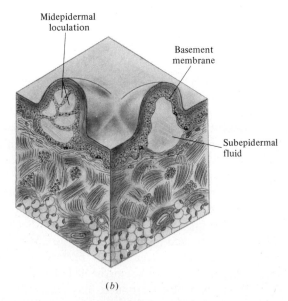

(*b*)

Figure 4-2 (*a*) Wheal; (*b*) vesicle; (*c*) cyst; (*d*) atrophy.

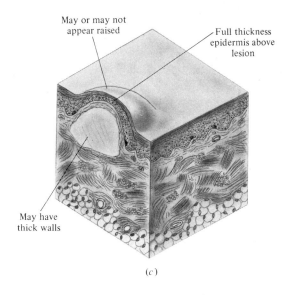

May or may not appear raised

Full thickness epidermis above lesion

May have thick walls

(c)

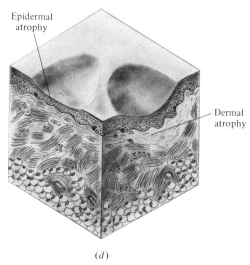

Epidermal atrophy

Dermal atrophy

(d)

Figure 4-2 For legend see opposite page.

are nonpulsatile and may or may not blanch on pressure. Such telangiectasias may be seen as the result of chronic sun damage, around scars, in certain light-sensitive diseases and collagen vascular diseases, and in certain skin tumors. They may also occur as a genetically determined disorder.

Severe inflammation, marked dilatation, or direct trauma to the blood vessels may cause blood to be present in the skin outside the blood vessels.

Tiny 1-millimeter collections of blood outside of the capillaries can sometimes be seen in the skin as purple-red dots. These are called *petechiae*
(Color Plate I*C*). Larger collections of blood in the skin appearing as
purple macules are called *purpura* (Color Plate II*A*). Sometimes massive
collections of extravascular blood in the dermis or subcutaneous tissue
cause large bruise-like lesions called *ecchymoses*. Ecchymoses gradually
change color as the extravasated blood products gradually decompose and
are absorbed back into circulation. Deep collections of blood from trauma
to large vessels in muscles or beneath fascial planes are called *hematomas*.
These are sometimes too deep to be seen on the surface of the skin, but
can often be palpated.

There are other pathologic mechanisms in the skin besides those in
which the blood vessels play the most obvious roles. Normally occurring
layers of the skin may thicken markedly. This thickening may be uniform
or irregular and may involve more than one skin component or layer. It
may be caused by viral infection within the epidermis or it may be a response to repeated trauma or pressure. If the skin is rubbed or scratched
repeatedly, the whole epidermis, including the stratum corneum, may
thicken into an elevated plaque with accentuated skin markings. This
change is called *lichenification* (Figure 4-3).

Thickening may also result from genetic flaws in cell kinetics, which
lead to increased rate of production of skin (as in psoriasis) or in decrease
or delay in the rate at which stratum corneum falls off (possibly a mecha-

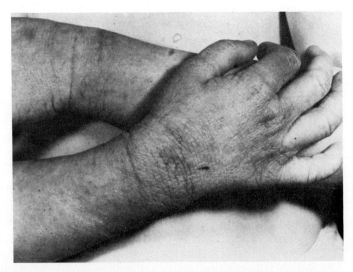

Figure 4-3 Lichenification. Thickening of the skin with exaggeration of the skin
lines results from frequent rubbing.

nism in some forms of ichthyosis). By careful inspection or by skin biopsy it is possible to determine what component of the skin is causing most of the thickness. This information is valuable in deciding the etiology of abnormally thickened skin.

Thickening of the stratum corneum is called *hyperkeratosis* (*hyper* too much, *keratosis* keratin formation). Such thickening is usually a response of the skin to repeated pressure or friction. Corns or calluses are local areas of hyperkeratosis. In some skin disorders, the hyperkeratosis is present over the entire surface of palms and soles.

Scale

A scale is abnormal stratum corneum which is present in such excess that the abnormal thickening and flaking can be observed grossly. It may be thin, silvery, and easily removed, or it may be thick, hard, and adherent. Scale may have very little color of its own but may transmit the erythema of the underlying skin, or it may have brown-black discoloration from pigment granules or from dirt and debris from the environment. The process of spontaneous shedding of scale is sometimes referred to as desquamation (Color Plate II*B* and Figure 4-4*d*).

Crust

Crust is simply dried-up serum on the surface of the skin. When skin is damaged, the barrier function of the stratum corneum is compromised, and serum or blood can ooze through to the surface of the skin. This fluid dries, coagulates, hardens, mixes with dirt and skin proteins, and forms a crust or scab. Some crusts are thin and crumble easily while others are hard and adherent. A superficial straw-colored or honey-colored crust is seen in impetigo, a superficial bacterial infection of the skin (Color Plate II*C* and Figure 4-4*c*).

Skin may also become thinner than normal. *Atrophy* may result from injury or inflammation, or may be the result of the gradual change of aging (Figure 4-2*d*). Atrophy may chiefly involve the dermis, or the epidermis, or both. When circumscribed dermal atrophy is present, the involved area appears depressed, as the epidermis dips down over the area of the decrease in the volume of dermis. Dermal atrophy may follow trauma or inflammation, and may accompany radiation dermatitis. When the epidermis is involved, the skin appears thin and almost transparent. Atrophy may occur in linear streaks (striae) as seen in pregnancy, Cushing's disease, and obesity.

The consistency of the skin may also be abnormal. *Sclerosis* is a hardening or induration of the skin, and is seen in morphea, scleroderma, and certain chronic dermatitides. On the other hand, loose, lax skin is seen in some genetic disorders. Rarely, people are born with focal sites of absence of skin.

Skin lesions may also be recognizable by the absence of a component of the epidermis. An *erosion* results when the upper part of the epidermis

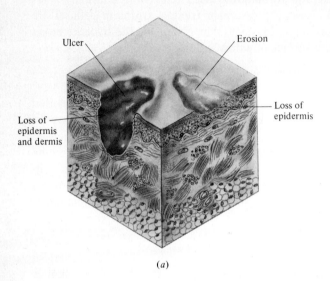

(*a*)

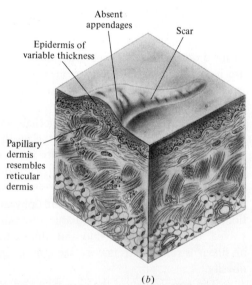

(*b*)

Figure 4-4   (*a*) Ulcer; (*b*) scar; (*c*) crust; (*d*) scale.

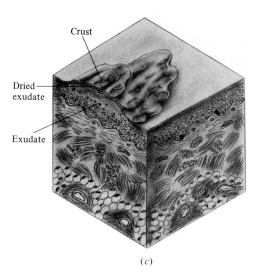

(*c*)

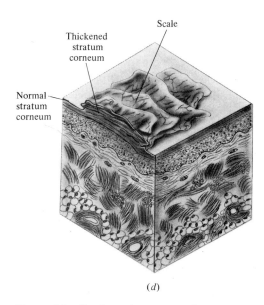

(*d*)

Figure 4-4 For legend see opposite page.

is missing, but the basal layer remains intact. Erosion may occur when the roof of a blister falls off. Since the stratum corneum is missing, fluid can escape and erosions are often moist or glistening. Erosions heal when the basal keratinocytes multiply, migrate outward, and replace the stratum corneum. No scarring results.

Ulcers

Ulcers are lesions in which the entire epidermis and upper dermis are missing (Figure 4-4*a*). Ulcers may result from trauma, decrease in cutaneous blood supply, tissue destruction by infection, neoplasms, inflammation, chemicals, and severe heat or cold (Chapter 12). If the ulcer is small, the epidermis at the edges of the lesion may grow over the defect as healing occurs. If the ulcer is shallow, the base of the epidermal appendages may remain unharmed. The epithelial cells along the walls of these appendages are capable of replicating, and migrating up, out, and over the skin to reepithelize the lesion. If the hair follicles and other appendages are absent, such epithelization is not possible. If no keratinocytes are present and the ulcer is deep, it may heal by scar formation (Chapter 5) rather than by replacement of normal skin.

Excoriations

Excoriations are the result of scratching. They are superficial excavations of epidermis which may be tiny crevices, fingernail-shaped lesions, or long linear scratches (Figure 4-5). They are visible signs of severe pruritus.

Anyone trained in recognizing skin disorders is aided in the diagnosis of skin diseases by noting the morphology, configuration or arrangement, distribution, and evolution of skin lesions. *Morphology* refers to the shape, size, form, and structure of individual lesions, as described above (macule, papule, vesicle, etc.).

Configuration or arrangement refers to the position of the lesions or parts of the lesion in relation to other lesions. Lesions may be linear, annu-

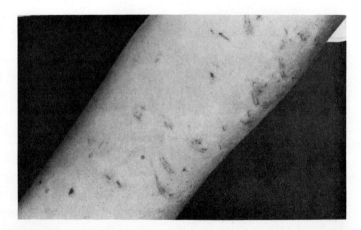

Figure 4-5 Excoriations. Linear abrasion and fingernail-shaped erosions result from vigorous scratching.

lar (ring-shaped), serpiginous (snake-like), or grouped. Lesions may also remain discrete and separate, or may become merged or confluent.

Distribution of lesions gives important clues to the diagnosis of skin lesions. Lesions may be generalized (scattered over the entire skin surface), or they may be confined to certain local areas of the body. Certain skin disease processes routinely involve palms and soles, genitalia, or mucous membranes. Involvement of sun-exposed areas suggests light-induced eruptions, and linear lesions, or lesions with straight borders, suggest contact dermatitis, externally induced skin lesions, or congenital dermatoses. Some skin diseases are localized to certain areas of sunlight exposure, trauma, or sites exposed to irritants or allergens. Acne occurs in certain areas because of the localization of sebaceous glands. Yeast infections of the skin occur at sites of moisture and occlusion, in body folds such as the axillae and between the buttocks.

Finally, it is sometimes necessary to observe the *evolution* of skin lesions; it may be necessary to observe how the morphology or distribution changes with the passage of time.

Diseases or disorders of the skin may be congenital (present at birth) or acquired (onset after birth). Both congenital and acquired disorders may or may not be hereditary (inherited from parents and ancestors). Existence at birth may be due to intrauterine infection or trauma and does not necessarily mean that a certain disorder is hereditary. On the other hand, when a disorder is not manifest until adult life, it can still be hereditary. Familial (affecting the different members of a family) disorders are most often hereditary disorders, but a common environmental factor or contagion may lead to familial occurrence of disease.

People may inherit a diathesis or tendency to develop a particular kind of skin disease, such as psoriasis, seborrhea, or atopic eczema. This means that such persons have inherited an abnormal constitutional state which causes them to react to certain environmental or internal stimuli by manifesting their particular skin disease. They may then have little or no trouble with, or symptoms of, that disorder or they may have a lifelong, severe, crippling disease.

PRURITUS

Pruritus, or itching, is an unpleasant, irritating cutaneous sensation which evokes a desire to scratch. This sort of complex reflex probably stems from a basic automatic instinctual or learned desire to remove any noxious agents from the surface of the skin. Irritating substances stimulate a motor response, which leads to their mechanical removal by scratching or rubbing away. Scratching and rubbing are excellent ways to exclude insects, debris, plant extracts, tree sap, and other noxious elements from hairy coats of mammals. Itching of the skin also allows man to quickly sense an irritating stimulus, and automatically attempt to remove it by rubbing it away. At the same time, as a response to the trauma resulting from scratching, blood flow to the area is increased as the dermal vessels dilate in response to the mechanical stroking. Any conscious awareness of the afferent aspect of this reflex arc is experienced as what we describe as itching.

Unfortunately, this protective mechanism designed to remove potentially dangerous agents from the skin surface can lead to damage of the skin. Potentially harmful agents may be sensed and removed, but scratching may damage the epidermis, remove the stratum corneum protective layer, and increase permeability to noxious substances. Many dermatoses and allergic phenomena release chemical mediators in the skin which cause itching. Scratching may then lead to skin damage.

In some ways, itching is related to pain. The same kind of small non-myelinated nerve fibers conduct itch sensation and pain. No itching can be elicited in analgesic skin, and skin which has a lower pain threshold frequently also has a lower itch threshold. Some stimuli which cause itching at low intensity may lead to pain at higher intensity. Pain and itch are nonadapting; i.e., the rate of impulse does not diminish rapidly with time after the initial impulse, but is relatively continuous.

The sensation of itching differs from pain in that pruritus can be elicited experimentally only from a stimulus in the lower epidermis or in the region of the dermoepidermal junction. Deeper stimulus causes only pain. Removal of epidermis abolishes itch but not pain. Pain and itch may be elicited by separate stimuli with distinct and repeatable thresholds. The sensations can be distinguished from each other and pain and itch may be experienced simultaneously from the same area of skin.

While all areas of the skin surface are capable of itching, the responsiveness to perceived impulses that are interpreted as itching varies, being greatest at the mucocutaneous junctions, the nostrils, the perineum, and the external ear canals. Almost any chemical or physical stimulus may produce pruritus if the skin becomes damaged. Vasodilatation, nerve stimulation, enzyme release, and mediators such as histamines, peptidases, kinins, and vasoactive polypeptides all may play a role in itching. Probably several different mediators evoke the same sensation. Itch threshold may be lower than normal, so that light stroking, minimal temperature changes, clothing, or other stimuli that would not normally do so, cause the sensation of itching. Such abnormal sensitivity occurs in and around skin which has just previously itched.

The natural motor response to the conscious or subconscious sensation of pruritus is to rub or scratch. Itching skin may be rubbed with the fingers or with other parts of the body. The fingernails may be used to cut, tear, or rub. A person with severe itching may be constantly in motion—scratching, twisting, moving about, rubbing against various objects around him. The signs of itching are, therefore, the marks left by this motor response. Excoriations may be punctate or linear, and may appear as erosions or as bloody crusts. Long linear parallel scratch marks may be present. Fingernails may become shiny and smooth as they become polished from the frequent rubbing. Rubbing or scratching the scalp or pubis may leave broken stubby hairs. Finally, lichenification may occur in susceptible individuals as a response to frequent rubbing.

Pruritus can be caused by any irritating substance that damages the skin (Figure 4-6). Foreign bodies, plastic or glass fibers, plant products, wool, insects, or other particulate matter on the skin surface may induce localized or scattered areas of itching. Excessive dryness can partially dehydrate the stratum corneum and lead to itching. Conversely, extremely high humidity can lead to sweat retention and pruritus, especially if occlusion of the skin is present. Many primary dermatoses are pruritic. Drug hypersensitivities may present as itching without an obvious rash. Intestinal parasites may cause generalized pruritus. Infectious diseases such as chicken pox, measles, or viral exanthens may lead to itching, but many infectious diseases manifested by a rash do not itch.

Finally, systemic diseases may lead to generalized pruritus. People

---

Dry skin

Drugs
  Opium derivatives, subclinical hypersensitivity reactions

Metabolic and Endocrine
  Uremia
  Obstructive biliary disease
  Diabetes mellitus (possibly)

Infestation
  Hookworm
  Onchocerciasis

Neoplasms
  Leukemia and lymphoma, especially Hodgkin's disease

Psychogenic
  Acute and chronic emotional stress
  Delusions of parasitosis

Figure 4-6 Causes of generalized pruritus without primary skin lesions.

with *diabetes mellitus* are prone to generalized itching. It has been postulated that pruritus in diabetics is related to decreased water content of the skin resulting from the deranged metabolism or that it results from the compromised microcirculation of the skin. The precise mechanism is not yet known. Local itching from *moniliasis,* especially in the anogenital region, is more common in diabetes.

Severe liver diseases, especially those associated with biliary obstruction, can be accompanied by severe generalized itching. Chronic renal insufficiency may lead to pruritus that is sometimes reversed by dialysis. Patients with leukemia, internal malignancies and lymphomas, especially Hodgkin's disease, may itch.

Several factors can worsen pruritus or cause borderline stimuli to be more likely to cause itching. Vasodilatation worsens itching. Therefore, heat and rubbing can be expected to make itching more severe. Tissue anoxia may increase pruritus. Stasis causes increased susceptibility to itching. Dependency and decreased blood flow may account for the fact that generalized pruritic dermatoses often itch more severely on the lower legs. Dryness also seems to increase the likelihood of pruritus.

It is not surprising that itching is a problem in venous stasis dermatitis. The skin over the lower third of the leg has a relatively poor blood supply which leads to local hypoxia. Venostasis and dependency lead to edema and vasodilatation. Rubbing causes increased vasodilatation and also lowers the itch threshold. A cycle of itch-scratch-itch is established and the scratching and rubbing further damage the skin, making the dermatosis more severe, leading to erosions, excoriations, postinflammatory hyperpigmentation, and areas of thickened skin, as well as shiny, atrophic, relatively anoxic skin.

Itching is frequently worse at night when there are fewer distractions to divert one's attention to other stimuli. As the natural diurnal temperature rhythm changes, there may be slightly more vasodilatation in the evening hours and people tend to be warm when covered in bed, which leads to further vasodilatation. The itching caused by *scabies* is markedly increased at night.

The major self-treatment of itching is scratching. Scratching converts the sensation of pruritus to that of pain and may at the same time damage or fatigue the receptor nerve. Frequently, however, excessive scratching or rubbing damage the skin, worsen many dermatoses, and cause itching to increase. "One scratch is too many, a thousand is not enough." A major step in treating such pruritus is to attempt to remove the itch stimuli and break the itch-scratch cycle. Avoid those factors known to increase pruritus.

Cool or cold causes vasoconstriction, and provides relief of itching.

Topical corticosteroids may reduce itching by reducing inflammation and leading to vasoconstriction. Menthol in potions causes a cooling sensation; camphor and phenol in lotions may partially numb the itch receptors. Local anesthetics will reduce itch, but they may lead to tearing of the skin by habitual scratching in the face of diminished sensation. Dryness can be corrected with soaks or lubricants.

Antihistamines administered orally or parenterally may lessen pruritus. Tranquilizers may allow a patient to be less agitated, overreactive, anxious, and hypersensitive to itch stimuli. Sedatives may encourage necessary sleep for the patient and a respite for the damaged skin.

REFERENCES

Ayres, S.: "The Fine Art of Scratching," *JAMA* **189:**1003–1007, September 1964.

Beare, J. M.: "Antipruritics," *Practitioner* **202:**55–61, January 1969.

Signs and Symptoms; Applied Pathologic Physiology and Clinical Interpretation, Fourth Edition, MacBryde, C. M., and R. S. Blacklow, eds.; Shapiro, A.: "Itching," J. B. Lippincott Company, Philadelphia, 1964, pp. 900–921.

Normal and Abnormal Reactions of Skin

The skin as reactor
Turnover time
Inflammation
Repair, regeneration, hyperkeratosis
Sunburn
Healing
Thermal injury (burns)
Immunity, allergy, hypersensitivity
Insect bites
Vascular reaction patterns
    Urticaria
    Erythema multiforme
    Vasculitis and purpura
Drug eruptions
Eczema
    Allergic contact dermatitis
    Other exogenous causes of eczema
    Endogenous causes of eczema
Primary irritant dermatitis
Interplay of reaction patterns

THE SKIN AS REACTOR

In one sense, the skin acts as our shell, a passive physical barrier and protective coating. It is a sheet of protein that holds the fluids and gels of the body in and keeps bacteria, radiation, and chemicals out. But the skin is more than a physical barrier. It is also a living tissue that repairs and replenishes itself and actively renews its outer layer.

The skin is still more. It can react.

As a functioning organ, the skin can respond to environmental stresses by performing specialized protective work. When the skin plays a role in temperature regulation, resistance to infection, foreign body rejection, hemostasis, and mechanical protection, it alters its physiology, growth patterns, and blood flow so as to minimize the damaging effect of insults of the environment. The skin has special activities which are reactions to potentially dangerous insults to the body. These cutaneous defense mechanisms take many forms.

Some of these cutaneous reactions to invasion or threat from the environment are nonspecific, simple responses of inflammation shared by other organ systems. Other responses of the skin are more specifically directed toward a particular kind of stress. Specific defenses respond to specific kinds of environmental aggressions. Moreover, the skin may react to stress in a way which makes itself better prepared to handle the same stress when it arises again. The defense reaction and the repair process occur in a way which make the skin more tolerant of the same damaging stress in the future. For example, friction causes a callus which can resist considerable further mechanical friction or pressure. The ultraviolet rays of the sun cause tanning and the resulting darker skin provides a better screen against any further sun damage.

The skin responses may take place mostly in the epidermis. The keratinocytes may make more keratin, divide faster, swell, or die sooner. The melanocytes may make more or less pigment. The stratum corneum may become thick or thin. Or the reaction may take place primarily in the dermis. The blood vessels may dilate and engorge. The fibrocytes may make more or less fiber protein or ground substance. The dermis may swell with fluid or become filled with cells which make their way out of the blood vessels and into the dermis itself. Reactions often involve both dermis and epidermis because their physiology is really inseparable.

Each reaction of the skin takes time. Some, such as hives, happen within seconds to minutes. Others, such as suntan, cyst formation, or healing, may take days. Callus formation may take weeks to months and some allergic reactions may cause symptoms intermittently for a lifetime.

Most of the reactions of the skin are alterations or magnifications of some of the normal cutaneous physiologic events discussed in Chapter 2. The normal and abnormal reactions of the skin are not always easily separated. The apparent purpose of each of the cutaneous defense responses is to minimize the destructive effect of injurious agents on our inner environment and on the skin itself. At times, however, the protective reactions themselves cause significant symptoms. Reactions may be exaggerated to the point of being counterproductive and even dangerous, as occurs in some allergic phenomena. It is not always clear where helpful, protective responses leave off and destructive responses begin. Itching may lead us to scratch and rub away noxious chemicals, but if the epidermis is torn away, more of the chemical is absorbed. Swelling of the skin dilutes injurious agents but excess swelling causes pain and loss of function.

Before examining some specific skin disorders, it is helpful to look at some of the general ways in which the skin reacts.

TURNOVER TIME

In adults, skin remains about the same size all the time. The number of cells and the thickness of the skin stays relatively constant. However, the skin is far from a static population of cells. As cells become keratinized and are worn off the outer coat, they must be replaced. There is a constant turnover of cells. Compared to the static cell populations of the musculoskeletal and central nervous systems, the turnover is rapid. The skin and mucous membranes, the bone marrow, and the gastrointestinal tract have similar rapid proliferation and high metabolic requirements.

When a basal cell divides, one of the new cells remains behind as the basal cell and the other is pushed upward into the spinous layer. As more cells divide, the spinous keratinocyte is displaced higher. It takes about fourteen days for this cell to be pushed all the way up to the stratum corneum. The dehydrated remainder of the cell then makes up part of the stratum corneum for another fourteen days before it is dislodged further onto the surface and is worn off as unnoticeable scaling. On the average, the whole trip takes a little less than a month. The skin "turns over" monthly in a continuous uninterrupted growth cycle.

A turnover of the cell population not only renews the stratum corneum as fast as it is worn off, it also automatically repairs any small physical defect or excavation caused by scraping, scratching, or tearing. The outward push also gets rid of any cells which happen to mature or keratinize abnormally. The constant outward current and sloughing could also help keep follicle and pore openings unoccluded. Renewal, repair, and the mechanical cleansing of this outward cell displacement continue automatically.

The rate of cell division and resultant outward displacement can be speeded if the skin becomes stimulated by rubbing, noxious chemicals, or irritating environmental factors. It follows that the transit from basal layer to stratum corneum would, therefore, be faster under such conditions. It takes a shorter time for cells to make the trip from basal layer to sloughing. The "turnover time" is shorter. If cells are being made faster and the skin stays the same thickness, cells must make it to the outside and fall off at a more rapid rate. Scraping, excess sunlight, abrasions, and minor irritation and injuries can also stimulate skin to be made faster.

In *psoriasis,* skin is made too fast because of poorly understood genetic factors. The cells divide frequently, pushing cells outward more rapidly and decreasing transit time. It may take as little as two days for a new daughter cell of a basal cell division to reach the stratum corneum. In as little as two more days the dead cell carcass, along with thousands of others, has fallen off as scale. The scaling is visible and, in fact, quite noticeable because of the large quantity of scale produced.

When skin is being made more rapidly, it does not necessarily desquamate at an equally increased rate to maintain the normal constant thickness. Skin which is being made too rapidly may thicken. It is also possible that skin may become thicker than usual because the stratum corneum falls off at a slower than normal rate. In some forms of ichthyosis, inherited disorders manifested by thickening of skin, the stratum corneum becomes very thick because it fails to fall off normally. Although the skin is manufactured at the basal layer at a normal rate, the skin appears quite thick, scaly, and dry because the cells remain in the stratum corneum too long. In other forms of ichthyosis, the epidermal cells are produced too rapidly. Skin cancers grow larger because the abnormal cells are being made faster than the cells in the surrounding normal skin. The tumors may become elevated if the cells do not mature and desquamate normally.

INFLAMMATION

Bacteria, viruses, heat, cold, solar radiation, chemicals, and electrical and mechanical trauma may injure the skin. The basic characteristics of the immediate response to injury of many kinds is the same in skin as it is in other organ systems. Whenever cells are injured or destroyed, protective responses, collectively called inflammation, begin. The purpose of the inflammatory reaction is to destroy, wall off, or dilute the injurious agent and then to get rid of the agent and any dead or injured cells. Inflammation is followed by repair.

When tissues or cells are injured, soluble chemical substances are released. It is these substances which initiate inflammation. These chemicals affect blood vessels to make them dilate and become more permeable. Cells and excess amounts of fluid can pass out of the altered vessels into the dermis itself. One of the mediators of inflammation is histamine. A firm stroke of normal skin causes certain cells of the dermis to release histamine. The histamine causes dermal vessels to dilate and to allow fluid to escape into the dermis. The grossly visible manifestations are a raised wheal (the fluid in the dermis) and erythema (the dilated vessels) at the site of stroking.

Capillaries in the skin, like capillaries elsewhere, normally allow water, salt, glucose, amino acids, and other small molecules to pass freely. When the mediators of inflammation act on these vessels and on the venules to make them more permeable, the large proteins which normally stay within the vessels may also escape into the dermis. These proteins create osmotic pressure which pulls water out of the vessels into the dermis. The rate of escape of fluid from tiny dermal vessels may be more than five times normal. This process continues for about twenty-four hours. The altered capillary endothelium permits white blood cells to leave the blood and pass through the vessel wall into the dermis. Polymorphonuclear leukocytes, lymphocytes, and monocytes may collect in the dermis and at times may even pass into the epidermis, working their way between the keratinocytes.

Polymorphonuclear leukocytes ("polys") are the first and most numerous cells to accumulate in acute inflammatory reactions. These motile, ameboid cells can phagocytize foreign material, such as bacteria, by actually engulfing or enclosing them within the cell body of the polymorphonuclear cell. The larger, longer-lived white blood cells, the mononuclear cells, provide the second line of defense at a site of injury. These cells, called monocytes or macrophages, can phagocytize larger objects, including dead polys. They possess proteolytic enzymes to digest foreign materials. The morphology of these cells is altered by the type and intensity of inflammatory reactions and they can fuse and divide to form giant cells to engulf larger particles.

When relatively large and insoluble foreign objects are present in the dermis, the usual sequence of inflammation is begun, but the vasodilatation, edema, acute polymorphonuclear leukocyte infiltration, phagocytosis, and resolution are all restricted and overshadowed by phagocytosis by mononuclear macrophages and by the focal accumulation of mononuclear cells which become so tightly packed as to resemble epithelial cells. Such "epitheloid" cell reaction is called a *granuloma*. The organisms causing tuberculosis, syphilis and leprosy, and certain fungi, stimulate the formation of granulomas. When initiated by inert materials, such a reaction is called a foreign body reaction, and the resulting accumulation of inflammatory cells is called a foreign body granuloma.

All the inflammatory responses are designed to get rid of the injurious agent. Increased blood flow brings warmth, which increases metabolism, a large number of white cells, which help to phagocytize foreign matter and to mediate immune defenses, and increased amounts of oxygen and nutrients to support the increased cell processes. The edema fluid dilutes any foreign substances. Sometimes the inflammatory processes become walled off in order to separate the injurious agent, and the dead cells and pus, from the rest of the body. In such cases, fibroblasts, white cells, and fibrin help form a separating wall.

REPAIR, REGENERATION, HYPERKERATOSIS

Repair follows inflammation. Dead or damaged cells are replaced by new cells. Fibroblasts can make new collagen and ground substance in the dermis. If the framework or stroma persists, surviving keratinocytes simply divide to replenish the basal layer, and then resume their orderly progression to differentiation and keratinization. Minor trauma can, in fact, be a stimulus for basal cells to divide more frequently.

One active response of the skin to the minor trauma of repeated pressure or friction is *hyperkeratosis* (thickened stratum corneum). Any kind of repeated minor trauma such as the rubbing produced by poorly fitting shoes, the mechanical stresses of barefoot running, the repetitious friction of guitar string plucking, the friction of sneakers, or the pressure caused by weight bearing over bony prominences, can lead to local thickening of the stratum corneum.

Hyperkeratosis extends beyond repair and renewal of the epidermis. It is a special overreaction to prepare better for more of the same trauma. Thicker skin can absorb more pressure and withstand more friction.

A *callus* is simply an acquired, slightly elevated area of hyperkeratosis, which appears at sites of pressure or friction. A *corn* (*clavus*) is a similar hyperkeratosis in which the thickening is more sharply demarcated. The keratin may form into a cone, core, or ball and lose the normal layering and skin markings of normal stratum corneum. Pressure may force a *clavus* inward, causing pain.

SUNBURN

An example of a more complex protective reaction of the skin, which combines several of the more basic defense mechanisms discussed above, is the cutaneous reaction to sun. These responses also demonstrate a system of defensive mechanisms, which not only diminish the injurious effect of an environmental insult and initiate specific repairs, but also stimulate additional measures, which improve the defenses against further sun exposure. Sunburn is an example of inflammation. Peeling is the result of increased epithelial turnover as a repair response. Tanning is a reaction which improves defenses against further sunburn.

Radiation from the sun provides the energy which sustains all life on earth. The heat from the ball of fire warms us, and the light provides us with a means of sensing our environment through vision. The photosynthesis mechanism in plants converts the sun's energy into our food. Sunlight acts on certain substances in the skin to manufacture vitamin D, which is necessary for the proper absorption and use of calcium in the body.

Yet some of the radiation of the sun is harmful to living cells. One-celled organisms, such as bacteria, can be killed by certain wavelengths of sunlight. Human skin receives painful burns if exposed to intense sunlight. Wrinkling and aging of the skin are accelerated by sunlight. Skin cancer usually occurs in sun-exposed areas, and is more frequent after years of prolonged sun exposure.

The sun radiates a broad spectrum of energy in the form of electromagnetic waves (Figure 5-1). The ability of this energy to cause chemical reactions, heat, and biologic effects depends on the wavelength of the energy. Therefore, this spectrum of energy and its effects on matter may be categorized by wavelength regions (Figure 5-1). Taken alone, this concept provides no complete understanding of the physics of radiation and matter, but it does allow us to separate and describe solar-induced biologic phenomena in a spectrum. In discussing the body's reactions to the sun, we must consider three wavelength regions: visible light, ultraviolet radiation, infrared radiation.

Visible light is simply that energy from the sun which stimulates the retina of the eye. The cells of the retina are sensitive to only a certain narrow range of energy. Great quantities of energy of wavelengths, longer and shorter than visible light, reach the earth, but since they do not stimulate the retina, they are invisible to us.

Wavelengths shorter than visible light are called ultraviolet because they begin next to the violet end of the color spectrum. Ultraviolet rays cause sunburn and suntan. They also play a role in wrinkling and aging.

Ultraviolet radiation itself can be arbitrarily divided into short (UV-C), middle (UV-B), and long (UV-A) wavelength ultraviolet (Figure 5-1). Such separation is helpful because the skin reacts quite differently to the radiation from each of these wavelength regions. Short-wave ultraviolet does not reach the earth because it is filtered out by the upper atmosphere. Short-wave ultraviolet (UV-C) kills bacteria and can cause mild sunburn, but since it never reaches the earth, it does not present a problem to man. At times, UV-C from artificial sources is used in operating rooms to kill the bacteria in the air. Such lamps, called germicidal lamps, can

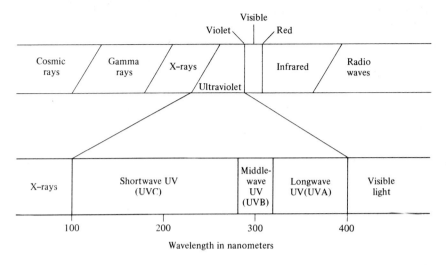

Figure 5-1 Electromagnetic spectrum with expanded scale of ultraviolet light.

cause conjunctivitis or sunburn and operating room personnel must be appropriately protected.

Middle-wave ultraviolet light (UV-B) reaches the earth. This is the part of the ultraviolet spectrum which causes sunburn. Although only a small portion of the sun's output is in the middle ultraviolet, these rays are very efficient in causing damage to the skin (Figure 5-2). These rays penetrate the epidermis, damage its cells, and pass into the dermis where they cause delayed dilatation of blood vessels. The resulting erythema (sunburn) takes several hours to begin and may last for several days.

Normally the long-wave ultraviolet light (UV-A) alone causes no noticeable changes in the skin. Although these wavelengths of energy may play some supportive or additive role in assisting the middle ultraviolet in causing sunburn or wrinkling, radiation with long-wave ultraviolet seems relatively innocuous when compared with the striking response of the skin to UV-B. However, in the presence of some drugs (psoralens, certain antibiotics including Declomycin®, many diuretics, occasionally others) or chemicals, or in some skin diseases, people become very sensitive to long-wave ultraviolet and erythema, exaggerated sunburn, or even blistering may result. Such people are *photosensitive.*

The skin repairs and renews itself after the insult of sunburn. Cells begin to divide more rapidly and are pushed to the surface more rapidly. The turnover time is thus shortened. Cells may be delivered to the surface so fast that their falling off (desquamation) is noticeable. People complain that they are "peeling." Despite this increased rate of desquamation, the

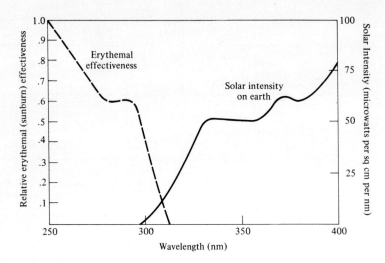

Figure 5-2 Relative output of sun and erythemal efficiency curve. The small region of 290 to 320 nm is the "sunburn spectrum."

skin ends up thicker than it was before the sunburn. A thicker stratum corneum is protective because it becomes more difficult for middle ultraviolet to penetrate the skin and cause sunburn.

As the epidermis if being made faster and the blood vessel dilatation of sunburn becomes less impressive, the melanocytes appear to be in a stimulated state. Their enzymes are more active. They make more melanosomes and make them faster. They deliver more melanosomes to the keratinocytes. In a few days, the skin begins to darken. This pigmentation, or tan, puts more melanin between the sun and the deeper parts of the epidermis. Because melanin absorbs the ultraviolet, less middle ultraviolet can penetrate to the cells of the lower epidermis and into the dermis, where it could strike the blood vessels, and cause more sunburn.

Just as the base-line color of the unexposed skin is inherited, so is the ability to tan. Many Irishmen, Scotchmen, or other Celtic people tan poorly, while most people of Mediterranean ancestry tan darkly and quickly. Blacks also tan, but it is less noticeable because their melanocytes are genetically programmed to produce large amounts of melanin without the added stimulus of sunburn. They are already well protected from the sun.

Although the warmth that we feel while in the sun is caused by infrared radiation, these rays do not cause sunburn. Sunburn is a delayed reaction caused by damage to the skin by UV-B (Figure 5-3). Infrared rays can pass through window glass. This is why we can feel warm when

Sun Rays	Ultraviolet			Visible	Infrared
Wavelength (nm)	Short 200-290 nm UV-C	Middle 290-320 nm UV-B	Long 320-400 nm UV-A	400-700 nm	> 700 nm
Physiologic and dermatological effect	erythema, conjunctivitis, bactericidal	sunburn tan* skin cancer, wrinkling, "aging"	drug-induced photosensitivity reactions, tan* IPD**	vision, IPD** minimal tanning	heat, sensation of warmth
BLOCKING AGENTS: Window Glass	Active eliminated	Active eliminated	No effect	No effect	No effect
Water in Air (Haze, clouds)	Active eliminated	Minimal block	Minimal block	No effect	Significant reduction
Ozone in Atmosphere	Active eliminated				
Water (1 foot deep)	Minimal block	Minimal block	No effect	No effect	Significant reduction
Umbrella	Active eliminated	Active eliminated	Active eliminated	Active eliminated	No effect
Most "commercial" Sunscreens	Minimal block	Minimal block	No effect	No effect	No effect
Benzophenones	Significant reduction	Minimal block	Minimal block	No effect	No effect
PABA, Esters of PABA, Cinnamates	Minimal block	Minimal block	No effect	No effect	No effect
Opaque Sunscreens, Pancake makeup	Active eliminated	Active eliminated	Significant reduction	Significant reduction	Significant reduction

Tan* = True melanogenesis, suntan
IPD** = Immediate pigment darkening

- Active wavelengths are essentially completely eliminated
- Minimal but definite block
- Significant reduction of the active wavelengths
- No significant effect

Figure 5-3 Sun spectrum and biologic phenomena.

the sun shines on us through the car or house window. Water or water vapor can filter out large quantities of infrared. On a hazy or cloudy day, less infrared radiation reaches the earth because it is filtered out by the water vapor in the air; therefore, we feel less heat on the skin. Because less heat reaches the skin, people tend to be comfortable in the sun much longer and tend to prolong their exposures. The result is that many bad sunburns occur on hazy days simply because people remain on the beach longer than usual. They feel less heat because less infrared is present but they get bad sunburns from too much UV-B (middle ultraviolet), both energy ranges being invisible.

UV-B does not pass through window glass. Although we can feel the warmth of sunshine through window glass, sunburn does not occur. Sunscreens are designed to block out or absorb the UV-B. For cosmetic reasons, most people prefer that visible light pass through the sunscreen. If visible light were also blocked, the sunscreen would be opaque and quite visible on the skin. Infrared, of course, passes through sunscreens.

The most commercially successful sunscreens are not very effective blockers of UV-B because most bathers do not want to avoid getting some erythema from the sun. They seek the "healthy glow." A slight redness and a tan are important status symbols. People get bad burns if the sunscreen is too inefficient or if exposures are excessive. It must be remembered that reflection from sand or snow adds to the ultraviolet dose arriving at the skin and that swimming and sweating remove most sunscreens. Sunscreens should be reapplied frequently if beach activities are vigorous.

The most effective topically applied sunscreens are those made from para-aminobenzoic acid (PABA) in alcohol, and creams containing cinnamates and benzophenones. These chemicals block UV-B; PABA remains on the skin despite moderate swimming and sweating, and transmits visible light. When the skin reacts to the damages we see as sunburn, one of the things it does is to generate the most efficient sunscreen, melanin. The process we admire as suntan is actually the skin manufacturing its own sunscreen.

Chronic exposure of the dermis to ultraviolet light over many years causes wrinkling and accelerates the appearance of aged skin. Wrinkling is often confined to sun-exposed areas. Since we subconsciously judge age by degree of wrinkling in the face, it is sometimes difficult to judge the age of older black people because of the absence of wrinkling of their skins. Their increased melanin has blocked out the years of ultraviolet bombardment.

Skin cancer development is related to sun exposure. It usually occurs in sun-exposed areas. Skin cancer is rare in blacks and is most frequent in light-skinned people (people with very little melanin) and in those with the most sun exposure (farmers, sailors, sun worshipers). Texas reports more skin cancer than Maine.

People's attitudes toward the sun influence the incidence of sunburn, wrinkling, and skin cancer. Several generations ago, it was a sign of prestige to be as white as possible. Only workers needed to be out in the sun. The nobility were proud of their fair skins. Today it is fashionable to be tan. It is now a sign of leisure to travel to beaches and islands. While it is unreasonable to avoid the sun, an attitude of moderation which includes use of effective sunscreens, and avoids prolonged, passive, purposeful sunbathing, will permit tanning, and help avoid the worst consequences of excessive sun exposure.

HEALING

When injury to the skin is sufficiently severe to interrupt the structural integrity of the skin, the defect cannot be overcome by inflammation, increased turnover, or thickening. Cell loss resulting in defects which extend into the dermis and/or result in areas of missing epidermis must be resurfaced. The complex reaction initiated by such defects is the process of wound healing. The word "wound" is a general word to describe any significant loss of integrity, continuity, or contiguity extending into the dermis, and resulting from cell injury, cell death, or from a mechanical disruption of the skin. Healing describes the process by which such a wound is resurfaced, reestablishes the continuity across the defect, and restores the ability to withstand tensile stress again.

Immediately after injury, the damaged cells, debris, serum, dirt, and clotting substances form a dried-up adherent plug or temporary cover called a scab or *eschar*. The surviving healthy keratinocytes in the area then begin to divide and migrate in to cover the defect with epidermis. During this process, called epithelization or reepithelization, basal cells adjacent to the wound are pushed laterally as well as outward as other basal cells divide. The cells that are pushed laterally remain as basal cells and divide again and again, pushing more cells over the wound's surface. Those cells which are pushed upward by the expanding cell population begin to differentiate and specialize to make keratin. Instead of dividing again, they keratinize to restore the stratum corneum. Epithelization is retarded or prevented by the presence of infection.

Wound healing depends also upon processes which occur in the dermis. Poorly defined forces seem to pull the two sides of a wound together, thus narrowing the gap in the defect. Such wound contraction is especially prominent after incisional injury. As fibrocytes seem to move into the defect and the approximating edges of the preexisting skin gradually pull toward one another, new collagen is laid down by the fibroblasts so that tensile strength returns. If sufficient framework persists, the dermis and epidermis act on one another in such a way that the skin is remodeled and repaired and appears normal again.

If the skin defect is large, if the edges are not approximated, and if excessive amounts of keratinocytes are destroyed, the resurfacing cannot take place directly. The defect is then temporarily filled with a vascular connective tissue called *granulation tissue,* which grows in from the surrounding dermis. This tissue may be gradually replaced by a dense, relatively avascular bundle of collagen known as a scar or cicatrix. Such resurfacing may end up with very thin or absent epidermis, no appendages, such as hair or sweat glands, and decreased innervation. In such cases, the framework is too much destroyed to support and direct normal remodeling.

THERMAL INJURY (BURNS)

Heat causes considerable increase in cell metabolism. Although heat also causes vasodilatation, increased blood flow may still not be enough to compensate for the high metabolic requirements. The presence of excess heat can lead to cell injury or cell death. Heat causes denaturation or coagulation of proteins and may inactivate or destroy enzymes essential for the survival of the cell. Dry heat causes desiccation or charring, while wet heat essentially boils the skin, which, like other tissues of the body, is mostly water. Such boiling results in an opaque, firm coagulation.

When intense heat is applied to the surface of the skin, it is the epidermis which suffers the greatest damage, with a progressive drop in the gradient of temperature-related changes at deeper levels. Burns of the skin can be classified by the depth and extent of tissue damage.

In first-degree burns, the epidermal cells remain morphologically intact and the only evidence of damage is pain, erythema, and edema. Healing takes place in days, without scarring.

In second-degree burns, there is coagulation and necrosis of epidermal cells, but the overall structure of the epidermis is maintained, except for collection of fluid within and beneath the epidermis. Clinically, this is manifested by pain, erythema, and blistering. Reepithelization takes place from epidermal appendages, and healing is complete in one to three weeks without scarring.

Third-degree burns result from destruction of epidermis and its appendages, as well as coagulation of variable amounts of dermis and subcutaneous tissue. Blood vessels coagulate and thrombose and the skin may appear as dry, marble-white to mahogany-colored, and hard. Ulcers, necrosis, and tissue sloughs leave defects which heal only over many months and with extensive scarring. Because nerve fibers are usually destroyed by the burn, there may be little or no pain and the burned area may, in fact, be anesthetic.

Scalds from hot liquids usually cause first- or second-degree burns, while flames, electricity, and hot metal usually cause a full-thickness injury. While thermal burns may happen very quickly, chemical burns which cause similar histologic changes may progress over minutes to days.

Immediate therapy of burns consists of cold packs or immersion of the burned area in static cold tap water until pain and erythema are reduced. There is no need to try to debride or remove adherent clothing on an emergency basis. The only indication for immediate vigorous therapy

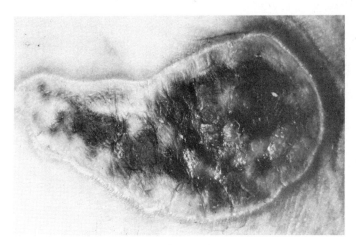

Figure 5-4 Severe third-degree burn. Full-thickness thermal damage results in skin that is hard and anesthetic.

is in the case of a chemical burn, where immediate and prolonged irrigation and exact antidotes may save considerable tissue.

Superficial burns may require no dressing or medication, although an emollient or lubricant is often soothing. Topical steroids may reduce inflammation. Although widely used, there is no evidence that topical antibiotics markedly reduce the incidence of infection. Topical anesthetics reduce pain temporarily but may sensitize the skin.

Second-degree burns are best treated with continuous saline soaks. Large blisters may be aspirated, but the roof of the blister should remain as a dressing. Elevation of the burned part may reduce edema. Gentle debridement may be begun on the second or third day. Topical or systemic antibiotics may be required if infection intervenes.

Third-degree burns, if extensive, require hospitalization and aggressive management (Figure 5-4). In no other medical and surgical problem is the vital role of the skin more obviously demonstrated than in a burn. The skin no longer holds fluids in or keeps microorganisms on the dry exterior. Serum leaves the body in great quantities and patients may die of shock if fluid volume, salt, and protein are not actively replaced intravenously. Control of sepsis requires expert use of topical and systemic antibiotics, meticulous nursing care, and careful control of the environment of the burn patient.

IMMUNITY, ALLERGY, HYPERSENSITIVITY

Inflammation as a basic reaction to injury is a defense mechanism shared by skin and many other organs. Changes in the epidermal growth in response to trauma or cell injury are responses seen in other organ systems which have epithelium, such as the gastrointestinal tract, respiratory tract, and genitourinary system. Although all of the skin and many other organs are capable of such reactions, responses are generally local. That is, only the area insulted responds. Areas not injured are not affected. In the simple inflammatory and epidermal reactions, the stimuli can be nonspecific, the reactions are local, and the skin and its vasculature is the only system involved.

The skin does, however, join with other organ systems to take part in more complex defense reactions, which are more generalized. The immune system is one such defense system. In immune reactions, the skin is only one of many sites of possible reaction and each defense reaction episode is initiated by a specific causative agent.

The immune system is one of the body's most advanced defense mechanisms. Immunity indicates protection against an invading substance brought about by the presence of antibodies. The invading substance which stimulates the production of antibodies and thereafter reacts with these antibodies is called an *antigen*. Bacteria, viruses, proteins, or drugs may act as antigens. Antigens are usually high molecular weight proteins and are usually complex enough to stimulate the production of several different kinds of antibodies, each kind in large quantity and relatively specific for that antigen. Antigens are agents that elicit the production of antibodies.

Antibodies are relatively large proteins called *globulins*. Since they render us immune, they are often referred to as *immunoglobulins*. Immunoglobulins can be divided into different groups, based on molecular size, physical properties, and biologic activities. Plasma cells and lymphocytes, both within bone marrow and lymph nodes, can manufacture antibodies. Invasion or introduction of the antigen into the body initiates the production of antibodies. Any future contact with the same antigen causes release, increased production, or activation of the specific antibodies. Each kind of antibody we produce in response to an antigen entering the body is very specific, and usually reacts only with that antigen. The antibody combines with or attaches to the antigen, rendering it less harmful by making a complex which is more easily phagocytized, more readily removed from circulation, less toxic, more readily precipitated out of solution, or made less effective in other ways. If the antigen is a bacterium or virus, the presence of specific antibodies may make us resistant to infection. The immune system is beneficial and necessary to maintain life.

Immunology is the study of immunity. Immunity (presence of protection because of the presence of antibodies) can be acquired naturally by exposure to diseases or antigens, or it can be acquired by vaccination. In both cases, immunity is "active" because the host actually manufactures its own antibodies. Immunity may be "passive" if previously prepared antibodies are injected into a host or passed on through the placenta to an offspring.

At times, the successful protective immune reaction is accompanied by symptoms in skin and elsewhere, caused by the antigen-antibody complexes. The host is protected from the most serious toxic or infectious nature of the antigen, but some of the antigen-antibody responses may cause vascular reactions, tissue swelling, or skin rashes. The symptoms of the immune response may even overshadow any ill effects which the antigen might have caused. The immune response may also be triggered by antigens which, in themselves, are harmless and nontoxic. A symptomatic "unnecessary" reaction of this kind is called a hypersensitivity reaction. It is immune-like because it is mediated by antibodies. It is not a part of protective immunity if it does not offer protection against an expected injurious effect of the antigen.

The same antibody system which provides life-saving immunity can also react to antigens which are not normally dangerous to the body. The resulting antigen-antibody combination may cause tissue responses which do not protect but are harmful to the host. The terms *hypersensitivity* and *allergy* are used interchangeably to describe a state of unusual reactivity to antigens which are normally harmless to the majority of individuals.

Various allergic (hypersensitivity) phenomena differ in mechanism, timing, the organs most involved, and severity. Hypersensitivity reactions are often classified by the time interval from introduction of the antigen until the onset of symptoms caused by the antigen-antibody combination. *Immediate* hypersensitivity reactions (occurring within minutes) include anaphylaxis and atopy, and are mediated by antibodies which circulate in the serum. *Delayed* hypersensitivity reactions (requiring hours to start and days to peak) include the tuberculin reaction and contact dermatitis, and are mediated by cells of the immune system.

Anaphylaxis is an immunologic tissue injury which happens almost immediately and which causes clinical symptoms within minutes. This reaction may be generalized and very severe. While any antigen could theoretically lead to severe anaphylaxis, the most common offenders are penicillin and serum products. Immediate and generalized pruritic urticaria may be the cutaneous manifestation of an anaphylactic reaction. The more threatening systemic developments are immediate and severe hypotension and marked bronchospasm. Death may result if epinephrine and supportive measures are not instituted immediately. The most important step is prevention. Careful questioning for past history of allergic responses should preceed any administration of medications, especially those given parenterally and those known to cause anaphylaxis.

INSECT BITES

The reaction to the bite or sting of insects is part inflammation, part immunity, and part hypersensitivity. Insects have been ubiquitous for millions of years. When the parasites bite or suck the skin, they inject anticoagulants and enzymes which make their blood meal possible. The predators inject substances which cause pain to ward off intruders or to cause paralysis of small prey. Sometimes the biting, sucking, or stinging parts break off and remain in the skin.

The bite, thrust, or stab itself causes minimal and usually grossly unnoticeable mechanical trauma to the skin. The injected chemicals and proteins are irritating to varying degrees and may cause immediate transient inflammation and pain. Usually the most bothersome symptoms which arise from insect bites are those resulting from allergy. In unusually hypersensitive persons, anaphylaxis follows an insect sting and may even result in death. However, most symptoms arising from insect bites are those which are the more delayed manifestations of hypersensitivity.

Hours to days after being bitten, persons who are allergic to some chemical left by the insect begin to note redness, swelling, and itching at the site of the previous bite. Those persons who have become more allergic will experience the worst symptoms while nonallergic individuals may not even notice the bites. This explains why only some family members of a household infested with fleas may be symptomatic. The delayed nature of the swelling and itching may explain why persons often do not see any insects at the time of their symptoms and why they may seem to continue to observe more new papules after exposure to the insects has ended.

Antihistamines given systemically may decrease the itching and swelling of insect bites, especially if given soon after being bitten. Topical steroids may slightly decrease the inflammation. Topical antipruritic compounds containing menthol or phenol may provide some symptomatic relief. Separating the insects from the host's environment or prompt exit of the host from the insect's environment is the best preventive therapy.

VASCULAR REACTION PATTERNS

A simple way to view many skin responses is to consider the reactions of the blood vessels of the superficial (papillary) dermis. Several clinical signs and syndromes are best explained by emphasizing vascular reactions. A few regular and repeatable sequences of microscopic vascular events are caused by many different stimuli. The clinical counterparts of these vascular reaction patterns are common.

A basic response of blood vessels to many different kinds of stimuli is a change in caliber by active constriction or passive dilatation. A brief, transient constriction may be followed by dilatation. The superficial vessels of the dermis often become dilated as a response to insult. The resulting redness (erythema) is simply the visible increase of blood within the capillaries of the dermis. Such redness may be associated with an increased *rate* of blood flow. Vasodilatation or erythema may be caused by pharmacologic agents, neurogenic stimuli, direct tissue damage, systemic disease, such as infection, and by increased body heat.

Urticaria

If the blood vessels of the dermis leak plasma, the result is that too much fluid accumulates in the dermis. The excess fluid outside the vessels spreads the fibers and mixes with the ground substance. A local, relatively acellular fluid (edema) accumulates in the dermis. *Urticaria* is simply transient erythematous and edematous swelling of the dermis caused by local increase in permeability of capillaries and small venules. This increased permeability is usually caused by the effects of histamine and other chemical substances directly on the vessel wall. Histamine is released into the skin by some of the cells in the dermis in response to various kinds of irritation, pressure, and chemicals. Allergic reactions can cause the release of histamine.

Urticaria is usually a sign of some kind of allergy or hypersensitivity. Hives may result from allergy to medications, infectious agents, or transfused blood products. Urticaria may be caused by food or by physical agents, such as sun, cold, or scratching, but such allergies are rare. Although hives may come and go for days to weeks, usually one single lesion does not remain at the same site for longer than twenty-four hours. While it is frequently difficult or impossible to find the cause of urticaria, most urticaria is temporary and often disappears after removal of the source of the allergy or after use of medications which compete with histamine (antihistamine).

Erythema Multiforme

Dermal vessels may be so deranged or altered that they do more than simply dilate or leak small amounts of fluid. If the insult or vascular reaction pattern is severe, the vessel may permit scattered lymphocytes and large amounts of fluid to enter the dermis so that the swelling in one site lasts for weeks. The pressure of the fluid may actually force up or lift the epidermis off the dermis, so that fluid-filled bullae are formed. The process may spread centrifugally so that other vessels become involved as the situation worsens. The original site of involvement may then improve or continue to worsen; the center of the lesions may look different from the periphery. Round, target-like, or "bull's-eye-type" lesions occur. Such vascular reactions are seen in *erythema multiforme*.

Erythema multiforme, frequently called EM, is a self-limited syndrome which is the clinical manifestation of a moderately severe vascular reaction pattern. The reaction probably results from hypersensitivity. Microscopically, fluid and cells pass out of the dermal vessels, and prolonged vasodilatation occurs. Clinically, the classic lesion is round with concentric central clearing or worsening, but as the name of the disease implies, the morphology can be quite varied (Figure 5-5). The lesions are generalized and may involve mucous membranes where transient blisters can leave erosions (see Chapter 12). Erythema multiforme may last six to ten weeks and then usually fades away. Stevens-Johnson syndrome is a severe form of erythema multiforme in which one or more mucous membranes are involved.

The first step in treatment is to try to find and remove the cause of the allergic response. The cause may be a drug, an infectious agent, including herpes simplex, or an innoculation. The antigen is often not determined and the process may recur. Fever and constitutional symptoms may be prominent. If the episode is unusually severe, and the mucous membrane involvement is marked, systemic steroids may be used to suppress the clinical symptoms.

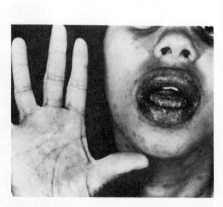
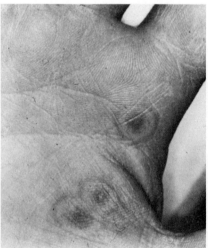

Figure 5-5 Erythema multiforme. (a) Severe generalized involvement including mucous membranes is often referred to as Stevens-Johnson syndrome; (b) close-up of target lesion.

Vasculitis and Purpura

If the reaction or the damage to blood vessels is even more severe, whole blood may pass through the vessels, resulting in purple-red discoloration of the skin (*purpura*). The vessel wall may become thickened, interrupted, or infiltrated with cells. Such severe changes in vessel walls, along with marked loss of fluid, white cells, or whole blood into the dermis, make up the reaction pattern called *vasculitis*.

Purpura from most causes is macular (cannot be felt) but when purpura occurs from vasculitis, the edema and cellular infiltrate in the dermis is so great that the lesions may be elevated and, therefore, palpable. Palpable purpura usually represents vasculitis. Vasculitis simply means "inflammation of the vessel." It can be caused by a hypersensitivity response (allergic cutaneous vasculitis) or may be caused by the presence of infectious agents such as bacteria or rickettsiae actually present in the dermal vessels. One of the clinical manifestations of sepsis (systemic infection) may be vasculitis.

One form of vasculitis, *erythema nodosum,* occurs deep in the subcutaneous tissue, most frequently near the tibial area in females. Erythema nodosum is probably also a hypersensitivity response. It begins as tender, erythematous nodules deep in the tissues; in time, these gradually flatten to look like a bruise or ecchymosis. The escaped blood products are finally resorbed, and the lesions heal without scarring. Some of the antigens which evoke the erythema nodosum type of vasculitis are streptococcal infection, tuberculosis, birth control pills, and other medications.

In the more severe of the vascular reaction patterns, the amount of edema in the dermis may lead to bullae or vesicles. These lesions may then fill with white blood cells, to become pustules, or with blood, to become hemorrhagic vesicopustules or hemorrhagic bullae. If any vascular reaction pattern or vasculitis is of such severity that the vessel can no longer function to supply oxygen and nutrients, the tissue normally supplied by that vessel may not survive. If the vessel is large enough so that the resultant cell death causes a tissue defect or visible lesion, such a lesion is called an *infarct*. Infarcts of the skin are often seen in patients with bloodstream dissemination of gonorrhea.

DRUG ERUPTIONS

Well over 1,000 drugs are in regular use in the United States. It is not surprising that some of these chemicals foreign to the body behave as antigens and cause hypersensitivity reactions. Allergic reactions to drugs often present as a rash. As many as 1 to 5 percent of inpatients will develop a cutaneous drug reaction during their stay in the hospital. The clinical manifestations of hypersensitivity to simple chemicals are usually confined to a skin eruption, but visceral organs may occasionally be involved.

Almost any drug may lead to a drug eruption. Drug eruptions may assume almost any morphology. Therefore, the possibility of drug eruption must be considered in the differential diagnosis of nearly every patient with a rash (see Chapter 11).

It is not known whether genetic factors make individuals more susceptible to drug rashes. However, persons with a family or personal history of hay fever, asthma, or atopic dermatitis are more likely to have serum sickness or anaphylactic reactions to certain drugs, especially penicillin. Exogenous factors may influence reactivity. Most patients with mononucleosis who take ampicillin get a drug rash. In general, however, it is not possible to predict which patients are likely to become allergic to a drug. It is known that certain drugs are more likely than others to cause allergic reactions.

While there are several mechanisms by which drugs may affect the skin, the most common drug eruption is caused by a hypersensitivity phenomenon in which the skin is essentially the only affected organ. The eruption is classically a bright red, semiconfluent, macular and papular, generalized, and bilaterally symmetrical rash of fairly abrupt onset. Usually when medical personnel talk of a "drug eruption" without other qualifying or descriptive terms, this is the rash to which they refer. A rash of this description may also be referred to as scarlatiniform, because of its similarity to the rash of scarlet fever, or exanthematous, because of its similarity to a viral exanthem. Such a rash may be accompanied by mild to moderate pruritus but often does not itch. The eruption may last several days to two weeks after the offending drug has been discontinued and may terminate with minimal desquamation.

The classic red, symmetrical, semiconfluent "drug eruption" appears as early as one to two days after initiating the offending drug or as late as seven to ten days after the drug has been discontinued. It is mediated by circulating antibodies different from those which mediate anaphylaxis (IgE), but similar to those which play active roles in immunization against many infectious diseases (IgG, IgM). These drug eruptions disappear several days after discontinuing the drug and may reappear if the drug is used again. If the drug is essential to the patient's therapy, it can be continued despite the rash. Under these conditions, the rash may remain, get worse, or disappear.

As is the case in any allergic reaction, drug allergies may present with cutaneous manifestations other than the classic red symmetrical rash. Urticaria can occur from drug hypersensitivity and, occasionally, drug-induced allergic reactions can cause eczematous, purpuric, or bullous erup-

tions. Erythema multiforme, erythema nodosum, and vasc[
caused by a drug. Hypersensitivity phenomena may also (
without obvious visible skin changes.

If previous sensitization has taken place, hypersensitivity eruptions manifested by urticaria may begin immediately after a drug is administered. Patients with such eruptions must be carefully observed because this type of drug eruption may signal anaphylaxis. Such immediate urticarial reactions should be carefully noted and recorded and the suspected drug should be avoided. The same antibodies which mediated the benign-appearing hives (IgE) may also mediate anaphylaxis with hypotension, bronchospasm, and death. Urticaria which appears later, after several days or weeks of drug administration, does not necessarily carry the same grave warning.

Most of what we know about the immune mechanisms of drug hypersensitivity phenomenon is drawn from the extensive research with penicillin. The mechanism for allergic reactions with other drugs may not be the same. Skin tests with penicillin may prove to be predictive. Those persons with immediate urticarial flare to certain of the penicillin breakdown products are most likely to experience anaphylaxis. It is much safer to administer the drug to persons not reacting to skin tests with any of the components of penicillin. Advances in skin tests and other methods of predicting reactions or selecting the likely candidates for anaphylaxis to penicillin are welcome, since several hundred deaths occur each year from penicillin administration.

ECZEMA

The terms eczema and dermatitis are often used synonymously, although the latter is a more general term suggesting no more than cutaneous inflammation. Eczema is one kind of dermatitis. Even so, eczema or eczematous dermatitis is not a specific skin disease but is a type of superficial inflammatory response of the skin with a certain sequence of morphologic changes and a characteristic histologic reaction pattern. This common complex of changes, called eczema, can actually be a response to various different stimuli.

The clinical appearance of eczema varies with time. Acute eczema appears as erythema and edema which frequently leads to vesiculation (formation of vesicles) (Figure 5-6). As the dermatitis progresses and the vesicles break, oozing, scaling, and crusting are present. Varying degrees of redness may remain as the dermatitis persists, but the most striking changes of chronic eczema are those which are the evidence of rubbing and scratching. Constant rubbing of the skin may lead to a characteristic

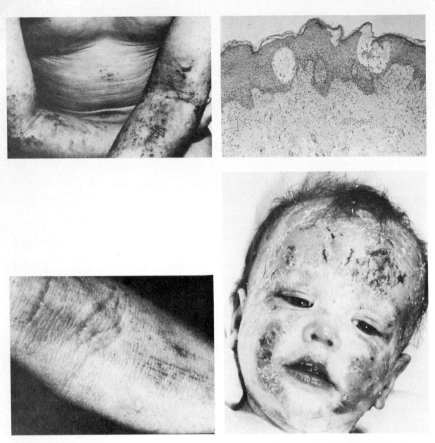

Figure 5-6 (*a*) Acute eczema. Weeping, vesiculation, and crusting; (*b*) photomicrograph of eczema; histologically there is excess fluid between the cells of the epidermis which may collect into microscopic vesicles; (*c*) lichenification results from rubbing, and linear abrasions from scratching; (*d*) chronic eczema; scaling, cracking, erythema, and thickened skin.

kind of thickening called lichenification (Figure 5-6). Skin markings are exaggerated and the skin appears to have an overall increase of thickness. Excoriations are often present. As the lesions heal, temporary hyper- or hypopigmentation may occur at the sites of involvement.

Histologically, intraepidermal vesiculation occurs during some phase of the development of all eczematous dermatitis. This characteristic edema between cells of the epidermis, called *spongiosis,* is the microscopic finding which unifies the concept of eczema. The affected cells are pushed apart by the edema and the stratum corneum may become poorly made, inadequately layered, stretched, or porous. Fluid actually pushes its way through to the surface of the skin, accounting for the weeping seen in acute eczematous dermatitis. Serum, dried proteins, dirt, and debris mix with the scale caused by increased cell turnover. Dermal vessels are dilated, accounting for the erythema. In more chronic stages, the most striking clinical and histologic feature may be the epidermal thickening—a later stage of the same cutaneous reaction.

Eczematous dermatitis may be associated with exogenous agents such as contactants which cause allergic contact dermatitis, with endogenous factors such as drugs, or with localized bacterial or fungal infections. A large group of eczematous dermatitides are of unknown etiology. Constitutional, metabolic, and immunologic factors often play a role, and some forms of eczema are hereditary (Figure 5-7).

The major symptom of eczema is pruritus. Eczematous dermatitis accounts for the highest morbidity of skin disorders in the United States. A high proportion of industrial absences, military disabilities, and as many as one-third of the visits to dermatologists are due to eczema. The cost of medications and hospitalizations, the compensation from business, and the loss of productivity are major problems. The emotional stress and itching suffered by eczema patients may be severe.

Allergic Contact Dermatitis

Allergic contact dermatitis is the most frequent eczematous dermatitis associated with exogenous agents. It is a manifestation of delayed hypersensitiv-

---

Exogenous Agents
Contactants (allergens)	Allergic contact dermatitis
Ultraviolet light	Eczematous polymorphous light eruption
Fungus	Eczematous response to dermatophyte infection

Endogenous Agents
Drug	Eczematous drug eruption
Altered epidermal constituents	Autoeczematization ("id")

Unknown Etiologies (possible hereditary factors)
Atopic dermatitis
Neurodermatitis, lichen simplex chronicus, prurigo nodularis
Nummular eczema
Dyshidrotic eczema
Stasis dermatitis
Seborrheic dermatitis
Eczematous pityriasis rosea

Figure 5-7 Causes of eczema.

ity. When the skin is exposed to a substance, a small amount may be absorbed. In a small percentage of persons, these absorbed molecules act as antigens. The person becomes sensitized or allergic to that substance. It requires anywhere from three to four days to three to four weeks for sensitization to occur (incubation time). Once the skin is allergic to the substance, further contact will lead to eczematous dermatitis. The eczema is confined to the sites of contact and usually occurs one to three days after the subsequent exposure. The eczema is the manifestation of the allergy. In some individuals, a large number of chemicals can act as antigens.

The configuration and distribution of the eczematous lesions give clues as to the contactant (source of antigen) involved. In those persons who are allergic, poison ivy causes linear eczema, because the plant streaks across the skin as the individual walks by. Persons allergic to certain metals may get eczema under rings or watch bands. Persons sensitized to leather may demonstrate sharply defined eczematous dermatitis only at sites where sandle straps cross the dorsum of the foot.

People can also become allergic to topical medications. Neomycin is a widely used topical antibiotic which may cause allergic contact dermatitis. Benadryl is an effective antihistamine used to suppress itching and diminish allergic reactions, when given parenterally. However, when used topically, it may be a sensitizer, causing allergic eczema at sites of application. When any skin lesion worsens or assumes an eczematous component after topical treatment, consider the possibility of allergic contact dermatitis to the medication or one of its preservatives or ingredients.

Treatment of allergic contact dermatitis begins by removing the antigen. The history given by the patient and the configuration and distribution of the lesions give the most evidence for diagnosis. Allergic contact dermatitis often has straight edges, linear lesions, and bizarre distribution which make it an obvious "outside job." At times, the doctor, nurse, and patient must engage in a combined detective-team approach to track down the offending antigen. Detergents, car seats, lipstick, sprays, deodorants, or one of hundreds of objects or chemicals handled daily may be blamed. In some instances, it is necessary to keep a diary to try to define the antigen. It is important to remember that the appearance of eczema is usually delayed by one to three days after the exposure to the contactant.

Patch testing (see Chapter 6) may assist in confirming the diagnosis. Substances from the patient's place of work or related to his hobbies may be tested to see if they cause allergic eczema. Sometimes a trial of one to two weeks away from work or hobby is followed by clearing of the dermatitis.

Topical therapy of acute and chronic allergic contact dermatitis is the same as for other eczematous dermatitides (see section on atopic dermatitis in Chapter 7). Two important additional factors must be considered. First, it is essential to discover and avoid the antigen. Secondly, systemic steroids are frequently justified for severe cases in otherwise healthy persons. Since the eczema episode after a single exposure is self-limiting, chronic treatment will not be necessary and the side effects of chronic steroid therapy are not encountered.

Other Exogenous Causes of Eczema

Allergic reactions to parental *drugs* can occasionally cause a generalized eczematous eruption. Scattered eczema may suddenly appear on the trunk and extremities of persons with *superficial fungus infections,* local severe eczema, or severe *stasis dermatitis.* It has been hypothesized that such an event results from absorption of altered products of skin, bacteria, or fungus from the site of infection which act as antigens to cause a more generalized eczematous rash similar to that which occasionally appears as a manifestation of drug hypersensitivity. Such a generalization of an eczematous dermatitis is often referred to as an "id" reaction or autoeczematization.

Endogenous Causes of Eczema

Seborrheic dermatitis often has a histologic pattern with elements similar to eczema, and clinically, seborrheic dermatitis occasionally has an eczematous component.

Patients with *atopic dermatitis* (see Chapter 7) have a decreased itch threshold and have prolonged bouts of pruritus and eczematous dermatitis; they have eczematous dermatitis in the antecubital fossae and popliteal spaces as well as the lateral sides of the neck. These patients often have family histories of asthma, hay fever, and eczema. The cause is unknown.

There are several other forms of eczema, often collectively called *neurodermatitis,* whose cause is not known. There is a wide range in extent of involvement. Small, transient, round lesions called *nummular* (coin-shaped) *eczema* may appear in one or several sites and last only days or weeks. Larger areas of eczema may be kept chronically active because of constant and persistent rubbing of pruritic areas, as seen in *lichen simplex chronicus* (circumscribed neurodermatitis). Generalized neurodermatitis also occurs. (These common eczematous dermatitides of unknown etiology are discussed further in Chapter 7.)

Eczema is a kind of dermatitis or superficial skin reaction which has a characteristic morphology and histology, and which has many causes. Contact allergy causes eczema. Less often parental antigens cause eczema. Some very common skin disorders whose cause is not known present as eczematous dermatitis. Constitutional factors contribute to the eczema of atopic dermatitis. Hereditary diathesis and emotional tension precipitate the eczema of neurodermatitis.

The chief complaint is itching. Treatment of all forms of eczema is similar and is based on reducing inflammation, avoiding irritants, reducing itching and scratching, and returning the normal hydration and barrier function to the skin. Specific treatment is outlined following the specific disorders which present as eczematous dermatitis (see Chapter 7).

PRIMARY IRRITANT DERMATITIS

Not all dermatitis caused by exposure of the skin to chemicals is allergenic in nature. Substances can simply irritate the skin. Such a reaction is called a primary irritant contact dermatitis to distinguish it from the allergic contact dermatitis described above. Most occupational and household contact dermatitis is simply irritation. The exact mechanisms by which the irritants provoke inflammation is not clear.

Contact dermatitis is any inflammatory skin response to substances in the external environment. There are two types of contact dermatitis. Primary irritant dermatitis is a simple nonallergic inflammation which occurs essentially in all persons exposed long enough to an injurious agent of sufficient concentration. Allergic contact dermatitis occurs only in the small proportion of persons who become sensitized (allergic) to a chemical from a prior exposure. It may take one to three weeks to become sensitized after the originating encounter, and then one to three days to manifest the signs of dermatitis, after a subsequent exposure.

The skin response in allergic cutaneous dermatitis is most likely to be the classic vesicular eczematous dermatitis, while the primary irritant response is more variable and is often just red, edematous, and scaling. The clinical appearance of the two reactions is, however, often very similar. Palms and soles are usually resistant to contact dermatitis of the allergic type because the stratum corneum is very thick and resists penetration. Otherwise, the distribution of contact parallels the extent of the exposure.

A great many substances can act as irritants to the skin, provided there is sufficient concentration and duration of contact. Most of the primary irritants are chemicals, although physical and biologic agents may cause a similar nonallergic contact dermatitis. Mildly irritating substances, such as soaps, solvents, and detergents, may require repeated or prolonged contact to cause visible or symptomatic skin changes. Strong acids or alkalies, on the other hand, will injure the skin immediately on the first contact.

Irritated skin becomes red and edematous. Scaling, weeping, or even erosions may occur if the irritation is severe. Pruritus is present and often persistent. Chronic irritation leads to a dry, stiff thickening of the skin, which may be accompanied by some hyperpigmentation, fissuring, or scaling. Such thickened skin may be more resistant to further irritation, but fissures may cause the skin to itch or burn more quickly on subsequent exposure. Just as with allergic contact dermatitis, it is essential to make the diagnosis of what primary irritant is causing primary irritant contact dermatitis because the most important step in therapy is simply avoidance of further contact. The patient must be questioned extensively about work, hobbies, medications, cosmetics, and soaps. In the case of allergic contact dermatitis, diagnosis can be confirmed by patch testing. Such tests are not helpful with primary irritants, since all persons exposed to sufficient concentrations of irritating contactants for long periods of time will demonstrate inflammation. Still, there is no substitute for extensive detective work on the part of physician, nurse, and patient in discovering the contactant causing either kind of contact dermatitis.

INTERPLAY OF REACTION PATTERNS

We have seen how sunburn, the response to ultraviolet light radiation, is a complex of several simpler cutaneous reactions to stress. The symptoms of an insect bite can also be divided into its several components: trauma, inflammation, immunity, and allergy. Many dermatoses actually represent interdependent and interreacting reactions. The constitutional host's predispositions, the etiologic agents, and the triggering factors are not always known, but the various elements of cutaneous response can usually be observed clinically and histologically in a manner that gives important clues to pathogenic mechanisms.

Chains of events can be long, compound, and complicated. Infection of skin can lead to inflammation and immune reactions. Hypersensitivity may develop. The products of infection may act as primary irritants, or may cause allergic contact dermatitis which leads to eczema. Acute eczema presents serum to the surface which in turn, provides moisture and food for infection. The disrupted stratum corneum is an inefficient barrier and the skin is more easily damaged by nonspecific irritants. Allergens penetrate more easily through damaged skin. Repair, regeneration, hyperkeratosis, and healing begin while insult and reaction continue. Pruritus leads to rubbing and scratching, which introduces new trauma factors.

Despite these complexities, many clearly defined clinical entities and skin diseases are recognizable and treatable. The exact cause of some of them remains unknown, but the sequence and nature of cutaneous responses is known. This provides a rational basis for treatment in most disorders, and, fortunately, logical rules for prevention in many others.

REFERENCES

Adams, R. M.: *Occupational Contact Dermatitis,* J. B. Lippincott Company, Philadelphia, 1969.

Artz, C. P., and J. A. Moncrief: *The Treatment of Burns,* W. B. Saunders Company, Philadelphia, 1969.

Baer, R. L., and H. Harris: "Types of Cutaneous Reactions to Drugs," *JAMA* **202:**710–713, November 1967.

Baker, H., and A. M. Kligman: "Technique for Estimating Turnover Time of Human Stratum Corneum," *Arch. Derm.* **95:**408–411, April 1967.

Bianchine, J. R., P. V. J. Macaraeg, et al.: "Drugs as Etiologic Factors in the Stevens-Johnson Syndrome," *Amer. J. Med.* **44:**390–405, March 1968.

Blomgren, S. E.: "Conditions Associated with Erythema Nodosum," *N.Y. J. Med.* **72:**2302–2304, September 1972.

Demis, D. J.: "Allergy and Drug Sensitivity of Skin," *Ann. Rev. Pharmacol.* **9:**457–482, 1969.

Epstein, W., et al.: "Epidermal Mitotic Activity in Wounded Skin," in *Advances in Biology of Skin, Vol. V,* Montagna, W., and E. Billingham, eds., Pergamon Press, New York, chap. IV, pp. 68–75.

Fisher, A. A.: *Contact Dermatitis,* Lea and Febiger, Philadelphia, 1967.

Lowbury, E. J.: "Prevention and Treatment of Sepsis in Burns," *Proc. Roy. Soc. Med.* **65:**25–27, January 1972.

Moncrief, J. A.: "Burns," *New Eng. J. Med.* **288:**444–454, March 1973.

Pruitt, B. A., and J. A. Moncrief: "Recent Advances in Burn Treatment," *Surgery* **68:**412–418, August 1970.

Reed, R. J., and C. H. Wallace, Jr.: "Basic Pathologic Reactions of the Skin," in *Dermatology in General Medicine,* Fitzpatrick, T. B., K. Arndt, et al., eds., McGraw-Hill Book Company, 1971, pp. 192–212.

Wernstein, G. D., and E. J. Van Scott: "Autoradiographic Analysis of Turnover Times of Normal and Psoriatic Epidermis," *J. Invest. Derm.* **45:**257, October 1965.

Wilson, R. D.: "Thermoregulatory Failure of the Burn Scar," *J. Trauma* **11:**518–521, January 1971.

Tools and Laboratory Tests Used in Evaluating and Treating the Skin

Inspection of the skin
  Technique
  Diascopy
  Wood's light
Diagnostic tests
  Rapid microscopic tests
  Patch tests
  Punch biopsy
Therapeutic tools and techniques
  Surgery and curettage
  Electrosurgery
  Cryosurgery
  Ultraviolet light therapy
  X-ray therapy

INSPECTION OF THE SKIN

Technique

Three essential requirements for making sense out of skin abnormalities or skin lesions are knowledge of skin pathology, adequate exposure of the skin, and a systematic or orderly approach to the inspection of the skin. Adequate lighting is essential. Lights should be placed so that there is no glare or shadow effect upon the patient's skin. In most instances the patient should be totally undressed but adequately draped so that the patient's modesty and dignity are preserved, yet any area is easily accessible for inspection. When patients are only partially undressed, examination proves to be inadequate, clumsy, and more time consuming. The skin of the naked and thoughtfully draped patient can be inspected quickly, completely, and professionally without any embarrassment to the patient.

It is important that there be an orderly sequence to the inspection of the skin. It is helpful to begin by looking at palms, fingernails, and the backs of the hands to prevent this informative and frequently forgotten area of the skin from being overlooked. The presence of palmar lesions and the nature of such involvement carries diagnostic information. The temperature of the hands, the sweatiness of the palms, the attitude with which the patient allows his hands to be turned, held, and inspected give many clues and messages. More importantly, taking the patient's hand immediately establishes some nonverbal, warm, and personal communication between the nurse or physician and the patient.

From that point on, it is advisable to begin with examination of the scalp and head, not forgetting to look into the mouth. Then proceed to a rapid inspection down over the trunk, looking into the axillae and groin, and being careful to look at pressure points on the buttocks and posterior shoulders. Conclude with an examination of the skin of the legs and feet.

It may be advisable to examine some small skin lesions with a magnifier or hand lens. Specific morphologic details of generalized rash or larger lesions can sometimes best be appreciated by looking closely at the magnified skin markings, or fine pattern of color changes. Such details as increased skin lines, follicular plugging, telangiectasia, and location of lesions in respect to hair follicles can best be appreciated with a hand lens. A small penlight or a lamp source held at an angle in a partially darkened room can detect slight degrees of elevation or depression of the skin by exaggerating shadow phenomena (side lighting).

Diascopy

When the skin or individual skin lesions are red because of increased blood within dilated dermal vessels, the redness can be diminished or made to disappear by putting pressure on the skin. Such external pressure simply collapses the blood vessels in the area and causes the blood to leave the dilated and open vessels and move into other parts of the dermis or subcutaneous tissue. If, however, the color in the skin is due to blood which has escaped outside of the vessels, direct pressure over the area does not diminish the color or make it disappear. Blood outside the blood vessels cannot quickly move elsewhere under the influence of pressure because it has no immediate channels for escape. Such examination of colored skin areas under the influence of pressure can be done simply by pushing on the skin with the finger. It is easier to observe the effect of such pressure if the object exerting pressure is translucent, so that the examiner may see through it. Such translucent objects are called diascopes. A hand lens, glass slide, or clear plastic instrument may be used to press gently on the skin and observe the effect upon the color of the skin.

Diascopy is also useful in separating the darkening of the skin caused by blood vessel dilatation from that darkening caused by increase in pigment. The erythema of blood vessel dilatation will disappear with pressure by the diascope, while the increase in pigment from tanning or other causes does not change with pressure. The increased pigment which is present in the epidermis is obviously not free to move about and leave the area of pressure.

When papules in the skin are caused mostly by edema and vasodilatation, they should seem to disappear when examined through the diascope. However, if papules are also caused by a dense accumulation of cells, some substance remains even though pressure is exerted on the lesion. After diascopy has excluded the redness of vasodilatation, it is possible to observe the underlying color of the lesion. With diascopy, very dense cellular lesions such as granulomas of the skin maintain a yellow or apple-jelly color, while noncellular papules usually seem to disappear completely.

Open vascular channels, such as those seen in erythema, spider angiomata, telangiectasia, some superficial hemangiomas, and simple red papules, can be made to disappear under the influence of pressure. Lesions in which the color is caused by blood outside the blood vessels, such as petechiae, purpura, and ecchymoses, or the lesions of vasculitis, do not disappear under such pressure. Color which is present in the epidermis, such as melanin or hemosiderin, does not disappear under pressure. Red papules which contain dense collections of cells may show some yellow, yellow-brown, or apple-jelly color after all the blood or redness has been pressed from them.

Wood's Light

The Wood's light or Wood's lamp is a high-pressure mercury lamp with a specially compounded filter of nickel oxide and silica which is designed to transmit only long-wave ultraviolet wavelengths. These wavelengths

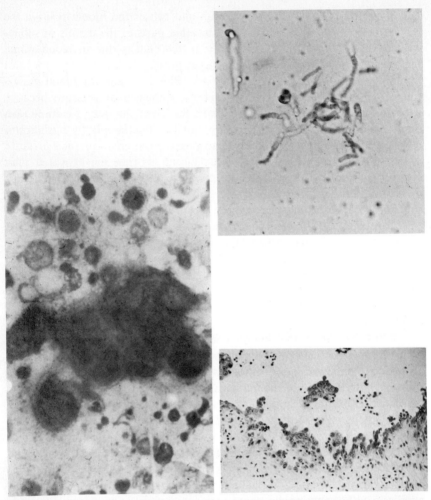

Figure 6-1 Rapid microscopic tests. (a) Hyphae seen in a KOH preparation support the diagnosis of superficial fungus infection (Chap. 7); (b) multinucleate cell scraped from the floor of a vesicle of herpes simplex (Chap. 7); (c) acantholytic cells; clumps of rounded, poorly attached cells float in the blister cavity of a patient with pemphigus vulgaris.

cause some substances to emit fluorescence which is visible and helpful in determining the fluorescing substance. Some superficial fungus infections of the scalp fluoresce a blue-green in the presence of Wood's light. *Erythrasma,* a superficial intertriginous bacterial infection, fluoresces a brilliant pink-orange or coral-red. The urine of some *porphyria* patients may fluoresce an orange-red when examined with the Wood's lamp. *Pseudomonas* infections may give off a yellow-green color under Wood's light before obvious signs of purulence appear. Such an examination is therefore useful in screening the skin of burn patients for the possibility of pseudomonas infections.

When subtle changes exist in epidermal pigmentation disorders, inspection in a darkened room with a Wood's light held close to the skin exaggerates the differences in degree of pigmentation present. Many nurseries use Wood's lights to examine the skin of newborn infants to identify the hypopigmented leaf-shaped macules indicative of tuberous sclerosis (a hereditary neurocutaneous disorder with potentially serious central nervous system malfunctions). While pigment which is present in the epidermis is exaggerated under Wood's light examination, pigment present in the dermis is not exaggerated. This permits a reasonable guess as to the site of melanin within the skin. Vitiligo, which usually represents a complete loss of pigment cells, is completely white under Wood's light examination, while pigment disorders which show some reduction, but not total loss, of pigment do not show such total absence of definable color.

DIAGNOSTIC TESTS

Rapid Microscopic Tests

There are several rapid microscopic tests which help in making diagnoses of skin lesions (Figure 6-1). Whenever a superficial fungus infection is suspected, scrapings obtained from the scales of a skin lesion, from the undersurface of the roof of a blister or from thickened nails can be collected on a glass slide. Potassium hydroxide, usually in a 10 percent concentration, dissolves away keratin and scales of the epidermis so that fungi can more easily be seen under examination with the light microscope. Hairs can similarly be examined for the presence of fungi which can be seen as long filamentous walled structures (*hyphae*) on microscopic examination. When infection is being considered, gram stain can be used to look for the presence of bacteria and to help in the identification of the organisms.

Using Wright's stain or Giemsa stain, microscopic examination of fluid and cells obtained from vessicles or bullae may be examined for the presence of multinucleated giant cells. Such cells are present in herpes simplex, herpes zoster, and chicken pox, and may be helpful in establishing the diagnosis of these conditions. Using the same stains one can look for the presence of acantholytic cells (epidermal cells which have become rounded and lost their spines or "prickly" nature) in the patients with pemphigus (see Chapter 12). Such examinations of cells from the bases of bullous lesions are sometimes referred to as Tzanck tests.

Patch Tests

Patch testing is used to validate a diagnosis of allergic contact sensitization and to identify and document the causative agent. It may occasionally be used as a screening procedure in persons with bizarre distributions of eczematous dermatitis. Since the entire skin of sensitized humans is allergic, this test actually reproduces allergic contact dermatitis in one small area, usually the back.

A patch test is a simple test in which an allergen (antigen) or a substance suspected of being an allergen is applied to the skin, occluded, and left in place for forty-eight hours. An eczematous response at the test site, which does not occur in an area similarly occluded but minus the antigen, is considered a positive reaction and suggests that the patient is indeed allergic to that compound. It is important to use concentrations of materials which are low enough so that primary irritant reactions do not occur. This ensures that the eczematous response is indeed caused by hypersensitization or allergy, and not simply by irritation.

Punch Biopsy

A punch biopsy of the skin is a rapid and simple test which often gives the physician valuable diagnostic information. A small, round, 4- or 6-millimeter punch which looks like a drill press or a tiny cookie cutter is firmly rotated against anesthetized skin. The cylinder of skin which has been cut is then removed, fixed, stained, and studied under the microscope (Figure

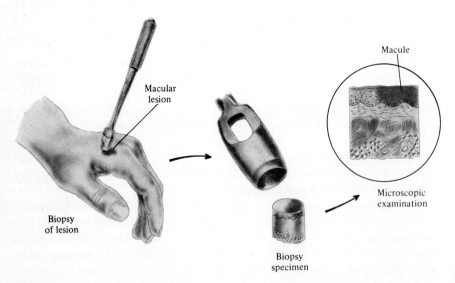

Figure 6-2 Punch biopsy of skin.

6-2). The site of the biopsy usually heals with a tiny scar and requires no special attention other than a small bandage for one day.

Biopsies, of course, may also be obtained by excision or incision of lesions. Wherever the panniculus (subcutaneous fat tissue) must be included in the biopsy specimen, it is best to excise an ellipse from the skin. Following this procedure, suturing is usually required for best cosmetic results. A shave biopsy simply removes with a scalpel blade that portion of any skin lesion which is elevated above the plane of the surrounding skin. This procedure is not only useful for obtaining material for diagnosis but also is often adequate treatment for benign epidermal growths such as nevi and seborrheic keratoses.

Punch biopsies are simple, quick, and safe. They are relatively painless and usually heal without complication and with minimal scar formation. They are frequently of great diagnostic help. In serious illnesses accompanied by skin changes, a rush biopsy can be ready for interpretation eight to twelve hours after it is obtained. This may be sooner than some chemistry laboratory tests are available and certainly precedes any bacteriologic or viral culture information concerning the patient's disease.

THERAPEUTIC TOOLS AND TECHNIQUES

Surgery and Curettage

When considering cosmetic results, punch biopsy is not the best technique for removing lesions greater than ½ centimeter. Larger lesions can be excised and the defect closed with suitable plastic repair. Skin cancers are often surgically removed. Many minor general surgical procedures are used on the skin to remove lesions, obtain material for histologic study, empty or remove cysts, drain abcesses, repair scars, or debride wounds (Figure 6-3).

Curettage is the scraping or scooping away of tissue with a circular cutting edge attached to a handle. When removing a lesion, one large scoop of tissue can be obtained for microscopic examination before the rest of the tissue is scraped away by repeated passes with the sharp edge of the curette. Friable tissue or dry crumbling lesions are easily removed in this manner, but the instrument is not sharp enough or strong enough to cut normal skin with ease. Most skin cancers are softer than the tough surrounding normal dermis, and the margins of the cancer can be detected with the curette by the change in feel from the softer, less resistant tumor tissue to the more resilient, tough, and firm dermis. Warts, keratoses, and basal cell epitheliomas may be treated by scraping until the lesion is gone. *Molluscum contagiosum* (Chapter 7) and *milia* can often be scooped out

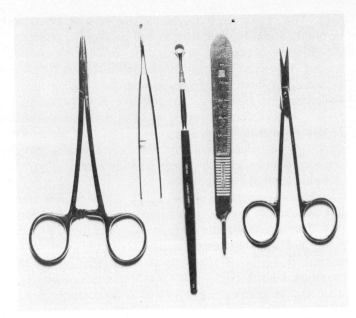

Figure 6-3 Tools for minor skin procedures. From left to right: hemostat, forceps, curet, scalpel handle, iris scissors.

of the skin. Some seborrheic keratoses can be crumbled away from the surface of the skin.

Electrosurgery

Small transportable electrosurgical units can deliver high-frequency alternating current which produces an electrical field around the tip of an electrode held against the skin. The high resistance (low conductivity) of the skin to electric current causes heat, dehydration, and mechanical disruption of cells. *Electrodesiccation* is a superficial destruction caused by a burst of electrical current onto the skin from an electrode held in the operator's hand. *Electrocoagulation* produces deeper and more severe destruction, better hemostasis, and more scarring. In the latter system, the patient is grounded and the treatment electrode delivers a charge into the skin, creating enough heat to "boil" and coagulate the tissue.

Benign superficial lesions such as warts, skin tags, and keratoses can be desiccated and cut away by electrosurgery. Skin tumors can be coagulated with electricity and then curetted away and small vascular lesions may be coagulated with electrosurgical units.

The heat provided by the procedure is partially self-sterilizing, making strict asepsis unnecessary. When alcohol is used to prep the skin, it must be allowed to dry completely before electric current is used, since alcohol is a flammable substance. Ethyl chloride sprays and some anesthetic gases are also flammable. Cardiac patients with pacemakers should not be treated with electrosurgery for fear of interfering with or deactivating the pacing device.

Cryosurgery

Skin lesions can be destroyed by freezing them. Cold injures the cells by poorly understood mechanical changes related to ice formation inside and outside of the cells, osmotic and electrolyte shifts, protein denaturation and solidification, and stasis of blood supply. Because of its good blood supply, the skin is relatively resistant to freezing. Although the skin does become solid at -1 to $-2°C$ it is necessary to bring the local skin temperature down to -18 to $-20°C$ for cell death or irreversible destruction to occur.

Two frequently used substances whose boiling point is well below that level needed to destroy tissue are solid CO_2 ($-78.5°C$) and liquid nitrogen ($-195.6°C$). Cotton tip applicators, saturated with liquid nitrogen, can be applied to the skin to destroy superficial lesions. Metal discs made cold with liquid nitrogen may be used with moderate pressure on the skin to obtain deeper freezing and more extensive destruction. Units are available which deliver a direct spray of liquid nitrogen to treat even larger and deeper lesions. A variety of benign and malignant lesions can be destroyed with cold injury. The procedure is rapid, easily done, usually requires no anesthesia, and leaves minimal or no scarring.

Many patients experience some pain after cryosurgery, and aspirin and sedatives may be necessary. An edematous response at the site of treatment begins within hours and peaks about one to two days later. Blistering may occur when deeper, more extensive lesions are treated. The most severely injured tissue can be expected to slough in two to three weeks, and healing is usually satisfactorily completed without complications within a month.

Liquid nitrogen cannot be kept in a completely airtight, stoppered container as it may explode. It must have some exit for evaporation. Specially made vacuum flasks are best for storage.

Ultraviolet Light Therapy

Ultraviolet light (UV) causes temporary suppression of the mitotic rate of the basal cells followed by a rebound increase in cell turnover. This latter stimulating effect may be related to the improvement seen in acne after repeated exposures to sunlight or artificial ultraviolet light. In a rapidly proliferating disease like psoriasis, the therapeutic effects of UV light may be more related to the temporary suppression of cell division. Chronic eczema is sometimes improved by UV light. It is commonly felt that it is the sunburn spectrum (UV-B) which is most responsible for the beneficial effects of sunlight and artificial UV in these conditions.

There are several sources of ultraviolet light for treatments, for clinical use, or for suntanning. The least expensive, most effective, most generally available source is natural sunlight. The inexpensive "sunlamps" emitting UV-B or sunburn spectrum are usually low-pressure mercury lamps or fluorescent bulbs. These are useful in home therapy. High-pressure, high-temperature mercury lamps which are larger, more expensive, and of higher intensity are frequently used in clinics, inpatient areas, and research laboratories.

Patients and personnel using UV sources must be carefully instructed to avoid harmful overexposures. Goggles must be used to protect the eyes. It is safest to use a dependable timer or to have someone else in the room during treatments. Low, suberythemal doses are used at first, and exposure times are gradually increased with each daily exposure.

Some artificial UV sources produce enough longwave UV to cause erythema after the administration of psoralens or photoactive dye substances. The longwave UV lamps ("black lights") which are ordinarily innocuous can be used in conjunction with psoralens to repigment vitiligo and, in conjunction with photoactive dyes, to photodestroy the DNA virus causing herpes simplex. The psoralens are very potent photosensitizers and should be administered only by experienced persons to avoid painful blistering reactions.

Germicidal lamps (shortwave UV, UV-C) are used in operating rooms, in tissue culture labs, over the doorways of surgical intensive care units, and in some wards. The shortwave UV radiation kills bacteria in the air and therefore reduces the rate of bacterial infection. The lamp can cause mild sunburn, itching, and some pigmentation if the skin is directly exposed for as little as a few minutes. The major danger for patients and personnel is a painful conjunctivitis which can occur after seconds of direct exposure to shortwave UV lamps. No one should ever look directly into these lamps or spend much time around the lamp without adequate protective garb or glasses.

X-ray Therapy

Many benign and malignant skin disorders can be treated with ionizing radiation. Such disorders as acne, warts, and eczema often respond very well to x-ray therapy. X-radiation is, however, used infrequently for these common dermatologic disorders. This decreased usage is partly because other means of treatment are easier, more effective, and less expensive.

More important, it is because of the growing awareness of the unfortunate late onset and long-term side effects of ionizing radiation. Chronic radiation dermatitis manifested by atrophy, telangiectasia, and pigment irregularity may become evident decades after initial x-ray therapy. This carries not only a serious cosmetic liability but an increased potential for skin cancer at the site of radiation. It is not lack of effectiveness that makes x-radiation increasingly unappealing, it is the serious permanent late side effects.

Still, x-ray remains a preferred therapy for skin cancer in certain parts of the body. It is a more efficient and less cosmetically destructive tool than surgery for tumors in certain areas of the central face, ears, and mouth. It is a reasonable therapy for skin cancer on older patients who may not tolerate surgery and whose life expectancy is such that late complications are not a serious consideration.

In addition, there are still those who suggest that if dosage, equipment, personnel, and total number of treatments are carefully and intelligently controlled and monitored, x-ray remains a key therapeutic tool for such problems as resistent cases of acne, hand eczema, or plantar warts. They believe that a limited number of superficial treatments do not carry a significant long-range danger. Sentiment is progressively shifting so that the moral and medicolegal burden of necessity of proof rests with those who continue to use x-ray for benign or chronic dermatoses. As better treatments for common skin disorders evolve, life expectancy gets longer, and fewer dermatologists are adequately trained in radiation therapy, its use may continue to diminish.

Although radiation does decrease size and activity of sebaceous glands, and improve acne, tetracycline therapy has made resistent, severe cystic acne less common. Although x-ray epilation (hair removal) was a moderately successful therapy of *tinea capitis* (scalp ringworm), the introduction of griseofulvin has made this therapy unnecessary. Although hemangiomas of infants can sometimes be sclerosed and reduced in size by x-ray therapy, it is now known that most of these raised strawberry hemangiomas gradually involute without therapy. *Hidradenitis suppurativa* may improve with x-ray therapy, after repeated failure of minor surgery, antibiotics, and drainage procedures. Many of these patients are now, however, being successfully treated by radical excision of the axillary vault.

REFERENCES

Arndt, K., and D. S. Feingold: "The Sign of Pyotr Vasilyewich Nikolsky," *N. Eng. J. Med.* **282:**1154–1155, May 1970.

Blank, H., and C. F. Burgoon: "Abnormal Cytology of Epithelial Cells in Pemphigus Vulgaris: A Diagnostic Aid," *J. Invest. Derm.* **18:**213–223, 1952.

Blank, H., C. F. Burgoon, C. D. Baldridge, et al.: "Cytologic Smears in Diagnosis of Herpes Simplex, Herpes Zoster, and Varicella," *JAMA* **146:**1410–1412, August 1951.

Brown, J.: "Erythrasma and Identifications with Wood's Light," *J. Am. Podiat. Ass.* **60:**322, August 1970.

Burdick, K. H.: *Electrosurgical Apparatus and Their Application in Dermatology,* Charles C Thomas, Publisher, Springfield, Ill., 1969.

Epstein, W. L., K. Fukuyama, and J. H. Epstein: "Early Effects of Ultraviolet Light on DNA Synthesis in Human Skin in Vivo," *Arch. Derm.* **100:**84–89, July 1969.

Goldman, L., H. Plotnick, and I. Balinkin: "Investigative and Clinical Studies with Diascopy in Dermatology," *Arch. Derm.* **75:**699–705, May 1957.

Knox, J. M., R. G. Freeman, W. C. Duncan, and C. L. Heaton: "Treatment of Skin Cancer," *Southern Med. J.* **60:**241–246, March 1967.

Robertson, W. D.: "Cryotherapy in Dermatology," *Ohio Med. J.* 64:1260–1263, November 1968.

Shelley, W. B.: "The Patch Test," *JAMA* **200:**874–878, June 1967.

Swartz, J. H., and T. Medrek: "Rapid Contrast Stain as Diagnostic Aid for Fungus Infections," *Arch. Derm.* **99:**494–497, April 1969.

Zacarian, S. A.: *Cryosurgery of Skin Cancer and Cryogenic Techniques in Dermatology,* Charles C Thomas, Publisher, Springfield, Ill., 1969.

Common Dermatoses of Otherwise Well People

Disorders related to sebaceous glands
   Acne vulgaris
   Acne rosacea
   Seborrheic dermatitis
Disorders of epidermal proliferation
   Psoriasis
   Other disorders of epidermal proliferation
Eczematous dermatitis
   Atopic dermatitis
   Nummular eczema
   Pompholyx
   Hand eczema
   Circumscribed neurodermatitis (lichen
     simplex chronicus)
Disorders of sweat gland occlusion
   Miliaria
Disorders of pigmentation
   Melasma
   Vitiligo
Miscellaneous disorders
   Pityriasis rosea
   Lichen planus

DISORDERS RELATED TO SEBACEOUS GLANDS

Acne Vulgaris

Acne vulgaris is an inflammatory disease involving the pilosebaceous follicle. Acne is so common that it can be considered a physiologic response to pubertal hormonal changes. Because of its high incidence, prolonged course, and familial predisposition, many patients and doctors are resigned to tolerating acne—letting the disease be "outgrown." This course may lead to unnecessary disfigurement in teenagers and young adults, and to permanent scarring. This "tolerated" acne causes embarrassment and self-consciousness at a time when identity development is critical.

Fortunately, acne is treatable. Much is known about the disease, and many forms of therapy have logic and a fair record of success. The microscopic sequences in the formation of lesions and several of the factors precipitating acne or causing it to flare have been identified. While it is not possible to cure acne, or prevent it from occurring in the first place, every patient can be treated, and can be expected to improve.

Acne seems to be more severe in people who inherit a tendency or diathesis to have acne. Although many acne patients have oily skin, the tendency to have acne is not clearly related to the fat content of the skin or to qualitative differences in sebum. Acne is not caused by chocolate, cokes, greasy foods, masturbation, or dirt. Acne may be one of the earliest manifestations of puberty and in girls may precede menarche by one or two years. However, acne may not begin until well into the third decade.

After remaining small and inactive throughout childhood, the sebaceous glands become large and very active as a physiologic response to the increased levels of male hormones which accompany puberty in both males and females. Acne lesions characteristically occur in areas of large and active sebaceous glands, especially in areas where the sebaceous glands tend to be quite large in proportion to the hair, into whose follicle the gland empties. These areas include the face, upper chest, and upper back. Acne can also occur in adults, but is not as common as in adolescents.

The characteristic lesions of acne are comedones, papules, pustules, fluctuant nodules, cysts, and scars (Figure 7-1). *Comedones* are noninflammatory dilated follicles formed by an expanding mass of sebum and keratin, which dilates, and ultimately obstructs the hair follicle canal. In the open comedo ("blackhead"), this keratinous material is readily evident in the widely dilated pore or follicle opening. The dark color of this material results more from the melanin in compacted keratinocytes than from dirt. In the closed comedo ("whitehead"), the keratin plug is less compact, and the follicle orifice narrower. The open comedo is most likely the advanced lesion and is derived from a closed comedo. The open comedo may be

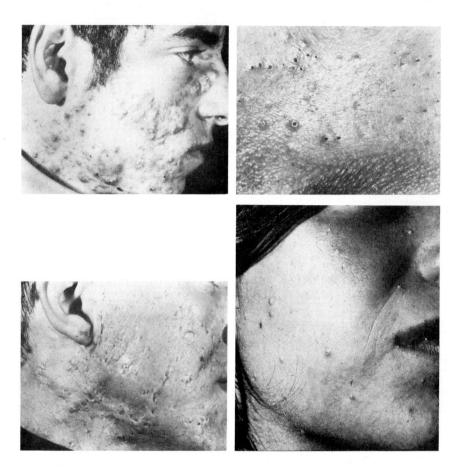

Figure 7-1 Acne vulgaris. (*a*) Moderately severe acne vulgaris; (*b*) comedones; (*c*) scars; (*d*) pustules and papules.

relatively inert while the closed comedo may lead to inflammatory lesions. Scars are usually small and wedge-shaped as if made by an ice pick, or may be crateriform with single or multiple openings; occasionally they may be linear depressions.

Larger inflammatory lesions of acne may be preceded by occlusion of the distal hair follicle canal. Rupture of the wall allows sebum, keratin, and bacteria to spill into the dermis (Figure 7-2). The erythematous papules and pustules of acne are formed by inflammatory responses to the products of the sebaceous gland which enter the dermis by way of the break in the wall of the hair follicle. Sebum is highly irritating to the dermis. An inherited weakness or defect in the follicle wall predisposes a rupture which may or may not be preceded by significant duct occlusion.

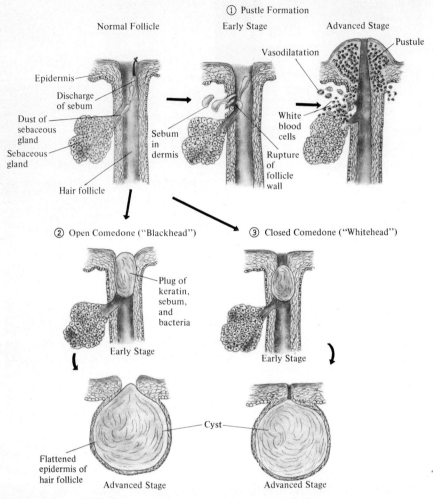

Figure 7-2 Acne vulgaris: formation of inflammatory lesions.

This altered follicle wall may be the most important hereditary component of acne.

Some of the bacteria which normally live in hair follicles are able to ingest the lipids of sebum. In order to use lipids as food, certain bacteria, *Corynebacterium acnes,* contain a lipase (enzyme capable of splitting fats) which breaks up the fatty acids of sebum into smaller molecular units. These shorter-chain fatty acids are much more irritating to the dermis than the original long-chain parent compounds. Sebum-containing fats altered by the bacteria enter into the dermis, leading to more severe inflammation.

Large papules become suppurative. The entire inflammatory process may be walled off, forming a cyst and, if the process is especially destructive, may lead to scar formation.

Some factors are known to precipitate or worsen acne in those persons who have the predisposition, and adequate levels of male hormone. External factors which are occlusive to the skin make acne worse. Occlusion may simply increase the likelihood of follicular pore occlusion and comedo formation. Resting the face in the hands may cause a focal flare-up of acne. Hair styled over the forehead or face may precipitate lesions in the covered areas. Greasy oil-base cosmetics tend to cause comedones. Soldiers remaining in hot humid weather get severe cystic acne underneath their backpacks. Sleep loss, severe physical stress, and emotional pressures seem to precipitate flare-ups of acne. Acne in students is often worse around exam time, and medical and nursing students often notice an exacerbation when they first become responsible for assisting in the care of hospitalized patients. Hormonal changes may cause a premenstrual flare-up. Certain medications, including systemic steroid and halogenated compounds, may cause acne lesions to appear. Acne may, in fact, be a sign of endocrine disorders such as Cushing's disease in which endogenous steroid levels are elevated.

Specific diets and eating habits seem to have little effect on most patients. One study showed that chocolate did not cause an increase in the number of lesions in teenage acne patients. Punitive parental pressure, guilt feelings about poor diet, and the social unacceptability of obesity which results from dietary excesses may, however, lead to emotional tension and a subsequent flare-up of acne.

The treatment of acne varies, depending upon the severity of the disease. It is important to consider the patient's perception of the cosmetic disfigurement involved. Some persons are highly concerned by even a single inflammatory papule while others seem to ignore and accept multiple pustules and cysts. The goal of treatment is not only the improvement of the appearance and self-confidence of the teenager but also the prevention of lifelong scars.

Keeping the skin reasonably clean and free of external occlusion is important; however, the excessive use of irritating soaps and topical antibacterial agents is not justified. Many of these agents are too drying, and the superficially located staphylococcal organisms they suppress probably play little or no role in the pathogenesis of acne. Abrasive soaps help to remove keratin, sebum, dirt, and the most superficial plugs. Such soaps contain particles of aluminum oxide, polyethylene granules, or other inert substances which mechanically irritate the skin, causing vasodilatation and stimulating increased cell turnover.

The so-called keratolytic agents such as sulfur, resorcinol, salicylic acid, and benzoyl peroxide are helpful when used topically in a frequency and concentration which leads to minimal erythema and desquamation. This dose varies from person to person, and from time to time adjustment of the frequency of application is necessary. If no scaling or dryness occurs, treatment will probably be ineffective. If the patient is uncomfortable, the frequency of application or the concentration of the medication should be reduced. It may be that these topical medications simply increase the rate of skin turnover and thereby act to cleanse and empty pores mechanically by a simple conveyor-belt or surface-slough mechanism. Physical agents such as ultraviolet light and applications of carbon dioxide or liquid nitrogen are sometimes helpful and may work by a similar mechanism.

Tetracycline in moderate dosage (½ to 1½ grams per day) improves pustular, papular, and cystic acne. Tetracycline inhibits the growth of *C. acnes*. Therefore, the enzymes made by these organisms are no longer available to change fatty acids of sebum to their more inflammation-producing breakdown components. After initial improvement it may be necessary to maintain patients on 250 to 500 milligram of tetracycline daily for long periods of time. Most patients tolerate tetracycline very well, but occasionally *monilial vaginitis* or mild transient nausea occurs. The tetracycline should be taken on an empty stomach because calcium in food, especially milk, binds the drug and prevents adequate absorption. Erythromycin, lincomycin, and other antibiotics are sometimes used for acne.

Simple mechanical procedures which empty comedones and drain suppurative inflammatory lesions hasten improvement, and large cysts can be made less inflammatory by intralesional injections of steroids. Acne in female patients may be improved by oral estrogens although an initial increase in acne is occasionally seen for several months before improvement is noted. Oral vitamin A has been used for some time in the treatment of acne although careful double-blind studies have not demonstrated clear evidence to justify its use. Topical vitamin A (retinoic acid) used in doses which cause minimal irritation seems to work at least as well as do the keratolytic agents mentioned earlier. Larger doses (higher concentration or more frequent applications) may cause considerable inflammation initially but may result in striking improvement of acne. The keratinization of the epidermal cells lining the distal hair canal wall may be affected in such a way as to make them less likely to rupture.

Most patients with moderate to severe acne can be treated with one or two topical keratolytic medications, tetracycline, and some mild form of physical or mechanical treatment. In the hands of an enthusiastic and skilled practitioner, the combination of minor acne surgery, intralesional steroid injection, and ultraviolet light is the most effective office therapy available. The vast majority of these patients can be expected to improve on this simple program. After the disease has remained inactive for several months, the ice-pick-like scars may be made less noticeable by dermabrasion. Larger scars require individual plastic surgery or injection procedures on each specific area.

Acne Rosacea

Acne rosacea is a chronic cosmetic disorder of unknown etiology in which acneiform lesions may be superimposed on permanent vascular dilatations of the face. It usually begins between the ages of 30 and 50, is more frequent in women but may be more severe in men, and is uncommon among highly pigmented persons. Gross and histologic appearance of some of these lesions may be similar to acne. It appears that acne rosacea is related to and dependent upon the presence of large, active sebaceous glands, because its lesions are often preceded by or coexistent with "seborrhea." However, no specific quantitative or qualitative abnormality of sebum and no precise etiologic role of the sebaceous glands has been demonstrated. Over the years many causative factors have been suggested, including bacteria, allergy, vitamin deficiency, hormones, tuberculosis, alcohol, caffeine, psychic factors, heredity, and a small mite called *Demodex folliculorum.* None have been shown to be the cause of acne rosacea.

The vascular component usually begins first. The central one-third of the whole face is the most strikingly involved, with relative sparing of the sides of the face. Blotchy or diffuse erythema comes and goes but eventually becomes relatively constant. Finally, telangiectasia becomes superimposed on the background of permanent but blanchable erythema. Papules and pustules may appear. The lesions look like acne vulgaris, except that comedones are unusual and cysts and scars are rare (Figure 7-3). The skin may feel cool and slightly oily. There is no pain or pruritus, but some patients complain of flushing or feelings of warmth.

Years of acne rosacea may lead to irregular, lobulated, bulbous thickening of the skin of the distal part of the nose. The resulting enlargement of the nose is accompanied by a purple-red discoloration and strikingly dilated follicles. This condition, called *rhinophyma,* is characterized histologically by vasodilatation, increase in sebaceous glands and connective tissue, and signs of chronic inflammation. A small percentage of patients with acne rosacea have ocular involvement with blepharitis (lid inflammation) or conjunctivitis. Keratitis is not common but when present may lead to corneal ulceration.

There is no specific treatment for the vascular component of acne rosacea. It seems reasonable to avoid stimuli which normally provoke facial vasodilatation, such as excessive sunlight, extremes of temperature, hot

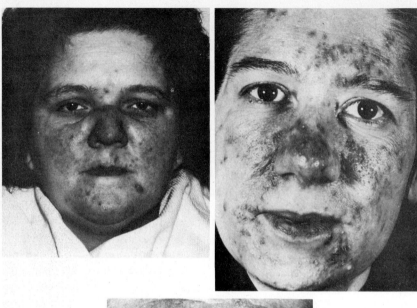

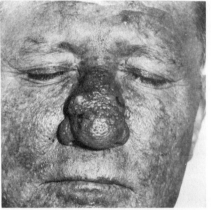

Figure 7-3 Acne rosacea. (a) Erythema, telangiectasia, and acneiform lesions of central third of face; (b) close-up of pustules and papules; no comedones are present; (c) rhinophyma.

liquids, spices, alcohol, and caffeine, although such avoidance has never been shown to be curative. The treatment of the acneiform component is essentially the same as that for acne vulgaris, except that irritating medications must be used with caution since they may increase vasodilatation. Ultraviolet light may similarly increase the redness. Tetracycline is often beneficial. Individual, large telangiectatic vessels may be electrodesiccated with a very small needle. Rhinophyma may be improved by surgically shaving, planing, abrading, or electrocauterizing away excess tissue under local anesthesia. Even with optimum therapy, complete clearing of acne rosacea is unusual, but progress of the disorder can usually be arrested and modest improvement achieved over several months.

Seborrheic Dermatitis

Seborrheic dermatitis is a common, erythematous, scaly eruption which occurs primarily in those areas with a high number and activity of sebaceous glands. This seborrheic distribution, which includes face, scalp, chest, and back, is the characteristic feature of the disorder. The cause is unknown. A constitutional predisposition seems to exist and some individuals have intermittent difficulties throughout postpubertal life. Emotional and physical stress may precipitate recurrences for unknown reasons.

Seborrheic dermatitis is seen in infants during the first months of life when sebaceous glands are functioning as the result of transplacentally derived maternal sex hormones. It then disappears until puberty and is a common disease throughout adult life. Despite this temporal relationship, the distribution, and the name of the disorder, no clear abnormality in sebaceous gland function has been demonstrated. Sebum in these patients has not been shown to be unusual in amount or content and has not been proven to be the cause of the disease. Some investigators have postulated that prolonged retention of sebum on the skin may act as an irritant or that components of sebum may be resorbed percutaneously to alter epidermal function, but this theory has not been documented.

Mild seborrheic dermatitis presents as only diffuse erythema with superimposed patches of dry scale and is most often seen on the scalp, eyebrows, presternal, and beard areas. Seborrheic dermatitis is the most common cause of a "butterfly" facial rash extending across the nose and over both cheeks. More severe involvement leads to dull red plaques covered with thick yellow-red semiconfluent scale (Figure 7-4). Body folds such as the nasolabial fold, postauricular fold, inframammary area, groin, and gluteal creases may become involved. Seborrheic dermatitis is a frequent cause of ear canal inflammation and of external ear dermatitis. Erythematous and scaling involvement of the eyelids (seborrheic marginal blepharitis) is common and may be associated with conjunctivitis.

The broadest definition of seborrheic dermatitis also includes minimal scaling of the scalp and the greasy, minimally erythematous faces of people with excessively oily skin who scale occasionally. Some persons would reserve the term "dandruff" for the flaking scalp and "seborrhea" for the excessively oily skin because there is little evidence of "dermatitis." Precision of terminology may not be essential until the etiology of seborrheic dermatitis is determined.

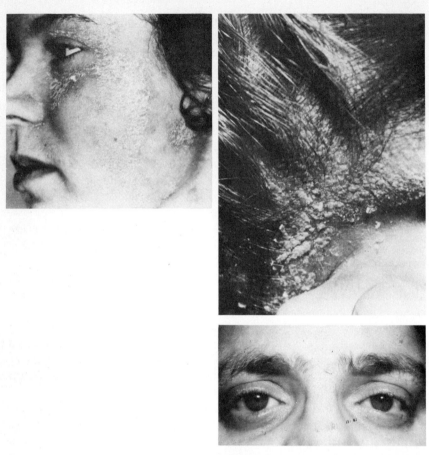

Figure 7-4 Seborrheic dermatitis. (*a*) "Butterfly rash"; (*b*) scale of moderately severe seborrheic dermatitis; (*c*) blepharitis. Scaling at margin of eyelids.

Seborrheic dermatitis is a chronic disorder, and treatment is symptomatic. The condition usually responds well to simple treatments but no permanent cure is known. Topical medications containing sulfurs, salicylic acid, resorcinol, and tars in various combinations are very effective and many are available. Shampoos add surfactants and detergents to these active agents and are effective when used two to three times per week. It is the scalp and not the hair which is being treated. The shampoo must remain in contact with the scalp for five to fifteen minutes in order to soften and loosen the scale. A second application of shampoo should follow rinsing. A final vigorous rinsing, with moderate scratching, removes the scale.

If lesions are extensive or inflammatory, a topical steroid is effective.

Topical hydrocortisone is often used for chronic or extensive seborrheic dermatitis. More potent steroids are effective but should not be used for prolonged periods of time because telangiectasia or skin atrophy may occur.

DISORDERS OF EPIDERMAL PROLIFERATION

Psoriasis

Psoriasis is a genetically determined chronic epidermal proliferative disease of very unpredictable course. Onset is most often in early adult life, but psoriasis may begin in infancy, in childhood, or in the aged. Once the disease becomes manifest, it may remain localized to a few sites and may be present only occasionally or it may cause intermittent or continuous generalized disease. All degrees in between these two extremes occur and there is no reliable way to predict the amount of difficulty to expect in a patient with newly discovered psoriasis.

The tendency to have psoriasis is inherited through multiple genes and no clear and simple pattern of heredity exists. In the United States, 2 to 4 percent of the population has psoriasis. Approximately 5 percent of psoriatics have an associated inflammatory arthritis, which usually involves the distal interphalangeal joints. This arthritis is occasionally severe and incapacitating. Serologic testing for rheumatoid arthritis is negative.

The lesions of psoriasis are elevated, erythematous, sharply circumscribed, scaling plaques which tend to occur symmetrically over areas of bony prominence such as elbows and knees (Figure 7-5). They also tend to occur on the scalp and trunk. Scalp lesions may be quite thick but usually maintain a sharp border. Active psoriasis may localize to the site of recent epidermal injury such as scratches, severe sunburn, surgical wounds, or other trauma. A characteristic and often overlooked site of involvement is within the intergluteal fold. A careful inspection of this area may assist in diagnosis. Almost any area of the body, however, may be involved in psoriasis. Occasionally, total body confluent erythema and scaling (exfoliative erythroderma) occurs, requiring hospitalization. About one-fifth of psoriatic patients note pruritus; it is rarely severe.

The scale appears to be thick. When examined closely, however, it is shown to be made up of uncountable numbers of thin micaceous (silvery), loosely adherent flakes which are easily removed and may accumulate in the patient's clothing or bed. Nail involvement may simply consist of punctate pitting of the nail plate, or more severe involvement may lead to subungual accumulation of scale and keratotic material. Marked subungual hyperkeratosis and severe matrix involvement may lead to markedly deformed nails.

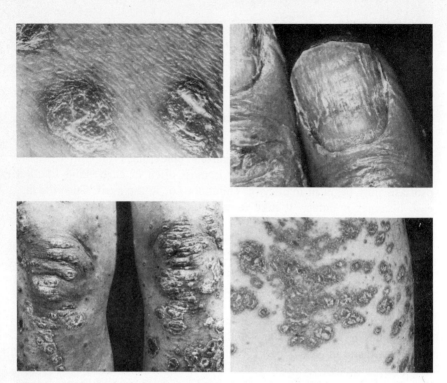

Figure 7-5 Psoriasis. (a) Typical plaque; (b) nail involvement; pits and deformed nail plate; (c) usual distribution—elbows and knees; (d) close-up of scale.

Factors causing flares of psoriasis are not well understood. There seems to be some correlation between moderately severe generalized psoriasis and alcoholism. It is not clear which problem is causal in such a situation. A similar relationship has been claimed with obesity. For unknown reasons patients given chloroquin may have a flare of psoriasis. In young persons, psoriasis may follow one to two weeks after a streptococcal pharyngitis. Emotional stress causes a flare in some psoriatics.

Microscopically there is marked epidermal thickening in psoriatic skin which is mostly a regular elongation of the rete ridges and a consequent elongation of the dermal papillae, showing capillary dilatation. There is increased evidence of mitotic activity at and slightly above the basal layer. Lymphocytic and histiocytic inflammatory cells are present in the upper dermis and polymorphonuclear cells may invade the epidermis (Figure 7-6).

The marked increase in the number of reproducing basal cells and the acceleration of the mitotic cycle of each cell which is seen in psoriasis combine to increase dramatically the *number* of cells produced. The transit time or turnover time is also markedly affected. After a basal cell of normal skin divides, it takes about 14 days for the daughter cell, which is pushed upwards, to reach the stratum corneum. It then takes an additional 14 days for this cell to pass through the stratum corneum and be sloughed as nonviable scale. In the regions of psoriasis, the entire transit time from the division of the basal cell to migration through the stratum corneum and sloughing as scale may be shortened to as little as three or four days. Psoriatics simply make too much skin too rapidly (Figure 7-6).

It follows, therefore, that the most likely mechanism by which the various treatments of psoriasis work is by retardation of the growth of epidermal cells. The agents which are most effective in treating psoriasis

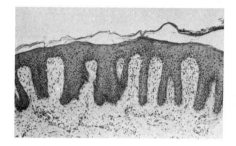

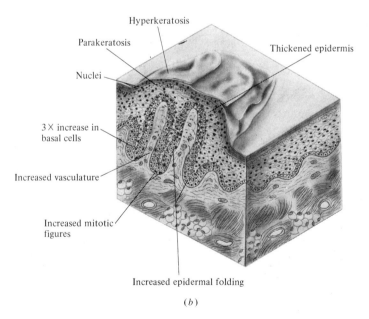

(b)

Figure 7-6 Psoriasis. (a) Histologic section of psoriasis (photomicrograph); (b) diagrammatic view of cell kinetics in psoriasis.

are those which are toxic to epidermal cells, especially those which affect cell replication. Systemic medications also impede cell replication elsewhere in the body, while those which are applied topically to the skin may have some selective effect on epidermis.

Although there is no permanent cure, most psoriasis is treatable. Most patients who are conscientious about applying their medications will respond. Optimism is not only well founded, it is a useful part of the treatment regime. Treatments include tar preparations, topical corticosteroids, mechanical treatments to remove scale, and antimetabolites.

Natural crude coal tar, wood and coal tars, anthralin, and other related compounds are frequently used. They are most effective when used in combination with ultraviolet light. An old, established therapy consists of applying crude coal tar to the entire body several hours before receiving ultraviolet light (Goeckerman regimen). It is a messy, smelly procedure which stains bedding, clothing, and tub, and is usually done as an inpatient procedure. In general, ultraviolet light, with or without tar, from artificial sources or from sun, is beneficial to most psoriatics, but overexposure should be avoided since sunburn can cause a generalized flare. There is evidence that long-wave ultraviolet light in the presence of photosensitizing agents may improve psoriasis.

Anthralin is a distillate of crude coal tar which, when added to a zinc oxide paste base and coated onto thick plaques, causes them to flatten within a few days. It may, however, be irritating to normal skin, and it does stain the skin and clothing. It is moderately difficult to apply and remove, but its effectiveness is such that it remains a useful treatment for especially thick and resistent psoriatic plaques.

Topical corticosteroids are beneficial, especially when they are applied under occlusion. The potent fluorinated compounds are most effective. Topical steroid application is frequently used in conjunction with other treatment programs. They are cosmetically acceptable creams and can be easily used by outpatients. Steroids are sometimes injected into psoriatic plaques with good results. Systemic steroids are frequently effective in clearing psoriasis, but the possible rebound worsening of psoriasis which follows a steroid-induced remission, and the chronic nature of psoriasis, makes such therapy impractical and dangerous.

Mechanical measures which macerate and remove scale and enhance penetration of medications are frequently necessary. These include salicyclic acid and other keratolytic agents, occlusive dressings, and baths. Mercury compounds are effective but may be allergenic in some patients and chronic use has been reported to lead to renal tubular damage. Propylene glycol in water removes scales in psoriasis and in other disorders of epidermal proliferation.

Mild scalp involvement can usually be managed with a tar shampoo. More severe involvement may necessitate adding keratolytic agents, occluding overnight with a shower cap, and using tar shampoo in the morning to remove the scale. Once the scale has been removed, topical steroids can penetrate the epidermis and reduce the inflammation of the scalp.

Antimetabolites, especially methotrexate, are very effective in treating psoriatics, but their use should definitely be reserved for resistant cases which do not respond to the usual measures. Toxicity to mucous membranes, bone marrow, liver, and gastrointestinal tract—adverse reactions of the antimetabolites—makes it clear that these medications should only be given by those with experience in their use. They are very useful when administered wisely, and when reserved for patients whose psoriasis remains a social and economic disaster despite optimum topical therapy.

Occasionally psoriasis begins or flares with vigor. Acute, severe, active psoriasis should be treated gently. Recently worsening, rapidly progressing lesions may be red, with little scale, and slightly tender. At this stage tars, keratolytic agents, and full erythema doses of UV should be avoided. If the lesions become irritated, they may worsen, and if the uninvolved skin is injured the flare may become more generalized and may last longer. A few days of rest, soaks, and topical steroids may quiet things enough to begin the more usual therapies.

Psoriasis is a chronic disease. The patient must learn to accept the possibility of repeated exacerbations. The attitude of medical personnel is a very important part of therapy. No one should register disgust in his facial expression or avoid touching the patient's skin. A long-term supportive attitude must balance encouragement with honesty. Patients become discouraged. The efforts they expend in home treatments must be recognized and praised. Support and optimism is required from family, doctor, and nurse. But it is essential to be frank with the patient about treatment requirements and prognosis. Most patients can deal with psoriasis if they remain informed, involved, and supported.

Other Disorders of Epidermal Proliferation

Keratosis pilaris is a disorder of unknown origin in which noninflammatory, fine keratotic papules occur at hair follicle openings (Figure 7-7). The asymptomatic papules usually are irregularly scattered over lateral aspects of the thighs and upper arms. The lesions give the skin a rough feel. Keratosis pilaris lasts for many years, is more prominent in a dry climate, and may occur more frequently among atopic individuals. Treatment is usually not necessary, but mild keratolytic agents in ointments or emollients make the papules less prominent.

Ichthyosis (from the Greek word for fish) refers to a group of heredi-

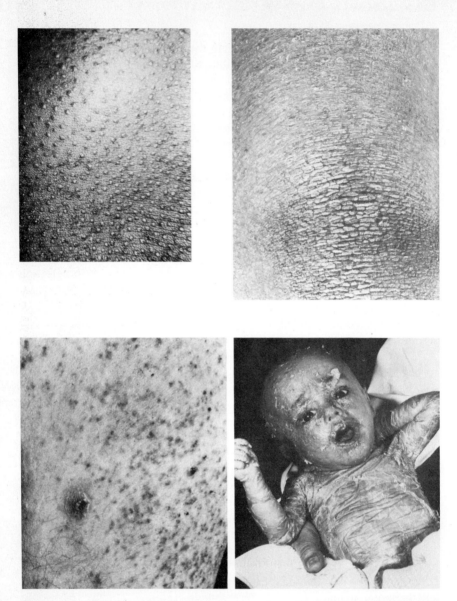

Figure 7-7 Disorders of epidermal proliferation. (*a*) Keratosis pilaris; keratotic elevations at hair follicles; (*b*) ichthyosis; marked thickening of stratum corneum; (*c*) Darier's disease; "dirty," greasy-brown hyperkeratotic papules scattered in a haphazard arrangement; (*d*) ichthyosis.

tary disorders in which an excessive amount of scale accumulates on the skin surface. The increased thickness of the stratum corneum may be associated with rapid turnover of the epidermis or with a normal growth rate. It is not known why the skin thickens, but it may be related to genetically determined increased transepidermal water loss or abnormal lipid metabolism in the skin.

Ichthyosis vulgaris, the most common and usually the least severe of the ichthyosiform dermatoses, is inherited as a dominant trait and may be noticed only as "dry skin" in adult life. The epidermal cell mitotic rate and turnover time are normal. For some reason the cells of the stratum corneum are retained and the skin thickens. In other forms of ichthyosis the cell turnover may be increased. Babies may be born covered with a thick membrane (colloidian baby), and the skin may look as if it were covered with fish or reptile scale. The alligator man in the circus has ichthyosis (Figure 7-7).

Darier's disease (keratosis follicularis) is a dominantly inherited disorder of keratinization manifested by asymmetric, small, firm papules scattered irregularly over the trunk, face, and flexor surface of the extremities. The dry, flesh-colored papules become tan to dark brown and greasy as they coalesce into plaques. More extensive involvement leads to vegetative patches, erosions, and crusts. Nails may become involved and mouth lesions occur. Sunlight may precipitate flares. The cause is unknown and the course is chronic (Figure 7-7).

Reiter's syndrome is a symptom complex of nonspecific urethritis, conjunctivitis, and asymmetric arthritis which occurs in young adult males. Skin lesions consist of hyperkeratotic scaling plaques of the scalp or extremities, pustules and erosions of the penis or scrotum, and conical hyperkeratosis and scaling lesions of the palms and soles. The cause is unknown. Many cases appear to be acquired venereally.

ECZEMATOUS DERMATITIS

Atopic Dermatitis

Atopic dermatitis is an eczematous disease with a characteristic distribution occurring in persons with a family history of allergic diseases. Affected individuals have varying numbers of certain associated stigmata relating to cutaneous vasculature, immunologic peculiarities, and a tendency to pruritus. Atopic dermatitis is one of several kinds of eczema (see eczematous dermatitis, Chapter 5) and cannot be separated from other eczematous reactions on the basis of the morphology or histology of any one lesion. The exact etiology of atopic eczema is unknown.

Atopy refers to a certain constellation of clinical presentations of human hypersensitivity which is hereditary. These include asthma, hay fever, and eczema (atopic dermatitis). Possibly some forms of urticaria, chronic hand eczema, and nummular eczema are variants of atopy. Although this atopic diathesis is familial, the exact mode of inheritance has not been established. Onset of any of these symptom complexes can be at any age, and patients may have one or all of the atopic manifestations.

Atopic hypersensitivity is characterized by a greater than normal tendency to develop certain antibodies after limited exposure to normally innocuous substances in the environment. These antibodies are of the skin-sensitizing type (IgE), are responsible for the urticarial reaction to skin tests, and can be passively transferred with serum to the skin of a normal person (Prausnitz-Küstner reaction). While these antibodies provide one label for the atopic diathesis, their definitive role in causing atopic eczema has not been demonstrated.

Although there is usually a family history of various forms of atopy, individual patients with atopic dermatitis may or may not have other manifestations of the atopic diathesis, such as hay fever or asthma. It is the tendency, or diathesis, to have eczema that is inherited. Environmental factors may never be sufficient to cause significant overt disease even though the abnormal susceptibility is present. The clinical manifestations are quite variable, ranging from minimal, occasional, localized eczema to severe, persistent, generalized disease. Symptoms of eczema are more common among male infants, children, and female adults. Atopic dermatitis appears to be more common in the well-developed countries of the world.

There are a number of anatomic and physiologic characteristics of the skin of persons with atopic dermatitis. They may have an increased number of skin markings of the palms which are noticeable as fine cross-hatched lines. An accentuated wrinkle or fold just beneath the margin of the lower lid of both eyes is called "Dennie's line." Both of these skin markings may be present from birth. Atopic dermatitis patients also have a tendency to have dry skin.

Physiologically, these patients have a marked tendency toward vasoconstriction of the cutaneous blood vessels. The skin, therefore, blanches readily. They may have pallor of the face and lowered temperature in fingers and toes. Stroking the skin may produce an immediate linear white reaction, caused by vasoconstriction of the stroked skin (white dermographism). Acetylcholine injected into the skin of atopic persons may produce a blanching reaction at the site of injection. By contrast, stroking or injecting acetylcholine into normal skin causes local vasodilatation and a red flare. Studies have also suggested that atopic eczema patients may have decreased sebum production and a tendency to sweat pore occlusion.

A symptomatic major and "historical" etiologic abnormality of atopic eczema has not been adequately explained anatomically or physiologically. This abnormality is a striking tendency to pruritus. The itch threshold is lowered so that minor stimuli such as exercise, lowered humidity, environmental temperature shifts, friction, and even stroking can cause itching. Rarely foods, inhalants, or pollens may initiate pruritus. Soaps, emotional tension, wool, and mild primary irritants can trigger bouts of generalized itching. Itchy skin with easily triggered and severe pruritus is the outstanding feature of atopic dermatitis. The itching leads to scratching and the scratching and rubbing are accompanied by the acute changes of eczema. Most of the clinical signs are secondary to scratching and rubbing. A generalized flare in an atopic child with one arm in a cast may lead to eczematous dermatitis over the entire body except under the cast.

Clinically, the cutaneous changes are those seen in other forms of eczema. The earliest and mildest findings are erythema and edema (Figure 7-8). This may progress to vesiculation and oozing with resultant crusts and scaling. Finally, if the process becomes severe or chronic, lichenification follows. Healing usually occurs without scarring but temporary hyperpigmentation or hypopigmentation may occur. Excoriations may be present at any stage during the process.

The first, or infantile, stage is not present at or soon after birth, but usually begins at the age of three to four months. Involvement characteristically appears on the cheeks and scalp and may spread to the extensor surfaces of the extremities. Erythema and dry scaling precede juicy-looking red papules, but frank vesiculation is rare in infants. Children and adults with atopic eczema differ from infants in that the flexor surfaces of the neck, antecubital fossa, and popliteal space are most frequently involved, vesiculation is more obvious during acute flares and lichenification is more striking. Onset can be at any age, and the disease may disappear at any stage and at any age. The most frequent story is one of exacerbations and remissions for two to three decades. As many as one-half of atopic eczema patients will develop some other atopic disease such as hay fever or asthma. Prognostication for any individual patient is difficult, and the spectrum of severity of symptoms varies from occasional itching of the antecubital fossa in wintertime to crippling illness, causing frequent hospitalizations, personality changes, and, rarely, secondary infections leading to death.

Pityriasis alba is an asymptomatic, superficial hypopigmentation which occurs as oval or irregular patches on the face, upper trunk, and proximal extremities of children and young adults. Variable amounts of erythema and scaling may be present. Signs of inflammation may be absent at the time of examination. Although seen most commonly in persons with atopic dermatitis, pityriasis alba is most likely a postinflammatory response to eczema of any cause. The overt manifestations of the causative eczematous process may have been minimal and not noticed by the patient.

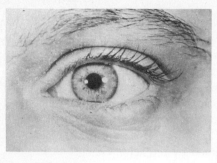
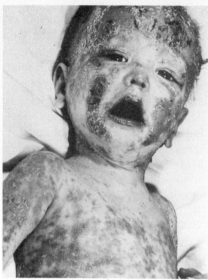
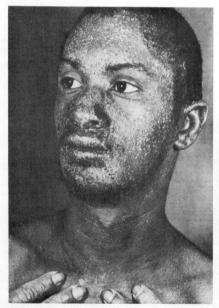
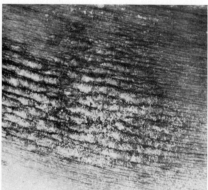

Figure 7-8 Atopic dermatitis. (a) Dennie's lines; an extra skin fold of the lower lid; (b) subacute and chronic eczema in childhood; (c) acute eczema in an adult; (d) striking lichenification; entire epidermis is thickened and skin lines are exaggerated.

The most important complication of atopic dermatitis is infection with either vaccinia or herpes simplex virus. A smallpox vaccination (vaccinia) or exposure to a recently vaccinated person may cause a severe infection in atopic eczema patients. Vaccinia viruses grow and multiply on the skin and probably spread from one cutaneous site to another by way of the blood stream. Sites normally involved with eczema become infected with the virus. Severe, confluent involvement may lead to prostration, fever, and much discomfort. Persons whose eczema has not been active for years may acquire the virus at sites of previous eczematous involvement. Vaccination is contraindicated in atopic eczema patients and their siblings.

Atopic persons exposed to fever blisters (herpes simplex) may similarly develop multiple sites of cutaneous infection with herpes virus. These two viral complications have traditionally been lumped together under the term Kaposi's varicelliform eruption, but are better labeled as eczema vaccinatum or eczema herpeticum depending on the infective agent. While morphologically and clinically similar, they can be distinguished by a Tzanck smear (see Chapter 6). Multinucleated giant cells are seen in herpes simplex but not in vaccinia virus infections.

Bacterial infection may also complicate atopic dermatitis. Secondary impetigo becomes superimposed on already compromised eczematous skin. The serum oozing onto the surface of the skin provides an excellent medium for bacteria. Deeper infections, including ecthyma, boils, abscesses, and cellulitis also occur, and otitis media is common in children with atopic dermatitis.

Contact dermatitis to topical medicines, especially neomycin, is more common in atopic patients. This is partly because these persons are more likely to be frequently exposed to such topical medications, but may also be due to a tendency to contact sensitization. This may also explain why there is an increased incidence of contact dermatitis to ragweed, nickel, formalin, and mercury. Dermatitic skin is also a less effective barrier in preventing antigens from passing into the skin.

Atopic patients appear to be more likely to have a hypersensitivity reaction after exposure to penicillin. The reaction may be severe and is often the anaphylactic type. The reason for this tendency to react to penicillin is not completely understood.

Atopic individuals are said to be tense, resentful, aggressive, restless, and hyperactive. It is not clear if this is a basic characteristic of the diathesis or the result of living with itchy skin. The problem of adjusting to eczema from early infancy is a sizable hurdle. Maternal attitude toward the child's skin is ambivalent at best and displays outright rejection at worst. Eczema upsets the normal physical intimacy between the mother and child. The infant who normally receives much of his early sensory

input from the stroking, cleaning, and snuggling of his mother, instead is
made to itch by any stimulus. The young child learns to manipulate his
parents by pleasing them when he controls his desire to scratch, or frustrating them when he excoriates himself. Throughout life, the eczema patient
itches when he is under emotional stress. Itching leads to scratching, which
produces more itchy skin. The cycle can lead to a patient's literally tearing
his skin.

Therapy must begin by avoiding the minor irritating stimuli which
trigger itching. The most common stimuli are listed above. A careful history
will disclose other individualized pruritus-producing factors which each patient notices about his environment. These factors should be avoided if
possible. Scratch tests or intradermal tests to individual antigens do not
usually give enough useful information to make them worthwhile. The environment should be kept at a constant temperature. Dryness can be
avoided by placing a cool mist humidifier in the bedroom during the dry
winter months. This helps to prevent the itching, scratching, and eczema.
The financial savings in medications and doctor bills make a room humidifier a good investment. The cool mist humidifier does not fill the room
with steam or fog and is essentially unnoticed. Excessive bathing should
be avoided.

Acute, exudative, eczematous dermatitis should be treated with cool
compresses, using water, saline, or Burow's solution. Wet open dressings
produce cooling by evaporation. Immersion in a bath containing oatmeal,
starch, bath oils, or tars provides temporary relief from itching. "Shake"
lotions are emulsions of soothing and drying agents in water which tend
to dry the acute weeping lesions. Application of a greasy ointment or a
water-in-oil emulsion while the skin is still wet will help hold water within
the stratum corneum.

The most effective and most frequently used medications for atopic
dermatitis are the topical steroids. They are the mainstay of therapy for
the subacute and chronic stages of the disease and their introduction has
greatly simplified management of eczematous dermatitis. They seem to reduce inflammation, cause some vasoconstriction, and diminish the pruritus.
Hydrocortisone is often effective. The more potent fluorinated and modified
steroid creams are even more effective. Frequent use of small amounts
well rubbed in appears more effective than a thick layer of medication
once or twice daily. Temporary intermittent occlusion increases penetration
of the medication. Atopic eczema patients, however, usually do not tolerate
occlusion for more than one to two hours at a time because of sweating
or pruritus. Topical steroids are also available in an ointment base to increase lubrication.

Topical tar preparations are also effective, but are messy. Topical
antipruritic agents containing menthol, phenol, or camphor may reduce

itching. Topical medications containing local anesthetics or antihistamines should be avoided because of their sensitizing potential. Topical antibiotics may help control secondary infection but if significant growth of pathogenic bacteria is present, then systemic antibiotics are indicated.

Systemic steroids usually bring dramatic relief but recurrence frequently follows their withdrawal. Because of the well-known complications, long-term use of systemic steroids in a disease as chronic as atopic dermatitis is not indicated. Occasionally severely involved patients are greatly benefited by and then successfully withdrawn from a short course of steroid therapy, but such a treatment approach is not usually appropriate. Rarely, a patient is so severely crippled by generalized atopic dermatitis that one can justify chronic steroid maintenance.

Antihistamines relieve itching and can produce sedation, which is especially helpful at night. Tranquilizers or sedatives are sometimes needed to quiet the agitated, scratching patient. During severe, generalized, acute flares, a change of environment, such as a brief stay in the hospital, often is remarkably effective in stopping an attack. With the change in environment patients often improve before medication is initiated.

Emotional stability is essential. Many flares are caused by nervous tension or a business or family crisis. Patients with a chronic, bothersome disease like atopic dermatitis may become severely depressed. More frequently, they become anxious, agitated, and tense, and may become exhausted from scratching, sleep loss, and hyperactivity. Family communications may weaken and break down, and reasoned optimism, reassurance, encouragement, and patience must come from medical personnel.

Nummular Eczema

Nummular (coin-shaped) eczema is characterized by scattered round patches of eczematous dermatitis on the dorsa of the hands, on the extensor surfaces of the arms, and on the legs and buttocks (Figure 7-9). It is a chronic, nonspecific reaction pattern without a known single specific etiology. Pruritus is present and may be severe. In children, it may represent a form of atopic dermatitis. In adults, it may be caused by irritants, atopy, dryness, or other factors. In the aged, it is almost always associated with dry skin. In all age groups, the course is chronic. Emotional stress may cause exacerbations. Topical treatments similar to those for atopic dermatitis usually work very well. Steroids injected into the lesions will rapidly eliminate them.

Pompholyx

Dyshidrotic eczema (pompholyx) is a common, relatively noninflammatory, recurrent, pruritic, vesicular eruption of palms and soles, of unknown

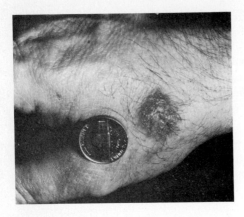

Figure 7-9 Nummular eczema. A round patch of acute eczematous dermatitis.

etiology. The original use of the term dyshidrotic, or "dyshidrosis," was to suggest a malfunction of the sweat ducts but this has proven to be a misnomer. Pompholyx is from the Greek meaning bubble and is a more apt term. Emotional stress tends to be a trigger factor. Pompholyx may be more common in atopic persons.

Tiny blisters occur most commonly along the sides of the fingers (Figure 7-10). These vesicles result from marked intercellular edema within the epidermis. When palms and soles are involved, the vesicles appear to be deeper because of the thick stratum corneum. Dyshidrotic eczema differs from the remainder of the hand eczema group in that the primary involvement is on the palm instead of the dorsum of the hand. The vesicles are also less inflammatory in the early stages, with less redness, weeping, scaling, and pain. Its recurring course may be one of the most chronic of hand eczemas. Pruritus is moderate.

Hand Eczema

Hand eczema is not a specific disease but is simply eczema of the hand. Its causes are as many as those for the eczematous reaction pattern of

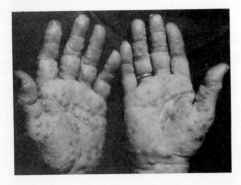

Figure 7-10 Pompholyx. Pruritic collections of tiny vesicles on the palms.

the skin. Hands get into everything. Hand eczema is most common in housewives, bartenders, cooks, food handlers, and medical personnel. It has many names, most of them referring to the profession of the owner of the hands rather than to the etiology of the eczema, e.g., housewive's eczema, surgeons' hands, dishpan hands. It is the most frequent dermatitis seen in industry.

The most common etiologic factors are low humidity, constant exposure to mild primary irritants, frequent hand washing, and atopic diathesis. Emotional and physical stress make people more susceptible. Scratching, rubbing, and minor trauma are additional factors. In addition, hand eczema is sometimes caused by specific disorders such as allergic contact dermatitis, fungus infections, lichen simplex chronicus, nummular eczema, or bacterial infections. Since many of the eczematous eruptions of the hands look alike, careful history, careful laboratory cultures, and microscopic examinations for organisms are usually more productive than is a physician's examination alone. A common cause of treatment failure is misdiagnosis, or failure to remove the cause.

Erythema, edema, vesiculation, weeping, and crusts are often accompanied by signs of scratching. Involvement usually begins and is most severe on the dorsa of the hands and fingers and then may spill onto the palms where painful fissures may occur. This acute stage is best managed by open wet dressings. The less acute stage is then treated with topical steroids. As improvement continues, the steroids can be occluded with plastic gloves to increase penetration. Rubber gloves may worsen the eczema. Pruritus may be severe and require systemic antipruritics. Extra care must be taken to avoid primary irritants such as soap, solvents, and detergents and to avoid possible sensitizing medications.

Circumscribed Neurodermatitis (LSC)

Circumscribed or localized neurodermatitis, also called lichen simplex chronicus or LSC, is a localized chronic skin disorder which results from repeated rubbing or scratching. It is, essentially, a patch of lichenification. Slightly more common in females and in Orientals, it is seen in all races, in both sexes, and at all ages.

Pruritus initiates the cycle. The itching may be constant or episodic and is frequently severe. It may originally be caused by stasis, insect bite, contact dermatitis, primary irritants, or any dermatosis. The itching may also begin in what appears to be normal skin without any known preexisting insult. Psychic factors may be involved.

Once rubbing and scratching have been started, the area is more susceptible to itch stimuli. Rubbing becomes a habit. Rubbing may be done subconsciously at bedtime, or when attention is diverted elsewhere, or scratching may be deliberate. Regular, almost ritualistic scratching sessions may be conducted daily, usually at bedtime. At times, wild frenzies of almost sensual pain and pleasure lead to actual tearing of the skin. Some patients use their heels to scratch, while others may use combs, pencil erasers, clothing, straps, or other articles.

In any case, the grossly visible lesion is produced entirely by rubbing and scratching, and will disappear when these activities stop. Patients with localized neurodermatitis seem to be persons who respond to rubbing with lichenification but there is no increased incidence among atopics or in atopic families. The circumscribed lichenified plaques may be infiltrated and firm in the center and covered with variable amounts of scale (Figure 7-11). Although histologic sections suggest intercellular edema, no obvious vesicles appear clinically. Hyperpigmentation often exists in the more chronic lesions.

The most common sites of LSC are the nape of the neck in women and the lateral aspect of the lower leg just above the ankle in men. The inner thigh, palms, and genitalia are frequent sites. Any area of the skin may be involved. Patients with localized neurodermatitis usually have only one lesion.

Treatment consists of discontinuing rubbing and scratching. It is difficult for patients to realize that they are the sole cause of the lesion. Some may deny scratching at all. Many patients harbor considerable hidden anger, and their rubbing serves as a useful outlet. Simply understanding the nature of the lesion may be enough to cause the patient to stop rubbing. Others need some mechanical assistance, such as finger cots to cover the nails at bedtime, occlusive dressings, or even a temporary cast to protect the lesion. Steroids containing medications, used topically, under occlusion, or, better still, injected intralesionally, hasten disappearance of the lesion. Lesions often reappear, as patients resume scratching.

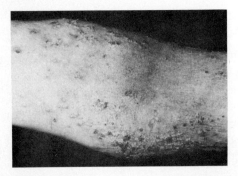

Figure 7-11 Lichen simplex chronicus.

DISORDERS OF SWEAT GLAND OCCLUSION

Miliaria

Miliaria is an inclusive term describing those disorders which occur when the free flow of eccrine sweat to the surface is impeded. The visible morphologic alterations resulting from sweat retention make up this group of disorders (Figure 7-12). The causes are multiple. Any injury to the eccrine sweat pore can lead to its obstruction. Inflammation from various dermatoses, maceration, sunburn, primary irritants, and bacterial colonization can cause occlusion of sweat ducts. The disorders arise most frequently when the environment is hot and humid, when sweating has been marked in rate or duration, and when prolonged occlusion is present. Fever or prolonged physical exertion may lead to miliaria.

Miliaria crystallina (sudamina) occurs when the sweat pore is obstructed within the stratum corneum. Within or just beneath the stratum corneum the retained sweat forms a vesicle, which appears as a tiny, very superficial, crystal-clear, tense bubble on the skin, with little or no surrounding inflammation. The lesions may be localized or generalized. Hundreds of tiny blisters may be present. The proportion of sweat ducts involved is usually not great and the blisters are asymptomatic and usually self-limiting, requiring no treatment.

Miliaria rubra (heat rash, prickly heat) is the result of obstruction of the sweat duct deeper within the epidermis (Figure 7-13). This results in some edema in the epidermis and an inflammation with vasodilatation, in the upper dermis. Therefore, the lesions appear as small, discrete, erythematous papules or papulovesicles. A hand lens may assist in diagnosis. Each lesion is located at a sweat pore, never at the hair follicle. Some diffuse erythema may radiate out beyond the papule. Itching, burning, or stinging is present (hence the alternate name, prickly heat). Symptoms and rash worsen with sweating.

Miliaria pustulosa, which frequently coexists with miliaria rubra, is a pustular variant of heat rash in which polymorphonuclear cells fill the papulovesicles.

If the obstruction of the sweat duct occurs in the dermis, an asymptomatic, noninflammatory papule forms beneath a sweat pore. This type of occlusion, called *miliaria profunda,* may involve a large number of sweat ducts and may lead to anhidrosis (absence of sweat delivery to the surface). A person with widespread involvement could have severe difficulty with temperature control during exercise or heat exposure. The absence of surface sweat to provide heat loss by evaporation could lead to high fever, tachycardia, headache, and collapse.

The best therapeutic approach to miliaria is prevention. Clothing

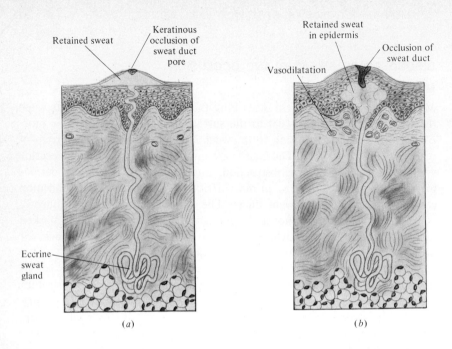

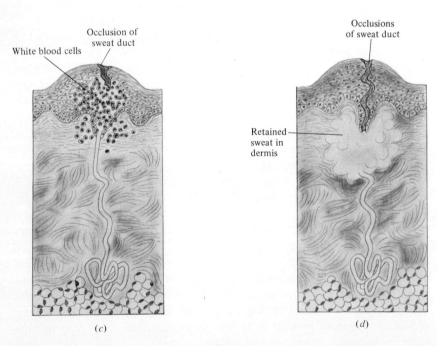

Figure 7-12 Miliaria. (*a*) Miliaria crystallina; (*b*) miliaria rubra; (*c*) miliaria pustulosa; (*d*) miliaria profunda.

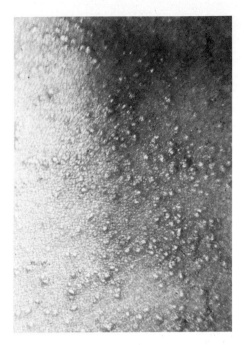

Figure 7-13 Miliaria rubra.

should be well ventilated. Bedridden patients should be turned frequently. Prolonged occlusions should be avoided. Exposure to excessive heat should be avoided, especially when the humidity is high or exercise is necessary. Once heat rash has started, the only effective therapy is the elimination of the need to sweat: less clothing, less activity, and less topical occlusive treatment. Air conditioning is therapeutic.

DISORDERS OF PIGMENTATION

Melasma

Melasma (chloasma, mask of pregnancy) is a macular, patchy hyperpigmentation of the cheeks and forehead occurring primarily in women who are pregnant or who are taking oral contraceptives (Figure 7-14). Occasionally men or nonpregnant women on no medication get melasma. Melasma is very prominent among Latin peoples. The pigment is normal melanin within the epidermis, and sun plays an important role in the pathogenesis. The lesions are asymptomatic and represent a cosmetic problem.

Treatment consists of topical application of hydroquinone to depigment the darkened areas gradually and reversibly. This chemical selectively lightens the hypermelanotic areas. Bleaches containing monobenzylether of hydroquinone should not be used because irreversible, total depigmentation results and creates another cosmetic problem. Sun exposure should

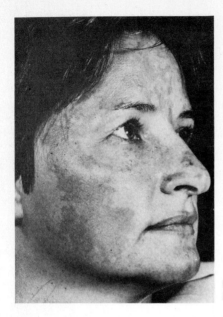

Figure 7-14 Melasma. Macular blotchy hyperpigmentation of face.

be avoided or an opaque sunscreen must be used because middle- (UV-B) and long-wave (UV-A) ultraviolet light will cause recurrence of melasma.

Vitiligo

Vitiligo is a genetically determined acquired patterned absence of melanin pigment of unknown etiology. One percent of all races have vitiligo. Vitiligo leaves the skin white and is therefore most noticeable in darker persons. Histologic examination of vitiliginous skin shows complete absence of melanocytes. The cause of the disappearance of the melanocytes is not known. Immunologic, chemical, and neural mediators have been hypothesized as causative. It has also been suggested that the melanocytes may "self-destruct" because of the premature rupture of certain normal enzyme packets within the cell. Multiple factors may be involved.

Nonpalpable white spots are noted around body orifices and over bony prominences (Figure 7-15). Pigment loss is usually symmetrical, slowly progressive, and permanent. Vitiligo may involve only a few tiny areas, or the entire exposed skin may turn white. Eye pigment is not involved. Erythema or itching may or may not precede the disappearance of pigment. Vitiligo may occur at sites of trauma. Most patients are otherwise normal, but vitiligo is seen in increased incidence among patients with hyperthyroidism, Addison's disease, pernicious anemia, adult-onset diabetes, alopecia areata, and morphea.

Vitiligo is a benign, noncontagious, cosmetic liability. However, in

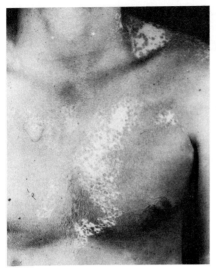
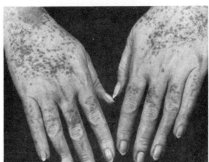
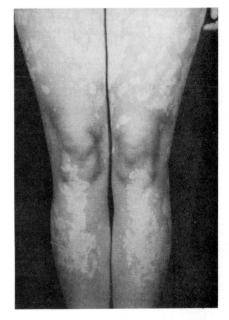

Figure 7-15 Vitiligo. (a) Moderate involvement; (b) perifollicular repigmentation after treatment with psoralens and ultraviolet light; (c) extensive vitiligo.

some cultures it is a severe social handicap and is referred to as "white leprosy." Persons with vitiligo are shunned, are not allowed in public swimming areas, and may not marry. Patients will spend much time and money in attempts to repigment their skin. Stains are used to paint white areas to match the surrounding uninvolved skin. These must be reapplied as they wear off the surface. Patients with extensive vitiligo may elect to bleach out the remaining normal skin chemically, in order to become all one uniform white color.

Prolonged and repeated exposures to sunlight or artificial sources of long-wave ultraviolet light, after administration of psoralens, a phototoxic medication, may cause gradual repigmentation in some patients. Under such stimuli, melanocytes may migrate into the white area from the periphery of the lesions and up from the bases of the hair bulbs within the vitiliginous skin.

MISCELLANEOUS DISORDERS

Pityriasis Rosea

Pityriasis rosea is a common, harmless, self-limited dermatosis which presents as multiple scaling patches on healthy young persons. It is believed to be viral in origin, but no etiology has ever been substantiated. Although the appearance of cases seems to occur in clusters in spring and fall, it can occur at any time. It rarely affects more than one family member and attempts at experimental transmission of the disease have failed. Males and females of all races are affected. Pityriasis rosea is uncommon in infancy and after age 50.

Characteristically, an initial single, larger lesion precedes the widespread appearance of smaller, multiple lesions. This first lesion ("herald patch") is an asymptomatic lesion with a diameter of 2 to 6 centimeters, usually on the trunk. It may precede the abrupt onset of the remainder of the eruption by days to weeks. The multiple lesions are usually 1 centimeter or less in diameter and most often are round or oval. Their color is pink to salmon, and they are covered with scales, which are wrinkled and crinkly (cigarette paper scale) in the center and more impressive around the periphery of the lesion (collarette scale). The oval lesions often line up with their long axes in lines of cleavage or in sweeping lines angling down and away from the center of the back. This may result in a necklace-like rash or a "Christmas tree" arrangement. The lesions, which may number over 100, usually remain nonconfluent (Figure 7-16).

Itching may be present but the rash is usually asymptomatic. The most common distribution is from ears to hips, but frequent exceptions occur. Pityriasis rosea usually disappears within eight weeks.

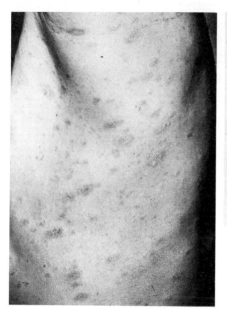 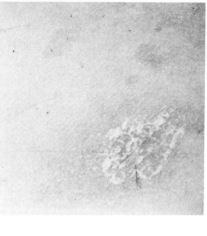

Figure 7-16 Pityriasis rosea. (a) Distribution in "lines of skin cleavage"; (b) close-up of a lesion; oval patch of erythema with fine scale about the edge.

All laboratory tests and cultures are negative in pityriasis rosea and the skin biopsy is not diagnostic. The diagnosis is based upon the appearance of the lesions. The herald patch may be mistaken for a superficial fungus infection. A KOH preparation of pityriasis rosea lesion is negative for hyphae. Widespread secondary lesions may be mistaken for secondary syphilis. Serology is negative in pityriasis rosea and is always positive in secondary syphilis.

Treatment is usually not indicated in a benign self-limited disease. Moreover, few treatments are effective. Sunlight may hasten the disappearance of the lesions. Antihistamines or aspirin have been reported to reduce pruritus, if present. Patients are usually satisfied to know they have a definite, well-recognized disorder which is benign and temporary.

Lichen Planus

Lichen planus is a pruritic inflammatory disease of unknown etiology manifested by violaceous, polygonal, flat-topped, raised lesions (pruritic, polygonal, purple, planar papules). The lesions which are initially discrete but which may become confluent occur most commonly on the flexor surface of the wrists, inner knees, ankles, oral mucosa, and glans penis (Figure 7-17). Tiny mucosal lesions are covered with superficial lacy white lines

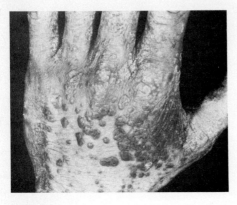

Figure 7-17 Lichen planus. Pruritic purple planar polygonal papules.

(Wickham's striae). Similar lines may be seen on skin lesions if immersion oil is applied to the skin lesions.

Itching may be severe but excoriations are uncommon. Lesions may appear at sites of trauma. Bullous lesions or hypertrophic lesions may also occur and the latter can be accompanied by significant hyperpigmentation. Histology is usually characteristic. Treatment is nonspecific and symptomatic. Topical steroids under occlusion are sometimes beneficial.

REFERENCES

Baden, H. P., and M. Pugliese: *Disease-a-Month,* "Psoriasis," Yearbook Medical Publishers, Inc., Chicago, 1973.

Bettley, F. R.: "Hand Eczema," *Brit. Med. J.* **11:**151–155, July 1964.

Brookes, D. B., R. M. Hubbert, and I. Sarkany: "Skin Flora of Infants with Napkin Rash," *Brit. J. Derm.* **85:**250–253, June 1971.

Cunliffe, W. J., J. A. Cotterill, B. Williamson, and R. A. Forster: "The Relevance of Skin Surface Lipids to Acne Vulgaris," *Brit. J. Derm.* 86:suppl **8:**10–15, 1972.

El Mofty, A. M.: *Vitiligo and Psoralens,* Pergamon Press, New York, 1968.

Farber, E. M., and R. P. McClintock, Jr.: "A Current Review of Psoriasis," *Calif. Med.* **108:**440–457, June 1968.

Freinkel, R. K.: "Antibiotics for Acne Vulgaris," *Ann. Intern. Med.* **71:**857–858, October 1969.

Freinkel, R. K.: "Pathogenesis of Acne Vulgaris," *N. Eng. J. Med.* **280:**1161–1163, May 1969.

Izumi, K., R. R. Marples, A. M. Kligman: "Bacteriology of Acne Comedones," *Arch. Derm.* **102:**397–399, October 1970.

Kligman, A.: "An Overview of Acne," *J. Invest. Derm.* **62:**268–288, 1974.

Leithead, C. S., and A. R. Lind: *Heat Stress and Heat Disorders,* Cassell & Co., Ltd., London, 1964.

Lipman Cohen, E.: "Pityriasis Rosea," *Brit. J. Derm.* **79:**533–537, October 1967.

Marks, R.: "Concepts in the Pathogenesis of Rosacea," *Brit. J. Derm.* **80:**170–177, March 1968.

Perry, H. O., C. W. Soderstrom, and R. W. Schulze: "The Goeckerman Treatment of Psoriasis," *Arch. Derm.* **98:**178–182, August 1968.

Roth, H. L., and R. R. Kierland: "The Natural History of Atopic Dermatitis," *Arch. Derm.* **89:**209–214, February 1964.

Zaias, N.: "Psoriasis of the Nail: A Clinical-Pathologic Study," *Arch. Derm.* **99:**567–579, May 1969.

Infection and Infestation

Life on the skin
  Skin ecology
  Infection
Bacterial infections of the skin
  Erythrasma
  Impetigo
  Ecthyma
  Bacterial folliculitis
  Furuncle
  Carbuncle
  Cellulitis
  Erysipelas
  Hidradenitis suppurativa
Fungus infection of the skin
  Candidiasis
  Dermatophytes
  Tinea versicolor
Virus infection of skin
  Warts
  Molluscum contagiosum
  Herpes simplex
Parasites
  Pediculosis
  Scabies

LIFE ON THE SKIN

Skin Ecology

The skin provides warmth, a place to live, and nourishment for a large population of microorganisms. Microscopic crevices, nooks, and crannies of the skin provide places to colonize. Water is available from sweat or insensible water loss. Amino acids, carbohydrates, and even some vitamins are available for food. Those organisms which can digest lipids have additional food available from sebum and epidermal cell fats.

By the time the infant's sterile skin has slid past the vaginal mucosa and spent a few hours in the newborn nursery, it has been invaded and colonized by all kinds of organisms until, gradually, an elaborate ecology system is established. The various microorganisms encountered transiently colonize the skin at the sites of contact, but gradually, because of special properties that vary greatly over different parts of the body, a characteristic flora develops by selection in the various body sites. Throughout life, microorganisms eat, multiply, compete for space, fall off, dry up, die, and sometimes spread to other human hosts. Mites live, mate, and have their offspring in the hair follicles of the eyelashes and face. Yeasts are found in the moist areas of the body. Fungi may quietly digest the dead stratum corneum of the foot. Viruses that use the skin as host do not multiply on the surface of the skin, but viruses which invade bacteria (bacteriophages) are plentiful on the skin's surface. Since viruses are parasites in living cells, those which parasitize skin have to invade into deeper levels of epidermis in order to replicate.

The predominant members of the skin world are bacteria. Gram-positive bacteria dominate the life on normal human skin. These abundant organisms can be divided into two groups according to their cell shapes: the cocci, which are spherical cells, and the bacilli or diphtheroids, which are rod-like. The cocci are mostly aerobic staphylococci. Streptococci are rarely found on normal skin, although throat carriers are common. Epidemiological and bacteriological evidence suggests that streptococci are spread to the skin of the host from the environment, from some nearby site, or from an infected person. The individual who then becomes a carrier is very likely to develop a skin lesion (a skin infection). Harmless species of staphylococci (*S. albus* or *S. epidermidis*) are major inhabitants of almost all regions of the skin. In fact, their presence may exert a restraining force on colonization from other organisms to which the skin is constantly exposed. This phenomenon, called bacterial interference, has been used to interrupt epidemics caused by pathogenic staphylococci. Artificially induced colonization of the nasal reservoir with harmless staphylococci may interfere with subsequent acquisition of other, possibly pathogenic, strains of staphylococci at that site.

Another of the skin cocci is *S. aureus*. Its usual home is the nostrils and, although present on the skin of up to one-quarter of normal persons, it is never dominant or abundant on normal skin. Two important properties of *S. aureus* are its ability to cause clinical infection and its capacity to acquire resistance to antibiotics. This bacterium can overgrow and replace the other cocci on damaged or dermatitic skin and also, if it penetrates into the skin, may cause folliculitis, boils, or abscesses. Normally, however, when present on the surface in its usual small numbers, it does not cause pathologic changes in the skin.

The gram-positive diphtheroids or bacilli are the other dominant residents of normal human skin and can be found on almost all regions of most persons. They can be separated into species on the basis of morphologic differences, oxygen requirements, and ability to utilize lipids as food. *Corynebacterium acnes* is one of the anaerobic (not requiring oxygen) bacteria which possess lipases and depends upon lipid for a food source. This bacterium plays a role in acne (see Chapter 7).

Gram-negative organisms are scarce on normal human skin, and modest growth can only be found in some moist, warm intertriginous sites. The relative dryness of the skin seems to limit these organisms which grow in such large numbers in the gastrointestinal tract.

The resident skin organisms develop some kind of balance or ecological system, with the skin providing food, water, and a place to reside. The absolute number of organisms and the ranking of numerical predominance varies from one body region to another. The trunk is a desert compared to the tropical rain forest of the axillae. The scalp is a shady protected area. The face with its microscopic layer of oily sebum provides food and greasy covering. The moist, warm perineum drains the cesspool of the anus and vagina. The ear canal is a dark, damp cave. In all these vastly different sites it is the relative number of organisms which change, more than the kinds of organisms. Although the proportion changes, the same few kinds of bacteria make up the residents of most areas.

Some bacteria reside on the uppermost stratum corneum. But since the most superficial flakes of flattened cells of the stratum corneum provide an unstable dry atmosphere, most colonies of bacteria are located down in the more protected, moist creases, crevices, nooks and crannies, the deep furrows of the skin markings, and the folds in the skin. The patulous sebaceous follicles of the face provide gaping holes filled with nutritious sebum for bacteria adapted to live in them. Normally, bacteria do not colonize the deepest levels of skin. Invasion deep into normal hair follicles is not routine. Eccrine sweat ducts are usually sterile. Bacteria do not invade and decompose apocrine sweat until after it is delivered to the skin surface.

Even though food, water, and housing are provided, we are not overwhelmed by bacterial colonization of the skin. In most sites, the depth of penetration is limited by stratum corneum. Cell kinetics provide a dumping system, as skin growth keeps pushing new sterile cells up from below. The skin is constantly being replaced, hair and nails grow outward, sebum is pushed out onto the surface. The skin's acid pH and the presence of fatty acids may discourage some organisms. The enzymes, metabolic products, or other unknown media changes provided by normal resident flora, discourage the colonization of unwelcome, strange, or pathogenic bacteria. Circulating immunoglobulins and delayed hypersensitivity play some unclear role in the defenses of the skin against certain organisms.

The most important factor limiting the growth and invasion of bacteria is simply the relative lack of water on the surface of the skin. As long as the skin maintains an intact and continuous layer as a relatively dry integument or cover, bacterial skin infection is unusual. If the skin is hydrated for prolonged periods of time, the bacterial growth increases and gram-negative organisms may begin to predominate. Burned skin loses its stratum corneum and outer epidermis. Serum and interstitial fluids are no longer held in. The skin is no longer dry. Bacteria may then overwhelm the host.

The populations are relatively stable but not static. The hands are constantly smearing colonies of bacteria from place to place. Organisms constantly settle on the skin from the air. Scales which fall off the body become airborne, providing a raft or flying carpet to carry bacteria to others.

Scrubbing the hands removes some surface bacteria but the colonies in the microscopic creases of the skin remain. Skin bacterial counts may actually be increased after showering or bathing. Increased skin temperature, dilatation of pores, and vigorous toweling may open the deep bacterial reservoirs and spread bacteria over the skin. Traumatized or dermatitic skin has a less effective stratum corneum barrier and may become moist, which results not only in the presence of more bacteria but also in a change of predominant organisms. Antibiotics in systemic or topical medications or in soaps or deodorants may selectively kill certain bacteria and permit others to predominate. Their use may, in fact, favor the growth of antibiotic-resistant organisms.

The bacteria usually found on normal skin are there because they are best adapted to the habitat provided by the skin. Staphylococci and diphtheroids are the dominant residents in most areas of the body of most persons of all races in all climates and with all kinds of habits of hygiene. They form a relatively stable community.

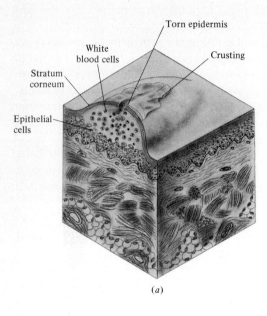

Torn epidermis

White
blood cells

Crusting

Stratum
corneum

Epithelial
cells

(a)

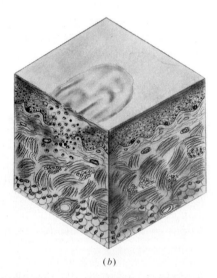

(b)

Figure 8-1 Superficial pyodermas. (a) Impetigo; (b) ecthyma; straw-colored glistening crusts on a background of erythema.

Infection

Infection occurs when the skin is invaded by microorganisms capable of producing disease, or when bacterial growth on the surface is sufficient to cause tissue reaction to the organisms themselves or to toxins generated by them. Moisture, obesity, skin disease, systemic steroids and antibiotics, chronic diseases, and diabetes mellitus may act as predisposing factors, but skin infections are also common among otherwise normal persons.

Bacterial infection occurs when the normal host-bacteria relationship is altered because of (1) the pathogenic properties of the organism, (2) the development of a portal of entry into the deeper layers of skin, or (3) other alterations in the ecology of the skin or in host-defense mechanisms. The signs of inflammation are largely those of the host response to the invasion of microorganisms. Breaks in the integrity of the skin may allow bacteria to invade the deeper, moist tissues. Already damaged dermatitic skin may be secondarily infected. Or the skin may be one of many organs showing signs of a systemic infection.

Pathogenicity (ability to produce infection or tissue response) of a bacterium is a complicated combination of many factors, most of which deal with its ability to protect itself against human host defenses and with its ability to liberate harmful irritating or allergenic substances. A bacterium species may simply be able to multiply extensively on the nutrients provided by skin. Some bacteria have surface components which discourage or delay their phagocytosis by white blood cells. Other organisms elaborate substances which assist tissue breakdown and local invasion and toxins which cause systemic symptoms.

Common bacterial infections which begin in the skin and are primarily limited to the skin are called pyodermas. The clinical characteristics of these infections vary, depending upon their exact anatomic site (Figure 8-1) in the skin and upon the magnitude and type of the attendant inflammatory response. *Impetigo* is a bacterial infection in the uppermost epidermis; *ecthyma* describes a similar infection which extends somewhat deeper. *Bacterial follicultis* is an infection of the hair follicles which may progress to deeper and more extensive furuncles (boils). An *abscess* is simply a collection of pus in a cavity which is formed by disintegration or necrosis of tissue.

BACTERIAL INFECTIONS OF THE SKIN

Erythrasma

Erythrasma is a superficial bacterial infection of the skin caused by *Corynebacterium minitissimum*. The bacteria invade and colonize the stratum corneum, thereby disrupting the normally compact cornified layers. It is a frequent cause of trivial asymptomatic infections of the groin or between the toes. Rarely, it becomes generalized. Erythrasma is more common in males, in hot, humid climates, in people living in close quarters, and in the aged. It also occurs more commonly in diabetics and in obese persons.

Well-demarcated areas of dry, finely scaling, brown to red skin slowly enlarge by extension of an irregular border. The most common site is where the scrotum comes in contact with the inner thigh. Axillae, inframammary folds, the intergluteal cleft, and toe web spaces are frequent sites also. When illuminated with a Wood's light (see Chapter 6) any site of erythrasma exhibits an orange-red to coral-pink fluorescence due to the production of porphyrins by the bacteria in the stratum corneum. Antibacterial soaps may diminish this fluorescence. Erythromycin taken orally for a week cures the infection.

Impetigo

Impetigo is a common, superficial bacterial infection of the skin (Figure 8-2). It is usually caused by Group A beta-hemolytic streptococci but coagulase-positive *S. aureus* is also frequently grown from the lesions and may represent a secondary invader. Impetigo is most frequent and most contagious among infants and young children, and is seen most often among lower socioeconomic groups. It can, however, occur at any age in persons of any status. Impetigo is more common in summer and early fall.

Impetigo begins as an erythematous macule on which develop fragile superficial vesicles, which break and leave red-based, oozing or glistening erosions topped with yellow-brown or golden yellow crust. This stuck-on crust may mat in the hair. After reaching a size of several centimeters across, the lesions may develop satellites which progress through the same sequence to develop the characteristic straw-colored crusts. Pruritus may be severe enough so that linear scratch marks surround the lesions. Histologically, there is a white blood cell–filled vesicle immediately beneath the stratum corneum which later breaks as the upper epidermis becomes a mass of fibrin, white cells, and debris. Stained material from the lesions show gram-positive cocci and culture may identify the specific organism involved. Most classic impetigo is caused by and grows out streptococci, but a more bullous variety of superficial infection in infants may be caused by and yield staphylococci. Mixed infections also occur.

At times, impetigo becomes superimposed on some other dermatitis. Any weeping eczematous lesion may be invaded by large numbers of bacteria, may become redder, slightly tender or pruritic, and colored with yellow crust. Frequently insect bites, scratches, burns, or abrasions precede the signs of superficial infection. Impetigo also appears to begin *de novo*

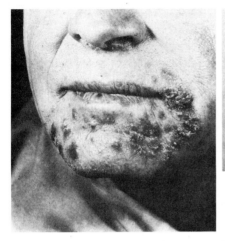
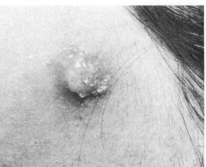
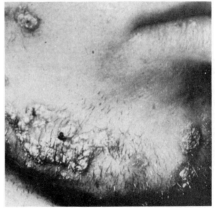

Figure 8-2 Impetigo. (a) Facial involvement; (b) bullous impetigo; (c) close-up of oozing and crust.

on normal skin but preceding minor trauma can never be ruled out. Small epidemics of impetigo may occur.

Rheumatic fever, which sometimes follows streptococcal throat infections, is not a complication of impetigo but acute glomerulonephritis may occur in as many as 1 to 2 percent of impetigo patients. Certain strains of streptococci are particularly nephritogenic, and in some parts of the southern United States, over one-half of all cases of glomerulonephritis are preceded by cutaneous streptococcal infection.

Treatment causes the lesion to heal more rapidly, reduces recurrence, and may lessen the risk of acute glomerulonephritis. If the lesion is larger than a fifty-cent piece, it usually requires systemic rather than topical antibiotics. Penicillin will eradicate the streptococci; specific synthetic penicillins are most effective against certain staphylococci; erythromycin is an acceptable alternate drug.

Experimental and epidemiological data suggest that a single injection of benzathine penicillin G is the best treatment for typical uncomplicated pyoderma in a nonatopic patient. Wet to dry soaks or gentle mechanical washing will remove the crust. Scarring does not occur. Family and medical people should wash thoroughly with bacteriostatic soap after treating patients.

Ecthyma

Ecthyma is a bacterial infection of the skin which extends deeper than impetigo. After a stage of vesicles or pustules surrounded by erythema, dry red-brown to yellow crust forms and attaches firmly over a true ulceration. Organisms and treatments are the same as in impetigo. Healing may take longer and occasionally scarring may result.

Bacterial Folliculitis

Folliculitis is infection in and around the hair follicles and can occur anywhere on the body. It is usually caused by staphylococci, but occasionally by other bacteria. Superficial folliculitis may begin as a small pustule at the follicular opening, surrounded by minimal erythema. Later, a crust forms which may be penetrated by a hair. Healing is uneventful. Deep folliculitis is surrounded by greater inflammation, lasts longer, and may lead to scarring and permanent loss of the hair of the involved follicle.

Predisposing factors include occlusion, friction, overhydration of skin, traction of hair, and exposure to oil or grease. Treatment begins by removing these factors. Topical hygiene with antibacterial soaps or hexachlorophene-alcohol rinses may help. Results from topical antibiotics are variable, and multiple or deep lesions may require systemic antibiotics.

Furuncle (Boil)

A furuncle is an acute, localized staphylococcal abscess around the hair follicle, which may extend down into subcutaneous tissue and which has a tendency to suppuration (formation of pus) and central necrosis. Since furuncles are probably preceded by a deep folliculitis, they are confined to hairy skin, although lanugo hair follicles may initiate the process. Furuncles occur at all ages. *S. aureus* is the most frequent cause and may produce toxins as it proliferates. Furunculosis refers to multiple or recurrent lesions.

Predisposing factors are similar to those of folliculitis. A high incidence of nasal and skin carriers of *S. aureus* is found among patients with furuncles. Persons with severe acne or seborrheic dermatitis may have fre-

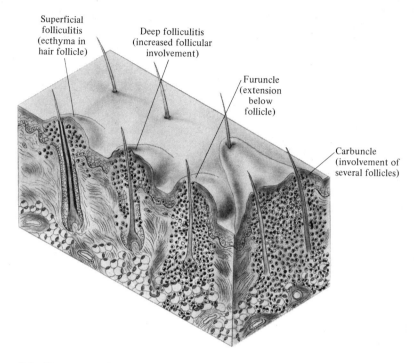

Superficial folliculitis (ecthyma in hair follicle)

Deep folliculitis (increased follicular involvement)

Furuncle (extension below follicle)

Carbuncle (involvement of several follicles)

Figure 8-3 Deeper pyodermas.

quent furuncles. Furunculosis may be seen with obesity, prolonged contact with grease or oils, diabetes mellitus, and chronic illness. Most patients with furunculosis have no other medical problems and many normal adults have several minor furuncles each year. Obstruction of hair follicles may precede lesions. Scratching, friction, pressure from belts, primary irritants, or lack of personal hygiene may predispose to furuncles.

Furuncles may occur on almost any part of the body, but most are on the face, the back of the neck, axillae, breasts, buttocks, perineum, or thighs. A sty is a furuncle of the eyelid margin. One or many lesions may be present. Each begins as a small area of painful induration in the dermis or subcutaneous tissue, and slowly enlarges to become an elevated, indurated, tender, tense mass with a 1 to 4 centimeter diameter. Histologically, this is a walled-off abscess filled with white blood cells, fibrin, and necrotic debris.

Intense, throbbing pain may be present. Malaise, regional adenopathy, and slight temperature elevation may accompany extensive furunculosis, but usually do not accompany isolated lesions. Over several days, the center of the furuncle becomes boggy and fluctuant, and a soft yellow or white head appears on the surface. Spontaneous rupture discharges thick, creamy yellow pus tinged with blood and is accompanied by relief of pain. Gram-stain and culture of pus show staphylococci. Healing then occurs over several additional days.

Although transient, asymptomatic bacteremia occasionally occurs, osteomyelitis or other distant foci of infection rarely occur. It is unusual for septic thrombophlebitis to accompany furuncles, but when this occurs in the central third of the face, it may lead to thrombosis of the cavernous sinus and death. The vast majority of furuncles heal without complications.

Small lesions usually require no therapy. Large or multiple furuncles should be treated. Warm compresses help relieve pain and may hasten the central pointing or maturation of the lesion. Incision or squeezing the lesion when it is hard and indurated is not helpful and may, in fact, cause the infection or inflammation to increase. However, once the center has become soft and filled with pus, it may be drained by puncturing or by incision. It should then be covered with a dressing, which should be frequently changed. Patient, family, and nurses should discard dressings carefully and should wash hands thoroughly after attending the patient.

If lesions are large, severely painful, multiple, on the central face, accompanied by adenopathy, or if the patient is ill, systemic antibiotics should be used. Semisynthetic penicillinase-resistant penicillins are best because of the possibility that the *S. aureus* is penicillin-resistant. Some persons have repeated episodes of furuncles. In these patients it is helpful to delay antibiotic therapy until one or more lesions are ready for drainage. The pus can then be cultured. After the organism has been identified and antibiotic sensitivity tests have been performed in the laboratory, a fourteen-day course of the specific systemic antibiotic is given.

The first and last steps of treatment are to prevent or correct any factors predisposing to furunculosis. In patients with long-standing recurrent furunculosis, rigorous personal hygiene is essential. Patient and family must bathe and shampoo daily with bacteriostatic soap. Nails should be clipped short. Razor blades should be discarded after each shave and the razor itself left in alcohol between shaves. Persons should have separate towels, washcloths, and sheets, which are laundered in boiling water and changed daily. Sometimes it is necessary to instill antibiotic cream or ointment into the anterior nose to stop recontamination with *S. aureus*. Bacterial interference treatment is successful at times. Recurrent furunculosis can be a very difficult therapeutic problem.

Carbuncle

A carbuncle is a complex of multiple interconnecting furuncles, which communicate by confluent extensions in the deep dermis and subcutaneous tissue. They tend to occur more frequently in adult males, and occur most frequently where the skin is thick. The lesions are large, painful, and covered by large areas of induration and erythema. It may take one to two weeks before fluctuance occurs and then the carbuncle may drain through multiple follicles.

Fever, malaise, leukocytosis, and adenopathy are more likely to occur than with simple furunculosis. Ulceration and scar formation usually follow the larger lesions. Treatment consists of bed rest, warm compresses, and systemic antibiotics. Drainage should be delayed until definite fluctuance occurs.

Cellulitis

Although the term *cellulitis* actually refers to any inflammation of cellular tissue, it is usually used more specifically to describe a diffuse, spreading, edematous, and sometimes suppurative inflammation within relatively solid tissues. Such a process is not as well defined or localized as an abscess and dissects widely through tissue spaces and cleavage planes. Some clinicians confine the use of the term to skin infection with a diffuse dermal and subcutaneous inflammation.

Bacterial cellulitis may occur as a complication of a wound or as an extension of other pyodermas, or it may appear to arise from previously normal skin. *S. aureus* and streptococci are the most frequent causative agents, but other bacteria may be responsible. Cellulitis is characteristic of highly invasive bacteria which produce enzymes. Beta-hemolytic streptococci can produce diffuse, rapidly spreading, deep-seated dermal inflammation which involves subcutaneous tissue. Exudate is scattered diffusely through the stromal planes.

Gradually extending induration, redness, and pain about a wound or pyoderma suggests cellulitis. As the erythema, swelling, and tenderness progress, malaise and fever may be present. The border of the lesion is indefinite. Without treatment, the lesion may progress to central suppuration, hemorrhage, necrosis, or gangrene. Rest, soaks, and systemic antibiotics are effective treatment.

Erysipelas

Erysipelas is a rapidly spreading, superficial cellulitis, which involves the dermis and superficial lymphatics. Although there is no sharp distinction between erysipelas and cellulitis, erysipelas is more superficial, and the name implies Group A beta-hemolytic streptococcus as the causative agent. The organism may gain access to the tissue by way of an abrasion, scratch, puncture wound, other pyoderma, or surgical wound. Any skin break, including herpes simplex, may be sufficient for access by the organism. In preantibiotic days, it was a frequent cause of postoperative infection and death. It is now less common and usually occurs in infants, the aged, and the debilitated, but occasionally it is seen on the face of an otherwise healthy person.

Rapid progression is a characteristic feature. Because the cellulitis is superficial, the expanding, palpable plaque of tender erythema has a sharp edge. Frank suppuration does not occur but the center of the lesion may develop blisters or crusts as a sign of secondary epidermal involvement. The patient is ill. Fever, elevated white count, headache, malaise, and other signs of toxicity are often present. Bacteremia is common. Death from sepsis may occur in untreated patients, but response to penicillin usually causes improvement within twenty-four hours.

Hidradenitis Suppurativa

Hidradenitis suppurativa is a chronic suppurative, scarring disease primarily of the axillae and anogenital regions (Figure 8-4). It is a bacterial infection of apocrine sweat glands and does not occur before puberty or begin after climacteric. It occurs most often in people who have the genetic diathesis for the disorder as well as for acne vulgaris. Women are affected more often than men. Obesity may be a predisposing factor.

Initial bacterial folliculitis leads to invasion of the apocrine duct and of the secretory tubule itself. Occlusion of the distal duct leads to dilatation of the proximal duct, further bacterial growth, and invasion of polymorphonuclear cells. Rupture leads to extension to adjacent apocrine ducts and glands. Pus may work its way to the surface, creating drainage tracts and fistulas. Healing is by fibrosis; the deep scarring distorts the microscopic architecture of the axillae and groin, making further infections more likely.

A period of painful red nodules in apocrine gland areas is followed by tender, diffuse, lumpy induration and finally by rupture and drainage of pus. Repeated episodes gradually increase the number of scars present. Large firm bands of scar tissue may bridge over depressed scars. After several years all the apocrine glands may be destroyed and apocrine sweating and the resulting characteristic odor is absent. The course is a chronic one.

Treatment of acute flares consists of specific systemic antibiotics, based on culture and sensitivity, and on careful surgical drainage of purulent cysts. Once antibiotics are administered raging inflammation can be quieted by short courses of systemic steroids. Between episodes the patient should avoid tight clothing, obesity, prolonged occlusion, and irritating chemicals. Those who do not respond to treatment can be considered for x-ray treatment or surgical removal of the axillary skin.

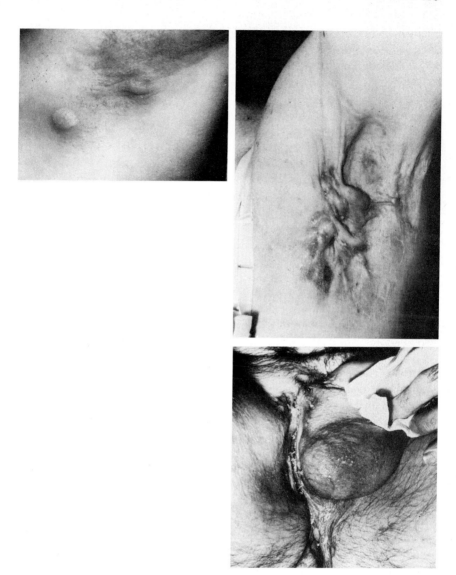

Figure 8-4 Hidradenitis suppurativa. (a) Acute inflammatory lesions; (b) chronic induration, scarring, and sinus formation; (c) groin involvement.

FUNGUS INFECTION OF THE SKIN

Fungi are primitive organisms which lack chlorophyll and have a firm, polysaccharide-protein cell wall surrounding the nuclei, food reserve, vacuoles, and cell fluids. Fungi are larger and more complex than bacteria. They may be unicellular, such as yeasts, or multicellular, such as molds.

Cells may join together in a line to form filaments called hyphae. Since they lack chlorophyll and therefore lack the capacity to manufacture their own organic materials, they must exist as either saprophytes (living on dead or decaying organic material) or parasites (living upon or within another living organism).

Fungi are ubiquitous. More than 100,000 species have been identified. Most of them are saprophytes. They play an essential role in the ecology by returning to the soil the nutrients extracted by plants. Some have useful physiologic specializations. Yeasts, which can transform sugar into alcohol and carbon dioxide, are indispensable to the brewery and the bakery. Many antibiotics, enzymes, and vitamins used in modern medicine are synthesized by fungi. On the other hand, large quantities of crops are damaged because of fungi pathogenic to plants; leather goods are subject to mildew, a fungus growth.

About 50 fungi are pathogenic to man. Some cause potentially serious systemic diseases, such as blastomycosis, coccidioidomycosis, cryptococcosis and histoplasmosis. Others are pathogenic primarily to skin, and cause such common disorders as ringworm and thrush. Many of the fungi that can survive on skin normally live in the soil or on animals, and only incidentally infect human skin. Others infect only man. The most common pathogenic fungi ingest only nonliving tissue such as keratin of stratum corneum, nails, or hair. Some cause few or no symptoms. Others invade the skin or elaborate substances which cause inflammation or hypersensitivity and lead to symptoms.

Fungal walls are relatively resistant to treatment with alkaline substances. Ten percent KOH hydrolyzes scales (dehydrated skin cells) and many components of human skin, but will not destroy the hyphae or spores of fungi. This provides a simple and rapid method of finding the fungi in tissues or exudates (see Chapter 6). Special media are used to grow fungi from infected specimens. The most popular is Sabouraud's media with chloramphenicol added to inhibit the growth of bacteria, and cyclohexamide to discourage the growth of nonpathogenic fungi.

Candidiasis

Candidiasis (moniliasis) is infection or inflammation caused by *Candida albicans,* a yeast-like fungus which may normally inhabit the gastrointestinal tract, the mouth, and the vagina. Although the yeast may occasionally be found in the moist perineum, or the skin between the toes, it is not a usual inhabitant of normal skin. Occasionally the commensal balance between organism and host is disturbed so that *C. albicans* causes inflammation. Rarely, generalized disease may occur, with sepsis and death, but usually the infection is limited to the mucous membranes, to mucocutaneous zones, or to moist areas of the skin. Much of the inflammation associated with such infections is due to an irritant toxin released by the organism.

Host factors which predispose to candidiasis include pregnancy, diabetes mellitus, or any debilitating chronic illness. Persons receiving antibiotics, systemic steroids, or birth control pills are more susceptible to infection with *C. albicans*. There is a circulating anticandidal factor in normal serum which helps to prevent invasion and infection by the yeast. This factor is reduced in infants up to six months of age and in patients with certain hematopoietic diseases resulting in increased susceptibility to candida infections.

A major requirement of the yeast is moisture. Therefore, moniliasis tends to occur in intertriginous areas, especially in the obese, and factors such as increased environmental temperatures, occlusion, and maceration tend to increase the incidence of infection. When infection occurs, the yeast may overgrow to such an extent that the colonies of organisms become confluent and can be seen as white plaques on mucous membranes. The clinical appearance of the inflammation differs depending upon the severity and the site of the infection (Figure 8-5).

Thrush is candidiasis of the mucous membrane of the mouth or vagina. Oral lesions begin as small white spots on the buccal mucosa or oropharynx and may extend forward to the lips or down into the esophagus. Lesions may occur at any age. Oral thrush appears about seven to ten days after birth in about 5 percent of newborns. Thrush may develop underneath dentures in older adults. White raised plaques on the mucosa coalesce to form extensive cheesy deposits which adhere relatively well to the mucosa; when removed, they leave erosions.

Although vaginal thrush is particularly common among diabetics, in pregnant women, and among those taking broad-spectrum antibiotics, it also occurs frequently in normal women. In severe cases, the vaginal wall may become red, edematous, and tender. An itchy vaginal discharge leads to involvement of the vulva. At times, involvement spreads to the labia majora, perineum, anus, and inner thighs. Pruritus is accompanied by pain on urination and intercourse. Candidal vaginitis and trichomoniasis may coexist.

Males may acquire genital candidiasis from an infected female. Males also get monilial intertrigo of the groin which characteristically may extend onto the scrotum. Since *C. albicans* normally lives in the gastrointestinal tract, primary perianal monilial intertrigo can occur in either sex.

Perleche (cheilitis, angular stomatitis) is a moist, erythematous area at the corners of the mouth which may be caused by *C. albicans*. Other

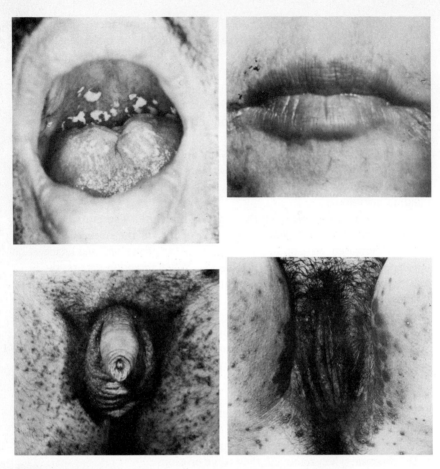

Figure 8-5 Moniliasis. (*a*) Thrush; white plaques of exudate on mucous membrane; (*b*) perleche; irritation at corners of mouth; (*c*) intertrigo; groin eruption accompanied by multiple satellite pustules; (*d*) intertrigo; angry red eruption of the groin.

causes include bacteria, drooling, habitual licking, cosmetics, or altered dental occlusion. Perleche may lead to discomfort by causing cracks and fissures.

Monilial *intertrigo* can occur in any moist, occluded area. The body folds behind the ears, between the buttocks, or the creases at the anterior, inner thighs may be involved. The web spaces between the fingers and toes may be involved, especially in persons who repeatedly wet their hands. The extra body folds of the obese person and the skin beneath pendulous breasts provide the moisture necessary for infection. Persons at bedrest for prolonged periods of time may develop yeast infections of the occluded surfaces of the back, especially if they have fever and night sweats in an overheated room.

Candidial intertrigo may be preceded by pruritus. Vesicopustules appear and rupture as they enlarge, leaving a denuded, intensely red base, surrounded and partially covered by shreds of white necrotic epidermis. All the denuded areas coalesce to form a pruritic, eroded, moist, angry red region which is aggravated in the creases of skin folds at the area of maximum occlusion. Outside of the slightly drier, minimally scaly border there are satellite pustules which are the newer lesions in a gradually expanding process. In addition to these small vesicopustules scattered just beyond the involved area, there is a striking contrast between the red, fissured, macerated, tender intertrigo and the adjacent normal skin.

Paronychia is an inflammation of the folds surrounding the nails, usually the posterior nail fold of the fingers. Infection of a mixed nature is often the cause. *C. albicans* and bacteria such as staphylococci, streptococci, pseudomonas, or others may be involved. Predisposing factors are trauma to the nail fold and repeated or prolonged exposure to moisture. Bartenders, cooks, dishwashers, laundry workers, housewives, and fishermen are prone to monilial paronychia. The thumb may be involved in thumb suckers, and the big toe in sweaty persons who wear airtight boots. A chronic paronychia may be somewhat tender; acute inflammation in the nail fold is very painful.

Diagnosis of moniliasis at any site is based on clinical appearance and confirmed by microscopic or culture examination. *C. albicans* frequently secondarily invades other dermatoses. Distinction between primary and secondary invasion is frequently not critical, since significant candida infection should be treated in any case. After treating the specimen with KOH, direct microscopic examination of scale, discharge, or white plaque material, or contents of a satellite pustule shows budding yeast (see Chapter 6). Culture on usual fungal or bacterial media shows colony growth in two to three days.

Treatment begins by investigating and eliminating the underlying precipitating factors. Besides avoiding all conditions that lead to constant or repeated moisture and maceration of the skin, it is important to initiate drying procedures actively. Intertriginous areas should be completely exposed to a heat lamp or fan several times daily. Loose clothing, air conditioning, powders, and topical medications which dehydrate the skin are also helpful. Specific therapy is the antifungal antibiotic, nystatin (Mycostatin). This nontoxic drug acts by direct contact and is available in powder, cream, vaginal suppositories, pills (to sterilize the bowel of monilia), and mouthwash. Nystatin alone usually cures mucous membrane moniliasis.

Dermatophytes

By precise definition, the word dermatophyte should include all fungi causing disease by invasion of skin, but common usage restricts the term to
those fungi causing ringworm. These fungi are essentially necrophilic; i.e.,
they restrict their food and habitat to dead keratinized tissue: stratum corneum of skin, hair, and nails. The dermatophytes can be divided into several species, depending upon the type of stratum corneum they prefer, their
natural habitat (soil, man, other animals), their microscopic and culture
characteristics, and the degree of skin inflammation their presence evokes.

Potentially pathogenic fungi of all kinds are ubiquitous in our environment. Although poor hygiene, poor nutrition, debilitating diseases, tropical
climate, and direct contact with the organism may increase the chances
of infection, the major determining factor seems to be a poorly understood,
variable, individual susceptibility. There is evidence of a serum antifungal
factor which inhibits dermatophyte invasion into living tissue. Acquired
immunity also occurs.

Tinea capitis (Figure 8-6a) (ringworm of the scalp) has been affecting the scalps of children since recorded history and is worldwide in distribution. Epidemic scalp ringworm is transmitted from child to child. Organisms can be cultured from barber's instruments, theater seats, hats, and
brushes. Prepubertal children are most susceptible, especially boys. Minor
trauma may be necessary to introduce the organism into the scalp.

The characteristic lesion is a round, sharply delineated area in which
the hairs are not absent, but are broken off at a level just above the skin.
The scalp may react with minimal erythema and slight dry scaling, or
it may react with a painful, deep, boggy, edematous inflammation called
a *kerion.*

Fungus infection of the beard may also occur. Infection may be superficial and mildly inflammatory and may appear as ringworm of the skin.
More severe beard involvement may cause pustular folliculitis, marked redness, kerion formation, or scarring with hair loss.

Tinea corporis (body ringworm) (Figure 8-6b) is a dermatophytic
infection of any nonhairy skin, usually seen in children, and most common
in rural areas and humid climates. Lesions are usually asymptomatic. Typi-
cally, it presents as a relatively flat, annular or arcuate lesion, with scaling
and erythema of its slowly advancing border and with central clearing. The
border, which may have fine vesiculation mixed with the dry scale, creates
a sharp contrast between involved and uninvolved skin.

Tinea cruris (Figures 8-6c, 8-7, and 8-8), or ringworm of the groin
area ("jock itch"), is often found in association with heat, friction, maceration, and obesity. It is seen most often in men, especially those who also
have tinea pedis. The morphology begins as that of tinea corporis but may

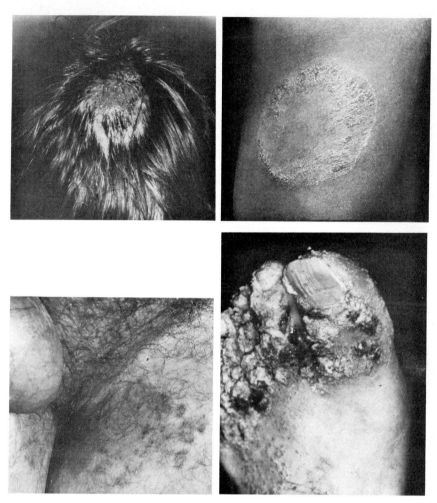

Figure 8-6 Superficial fungal (dermatophyte) infection. (a) Tinea capitis; (b) tinea corporis; (c) tinea cruris; (d) tinea pedis; extensive scaling and hyperkeratosis. Most tinea pedis is not this severe.

be modified by rubbing, scratching, maceration, or friction with tight clothing.

Tinea pedis (ringworm of the feet) (Figure 8-6d) is the most common of the superficial fungal infections and probably affects half of the adult population at some time during their lives. It is unlike tinea capitis in that it is a postpubertal disease. Tinea pedis is more common in tropical climates and in summertime. Simple contact with the fungus which is found in socks and shoes, on floors, and elsewhere, is probably not

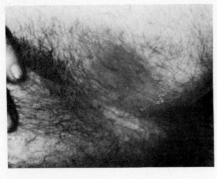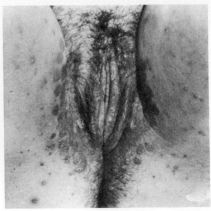

Figure 8-7 Close-up of border of "jock itch" or groin itch. (a) Tinea cruris; well-demarcated scaling border, with central clearing and sparing of crease and not extending onto genitals; (b) candidiasis; indefinite border with satellite pustules, increased erythema in inguinal crease, and extension onto genitals.

enough to contract infection. Minor trauma to the skin of the foot and individual susceptibility are probably necessary for infection to occur.

Tinea pedis usually causes only mild interdigital scaling and maceration but it may lead to widespread scaling of the sole with thickening of the heel and extension up onto the lateral foot. Occasionally inflammation is severe, with erythema and possibly blister formation. Pruritus is common. Fissures may be painful and may lead to secondary bacterial infection. Some persons with tinea pedis also note mild thickening and scaling from fungal infection of the palms.

More than one-third of those patients with dermatophyte infection of the skin will note fungal infection of the nails (*onychomycosis*). Toenails are more commonly affected and may become brittle, thickened, broken, and distorted, with a white or yellow discoloration. Nails may be almost totally destroyed. Several nails may be involved. The major complaint is usually the unsightly cosmetic appearance but tenderness occasionally develops and jagged edges of nail may catch on socks or clothing.

Wood's light causes fluorescence of some of the organisms causing tinea capitis. Microscopic examination of scales, nail fragments, or hairs treated with KOH confirms the diagnosis of fungus infection. Culture defines the species of dermatophyte.

The usual oozing, blistering, or edematous lesions should be treated with cool compresses until they are less inflammatory. Specific antifungal medications may be irritating to highly inflamed skin. Topical medications containing haloprogin or tolnaftate usually cure the dry, uncomplicated, superficial tinea corporis in one to three weeks. Scaling and thickening

	Tinea Cruris	Moniliasis	Eczema
Etiologic agent	fungus	yeast	itching and scratching
Surface	dry, scaly, erythematous	angry red, moist	chronic eczema, lichenification
Symptoms	pruritus	pruritus, pain	severe pruritus
Area of maximum occlusion (skin fold in crease)	relative sparing	maximally involved	relative sparing
Border	well-demarcated scaling border ahead of central clearing	may be well demarcated ± satellite pustules	not well demarcated
Scrotum	often spared	often involved	may be involved and be thickened
Microscopic examination (KOH)	hyphae	hyphae, budding forms, blastospores	negative

Figure 8-8   Clinical manifestations of common groin eruptions ("jock itch").

of palms and soles may be reduced with keratolytic or primary irritant medications such as salicylic acid used in combination with one of these specific topical antifungal medications.

Griseofulvin is an antifungal antibiotic which is itself a metabolic product of certain species of fungi. It is highly effective against dermatophytes but has no effect in treating candidiasis, tinea versicolor, or bacterial infections. Griseofulvin is best absorbed from the gastrointestinal tract after a fatty meal and diffuses to the epidermis in the extracellular fluid to become concentrated in the horny layer. Tinea corporis or tinea pedis which is extensive or is resistant to topical therapy responds to three to four weeks of griseofulvin. It is especially effective in tinea capitis and has made x-ray epilation treatment unnecessary. It is the only effective treatment of onychomycosis.

Griseofulvin may reduce the effectiveness of oral anticoagulants by increasing the liver's enzymatic inactivation of the anticoagulant. When patients are started on griseofulvin, a higher dose of anticoagulant drugs may be necessary to maintain the same level of anticoagulation. More importantly, when patients have been on both drugs simultaneously and the griseofulvin is discontinued, bleeding may result from over-anticoagulation effect. It has also been noted that phenobarbitol given concomitantly with griseofulvin may decrease its antifungal effectiveness. Griseofulvin should not be used in patients with porphyria.

Fungal infections of nails should be approached with the understanding that topical therapy almost never cures the fungus, that griseofulvin therapy is expensive and may take longer than a year, and that relapse after such therapy is not uncommon. Results may be improved by surgical avulsion of the affected nail prior to initiation of oral griseofulvin, but many patients consider this a drastic therapy for a cosmetic disorder.

In treating all fungal infections, it is best to avoid environmental factors which enhance heat, moisture, maceration, and trauma. Towels, clothing, and sheets should be changed frequently, and well laundered in hot water. Footwear should be nonocclusive and should fit well. Reasonable hygiene is important but it is not possible to totally avoid contact with pathogenic fungi.

Tinea Versicolor

Tinea versicolor (TV) is a common, chronic, asymptomatic, superficial fungal infection which most often involves the upper trunk and shoulders of young adults. The name versicolor describes the variability in color of the semiconfluent, superficial, bran-like (furfuraceous) scale which may be darker or lighter than the surrounding uninvolved skin (Figure 8-9). The lesion may be more obvious in summer when the uninvolved skin

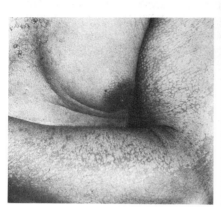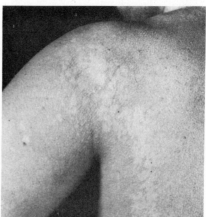

Figure 8-9   Tinea versicolor.

is tan. Inflammation is minimal or absent because the fungi never penetrate deeper than the outer stratum corneum. TV is usually not pruritic, and is only of concern cosmetically. It is frequently not noticed by the host.

The disorder may be more common in patients with Cushing's disease or in persons taking exogenous steroids, but the vast majority of affected persons are normal. Face, neck, or extremities may be involved, but most cases are confined to the upper trunk. Scale may be tan, white, pink, or brown. It is usually the same color on one patient at one particular time but may change shades slightly from time to time. Early lesions may have a perifollicular distribution but they usually extend and merge into annular lesions which eventually become large, semiconfluent, map-like areas of macular desquamation. The lighter lesions must be distinguished from vitiligo which differs in that it is totally amelanotic (totally white because of zero pigment) and from pityriasis alba which usually occurs in atopic individuals along with a history of some inflammation at the site of hypopigmentation.

Wood's light examination may intensify the differences in color between affected and unaffected areas, and occasionally the scale shows a copper-orange fluorescence. Microscopic examination shows a characteristic picture of hyphae and spores. The organism involved, called *Malassezia furfur,* may be a variant or a different growth phase of a yeast-like organism which is frequently found on normal skin.

Selenium sulfide suspension (Selsun) is the most satisfactory topical agent, but salicylic acid, sodium hyposulfite, and other topical antifungal agents have been used with success. Although the fungal infection may be gone after several days, the tinea versicolor-induced differences in color or pigmentation of the skin may last until the next summer tan is obtained. Recurrences are common and probably result from a high individual susceptibility and reinfection or from inadequate treatment. After a vigorous shower and use of a brush or washcloth, the medication should be applied and left on overnight, on several different occasions. Unlaundered underwear, sheets, and socks should not be used after treatment because reinfection may occur.

VIRUS INFECTION OF THE SKIN

A virus is a submicroscopic organism which is capable of multiplication only within a living susceptible host cell. Therefore, these organisms, which are considerably smaller than most bacteria, are obligatory parasites. When the virus enters the cell, it interacts with the cell's genetic and metabolic machinery in order to insure its own replication. Such interaction may or may not have pathologic consequences for the host cell. If no observable host cell changes occur, the infection is subclinical or latent. On the other hand, cell morphology and physiology may be changed and may lead to inflammation resulting in illness or lesions, or the host cell may die.

The intact virus has a core of its own genetic material which is either ribonucleic acid (RNA) or desoxyribonucleic acid (DNA). An outer coat of protein protects the core during transit from one cell to another. It is this coat which is an antigen and which stimulates immune responses from the host. Multiple, nonimmune defense mechanisms and substances also help to keep viruses from entering cells and replicating. The stratum corneum or horny products of nail and hair cannot be infected by a virus since live cells are needed to support its reproduction.

Skin lesions may result as a manifestation of systemic virus infections, such as measles and chicken pox, or the skin and mucous membranes may be the primary site of multiplication of such viruses as herpes simplex. Finally, some viruses, such as warts or molluscum contagiosum, seem to have their pathologic effects limited to the skin.

Warts

Warts are circumscribed new growths which are due to hypertrophy of the epidermis, induced by infection of the living epidermal cells by a specific virus. Warts are benign intraepidermal tumors of the skin. The skin cells grow and multiply excessively as a result of being infected with the human papilloma virus. While the lesions are not particularly contagious, they can be spread to new sites on the host by accidentally inoculating the virus into the epidermis by way of a scratch or puncture (autoinoculation). After an incubation period of one to several months, the new lesions may begin to appear. While warts may appear at any age, the highest incidence is during the second and third decades.

The morphology of the wart differs from one site of the body to another. The same virus causes a different kind of response on mucous membranes than it does on the adjacent skin. The wart on the finger looks quite different from the wart on the sole of the foot. Warts in moist areas differ from those of dry skin. The appearance of warts in various body regions is so varied that different names are usually used to describe the tumors (Figure 8-10).

Verruca vulgaris (common wart) is a small, elevated, circumscribed, painless, flesh-colored, hyperkeratotic papule. These lesions appear most commonly on the dorsa of the fingers and hands and can be especially bothersome if massed around the nail folds. Black dots may be seen scattered through the semitranslucent lesion. The dots are caused by hemosiderin (blood) pigment in thrombosed capillary loops. Common warts have a rough surface because of numerous tiny irregular papillary projections of keratin. When the adjective "verrucous," meaning wart-like, is used to describe the surface characteristics of any lesion, it refers to similarity to verruca vulgaris.

Flat warts (plane wart, verruca plana) occur as multiple, 1 to 3 millimeter, slightly elevated, circumscribed papules most often seen on the face or neck.

Filiform warts (verruca filiformis) are slender, thin, finger-like projections, which usually occur on the face, neck, axillae, or shoulders.

Plantar warts (verruca plantaris) are simply warts which grow on the plantar surface of the foot. They grow inward because of pressure from walking or standing. When virus infects the living keratinocytes, the usual response of epidermal thickening occurs. The thickened epidermis causes pain as it is pushed into the foot by normal weight-bearing forces. The normal skin markings of the skin of the foot do not transverse the lesion, but are interrupted by the firm, flat, or slightly elevated hyperkeratotic plantar wart. The lesions are shaped like a cone with the apex pointed inward and the base at the surface. Paring down the lesion reveals black dots (thrombosed capillaries). Pressure on the lesion may cause pain.

Plantar warts must be distinguished from calluses or corns. While skin markings are interrupted by warts, they are intact and often exaggerated over a callus. A callus causes less pain on squeezing or pressure. When pared with a sharp blade, the callus lacks the black dot appearance of thrombosed capillaries, and is not cone-shaped.

Condyloma accuminata (moist wart, genital wart, venereal wart) are fleshy, nonhorny, cauliflower-like epidermal growths in moist areas. The host response to the wart virus in such areas as the genitalia, anus, axilla, or nipple is such that the wart assumes the appearance of clusters of small, highly vascular, pale, or pink digitations. If the lesions extend onto dry skin, the wart assumes the morphology of verruca vulgaris. Transmission of the virus by sexual intercourse is possible but nonvenereal acquisition of condyloma accuminata also occurs. These lesions may become quite large and painful. They may interfere with intercourse, urination, or defecation.

Therapy   Destruction of the benign tumor and the wart virus is an easy task. They are susceptible to injury by cold, heat, electricity, or chemicals and can be cut off. The real difficulty in treatment is the prevention of excessive damage to surrounding normal skin and the prevention of

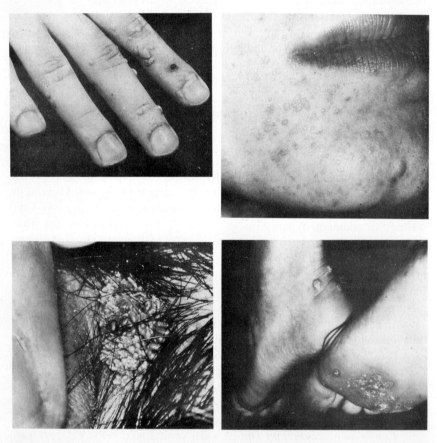

Figure 8-10 Warts. (a) Verruca vulgaris (common wart); (b) verruca plana (flat wart); (c) filiform warts; (d) plantar warts; (e) condyloma accuminata (venereal wart); (f) multiple warts around paronychia.

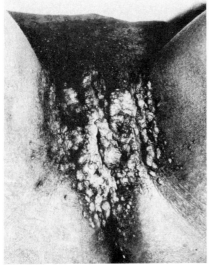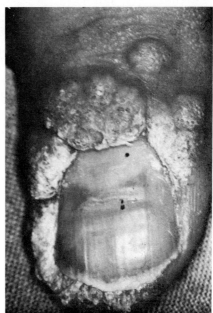

FIGURE 8-10 For legend see opposite page.

scars. This is where the art, debates, and wide range of preferences of wart treatments come in. To complicate therapeutic decisions even more, it must be remembered that most warts are asymptomatic and that most warts will disappear without treatment if left alone for one to two years. Reasons for treatment are cosmetic considerations, prevention of spread by autoinoculation, pain because of location (anogenital, plantar), and psychological considerations. Large digital warts may get in the way and often catch on clothing or other articles.

Surgery and electrodesiccation are effective but painful and often leave scars. Cryosurgery with liquid nitrogen usually is effective without scarring but may require more than one treatment. Cantharidin causes a painful intraepidermal blister which lifts the infected epidermis, causing the wart to fall off. Keratolytic agents and primary irritants may eventually slough the wart if used repeatedly. Condyloma accuminata warts are best treated with 25 percent podophyllin which can be made up in tincture of benzoin to keep it localized to the lesion. Podophyllin can be irritating to normal skin and the treated area should be washed thoroughly four to six hours after treatment. Repeated weekly applications may be necessary.

The excellent results claimed from psychotherapy are hard to evaluate in a disease such as warts, which can disappear spontaneously. Working with children with bilateral hand involvement, some investigators have been able to use suggestion therapy to make verruca vulgaris lesions disappear from one hand and not from the other. After further hypnosis or suggestion, the other hand may then be cured. Until more is known about this phenomenon, it seems best to assume that whatever modality is employed, self-confidence and optimism will be useful on the side of the therapist.

Molluscum Contagiosum

Molluscum contagiosum is a benign epidermal tumor caused by a virus which forms a characteristic firm, waxy, umbilicated papule (Figure 8-11). It may be spread by direct person to person contact or by autoinoculation, and may be solitary or in clusters. Most lesions are rarely larger than one to several millimeters in diameter. Rarely, they may also become generalized in atopic individuals.

Molluscum contagiosum is seen primarily on the faces or trunks of infants and children, or in the pubic area of sexually active young adults. Usually few in number, most lesions are asymptomatic. Diagnosis is made by clinical appearance and by examining the contents of a papule smeared on a glass slide. The stained specimen reveals oval, smooth-walled, homogeneous masses called molluscum bodies.

The lesions may be removed by a curette, light desiccation, or cryo-

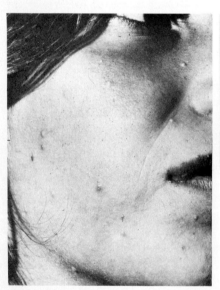
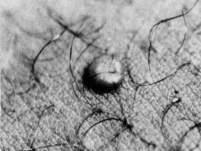

Figure 8-11   Molluscum contagiosum.   (a) Multiple lesions; (b) close-up of single lesion.

surgery. They may disappear in several months if left alone, but this carries the risk of spread to host and others by repeated accidental inoculations.

Herpes Simplex

Herpes simplex is a spectrum of infections caused by the virus, Herpesvirus hominis. *H. hominis* may be one of the most widespread pathogens of human beings. The virus is almost universal in distribution and more than 50 percent of humans have antibody evidence of having been infected at some time. Infection may cause the common fever blister, or it may lead to severe, painful infection of the mouth, genitalia, or eye (Figure 8-12). The range of clinical manifestations of infection goes from absence of any signs or symptoms to severe illness or death and depends upon complex host-virus relationships.

H. hominis normally infects only human beings. When entering into the cell, it may remain there in a latent or quiescent manner or may completely dominate the cell's reproductive machinery, leading to the death of the cell. The skin and mucous membranes are the major tissues invaded and infection is within the living cells of the epidermis. The protein coat of the virus acts as an antigen and stimulates production of antibodies to the virus.

There seem to be two distinct types of herpes viruses which differ biologically, morphologically, and antigenically from one another and which tend to differ in their habitat and pathogenesis in man. While type 1 seems to be more frequently recovered from nongenital herpes simplex, type 2 herpes virus is most often associated with genital lesions, and is, therefore, often spread through sexual contact as well as from mother to newborn during delivery. There is seroepidemiologic evidence that type 2 herpes may be associated in some way with cervical carcinoma.

The mechanisms and mediators of the host-cell virus relationships are not known. The clinical syndromes which result from a first encounter with the *H. hominis* virus differ from those caused by later reinactivation of virus which has been living in cells for months to years since its original penetration.

The usual manifestation of cutaneous involvement is grouped vesicles or vesicopustules on an erythematous base. On mucous membranes, the roof of the vesicle is frequently absent, leaving grouped erosions surrounded by erythema.

The first encounter with herpes may occur by an inoculation of the virus into any site of skin or mucous membrane or by infection of a cut or scratch. Antibodies to the virus are not present at the time of the initial infection of the host. Antibodies develop during the course of the infection. This primary infection may be completely asymptomatic or it may be quite severe. When lesions are present, they appear as grouped vesicopustules surrounded by edema, tenderness, and erythema. Such a lesion, called primary cutaneous inoculation herpes, usually crusts and heals within one to two weeks. If the viral infection is extensive, a striking confluent sea of vesicles covering large areas may be surrounded by erythema. Adenopathy and fever may develop. Swelling and secondary bacterial infection can cause severe pain.

Mucous membranes are particularly susceptible to primary infection. The virus can probably penetrate the intact mucosa. Gingivostomatitis is a common manifestation of primary herpes infection in infants and children. Transient vesicles in the oral cavity quickly change into erosions and may coalesce to involve large areas of the gums, lips, and oral mucosa. Fiery red erosions are covered with variable amounts of intact epidermis, serum, and purulence. Lesions often extend into the posterior oropharynx and out onto the skin. Edema and tenderness prevent eating. Children often drool to avoid swallowing, and the saliva mixed with the necrotic outer epidermis and serum has a foul odor. Tender regional adenopathy is present and the child often feels ill for seven to ten days.

In adolescents and young adults, the virus may be introduced venereally. In this age group, primary herpes appears as severe vulvovaginitis, cervicitis, balanitis, or urethritis. Pain and incapacitation may necessitate hospitalization. The morphology of the lesions is the same as that seen in the mouth. When lesions spill onto the skin, they have the characteristic grouped vesicles on an erythematous base before they become confluent. By giving mouth care to patients, nurses and dentists are prone to incidences of primary inoculation herpes on the fingers (herpetic whitlow). Viral tonsillitis, pharyngitis, or rhinitis may occur with primary herpes simplex. Asymptomatic involvement of internal organs probably occurs on occasion. Although primary herpes simplex is sometimes quite severe and painful, it usually heals without serious sequelae.

Primary herpes simplex may, however, cause serious disease. Herpetic keratoconjunctivitis may permanently compromise vision. Meningoencephalitis can result from a herpes infection. Eczema herpeticum (see Chapter 7) is a form of primary herpes simplex. Newborn and debilitated patients may be overwhelmed with a widespread fatal herpes infection. Infection of the newborn carries such risk of serious complications or death that Cesarean section should be considered when a woman is discovered to have a vaginal infection late in pregnancy. This prevents the fetus from coming into direct contact with the infected mucosa.

Recurrent herpes simplex occurs when latent or quiescent virus, acquired months to years previously, becomes reactivated. The original infection may have been asymptomatic or may have been documented by mild or

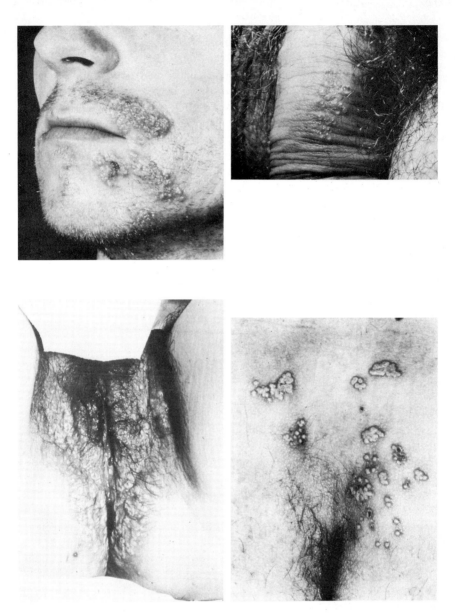

Figure 8-12 Herpes simplex. Grouped vesicles on an erthematous base. (*a*) Recurrent lesions of mouth; (*b*) herpes progenitalis; (*c*) primary lesions of vulva; (*d*) close-up of grouped configuration.

severe primary herpes simplex. Recurrent herpes simplex lesions tend to be small and to occur repeatedly in the same site; they are self-limiting and maintain the characteristic grouped vesicles on an erythematous base. Tender adenopathy often occurs in recurrent herpes simplex that has not been secondarily infected with bacteria.

The host has antibodies against *H. hominis* at the beginning as well as during and after the recurrent herpes simplex symptoms. The host factors which trigger the reactivation of latent viruses or prevent spread beyond the site of reactivation are not known. It has been noted that, in some persons, sunburn, fever, and severe emotional or physical stress frequently and regularly precede recurrent herpes simplex. Any cutaneous or mucous membrane surface may be the site of recurrent herpes simplex. The most common sites are about the lips (fever blister) or on the external genitalia (herpes progenitalis). Often pain, burning, or tingling precedes the appearance of the vesicles by hours to days. The lesions crust and heal over a seven to ten day period. There may be recurrences once in a lifetime or every few weeks for years. It is not certain which of the host cells harbor the latent virus between recurrences.

In both the primary and recurrent infections, the virus is present within the cells of the midepidermis and within blister fluid. *H. hominis* can be cultured from the lesions. The lesions of herpes simplex are infectious to other people. Light microscopic examination of the base of the vesicles shows multinucleated giant cells. Biopsy is usually not necessary for diagnosis because the lesions are so clinically characteristic. A knife blade scraped across a recently denuded area will provide enough material to search for multinucleated giant cells. Such cells are seen with herpes simplex, herpes zoster, and varicella. Serologic tests are available for use in difficult diagnostic problems.

Treatment for herpes simplex is primarily directed at the symptoms. There is no safe, specific, convincingly effective antiviral chemotherapeutic agent. Also, there is no clearly successful prophylactic therapy against recurrent herpes simplex.

Systemic analgesia may be needed for the severe pain of the primary infection. Topical anesthetics may be necessary to permit eating, urination, or defecation when mucous membranes are severely affected. Tetracycline mouth rinses may prevent secondary infection. Sitz baths often provide some relief of genital lesions.

Recurrent lesions may dry up more quickly with topical medications containing aluminum acetate. Some persons note that, if treatment is initiated early enough, repeated application of topical steroid to recurrent herpes simplex lesions will decrease severity and duration of symptoms by limiting inflammation. Care should be taken not to apply steroids near the eye because of the possibility of increasing the host's susceptibility to herpes keratitis. Dyes which have the capacity both to bind to DNA and to absorb light energy have been used in an attempt to photodestroy the DNA virus. This treatment by dyes has been reported to prevent further episodes of recurrent herpes simplex. Iododeoxyuridine (IDU) is an antiviral agent which inhibits the synthesis of the DNA of the virus. It appears effective in treatment of herpes of the eye and has been used in serious systemic viral infection with variable results.

PARASITES

Humans are host to many kinds of parasites. On a worldwide scale, parasitic diseases are a major medical and economic problem. The skin is the source of entry for many of these organisms and the major place of abode for others. The skin can also be injured by animals. Sea creatures such as jellyfish, sponges, and sea urchins cause characteristic patterns of injury and inflammation. By biting, stinging, and laying eggs in the skin, many insects cause inflammation and hypersensitivity reactions; they also carry diseases to human beings. Throughout recorded history, people have been itching because of lice or mites which are present on the skin.

Pediculosis

Blood-sucking lice are wingless insects which are obligate parasites; some of them are host-specific for man (Figure 8-13). They obtain nutrition by sucking blood from the skin, leave their eggs and excrement on the skin and are passed from person to person. During times of crowded, unsanitary conditions, the incidence of pediculosis is quite high, but the disorder is not rare among the highly civilized.

The head louse and body louse are both types of *Pediculosis humanus*. The female is a 3- to 4-millimeter oblong creature with legs adapted for grasping hair. She lays about eight eggs each day which hatch in about eight days and require another eight days to mature into adult lice. The eggs are firmly attached to a hair or a thread of clothing. These oval egg capsules, frequently called "nits," can easily be seen with a hand lens. The adult male is slightly smaller than the female. The head louse and body louse differ slightly in feeding habits and physiology, but are capable of interbreeding and look very much alike. The body louse may have developed from the head louse when humans began to wear clothes and cut their hair. The head louse is usually confined to the scalp or beard and as few as ten insects may be found. Itching is severe, and scratching may be so intense that excoriations, secondary bacterial infection, edema, and adenopathy obscure the diagnosis. Nits are seen near the base of the hair.

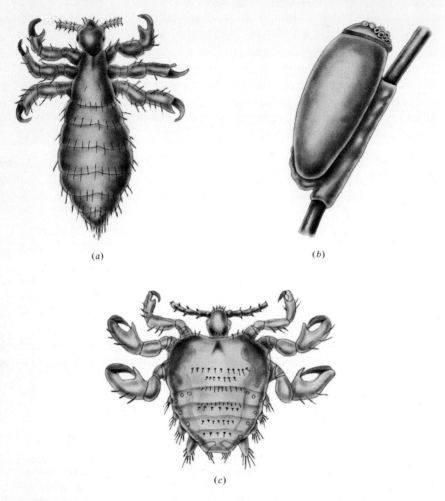

(a)   *(b)*

(c)

Figure 8-13 Lice of man. (*a*) Pediculosis humanus var. capitis; (*b*) nits; (*c*) phthirus pubis.

The infestation may be spread to others with combs, caps, brushes, or towels.

The body louse usually resides and lays eggs in clothing, especially those inner seams that touch the skin of the waist and upper back. It moves to the skin only for a blood meal and then returns to the clothing. Although it normally feeds at frequent intervals, the body louse can survive up to ten days between meals. Eggs can survive slightly longer and then the young lice must begin to find a place to feed. In any case, garments which have been stored for one month will not be infested. The louse can be transferred from one person to another by direct contact or by way of clothing, bedding, or towels. Occasionally, outer garments also carry living insects.

The pubic louse, *Phthirus pubis,* differs in appearance and habits from *P. humanus.* The pubic louse is rounder and has large claw-like pincers on its legs, which make it resemble a tiny crab. The primary habitat is the region covered by pubic hair, although occasionally it infests eyelashes. These crab lice cling constantly to the skin without leaving, feeding intermittently, and laying eggs which appear as nits. *P. pubis* is most often spread by sexual contact and is, therefore, considered by some to be one of the most common venereal diseases. It can also be contracted by contact with bed clothing, towels, or toilet seats.

When feeding, lice inject saliva and enzymes into the skin and suck blood, leaving a tiny pinpoint area of redness or purpura. After forty-eight hours, this site shows edema and pruritus which lasts for days. It is most likely that the saliva, head parts, and feces of the louse act as antigens to cause a somewhat delayed hypersensitivity response which accounts for the severe itching and the individual variation in pediculosis-induced pruritus. Rust-colored specks of blood-tinged excrement can often be seen. Pinpoint erythema, raised macules, pinpoint excoriations, and long parallel linear scratches may be followed by crusts, secondary infection, and adenopathy. Chronic infestation can lead to sleeplessness, weight loss, fever, and leukocytosis.

Diagnosis is made by finding the nits or lice on a patient with the above findings and a complaint of pruritus. Topical treatment is effective. Gamma benzene hexachloride (Kwell®), a pesticide also known as Lindane, is effective. It is available as a shampoo, cream, or lotion to treat the various parts of the body affected. Repeated treatment may be necessary. Clothing, linens, and towels should be dry-cleaned or washed in hot water. Benzyl benzoate and DDT are also effective therapy. Eyelash involvement can be treated by combing out the nits, and then applying 0.25 percent physiostigmine (Eserine®).

Scabies

Infestation with and sensitization to the itch mite, *Sarcoptes scabiei,* causes severe itching (Figure 8-14). The fertilized female mite pierces the stratum corneum, and burrows into the skin. She leaves three to four eggs per day in the tunnel in the skin, which hatch three to four days later. The burrowing itself probably causes no symptoms but later allergic reaction to eggs, feces, and mite parts causes redness, swelling, itching, and even vesiculation. By this time, the organism has burrowed further to a new site, beyond what looks like the end of the serpiginous inflammation. After sensitization

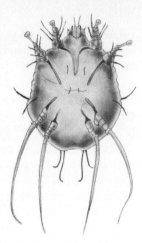

Figure 8-14 Sarcoptes scabiei.

is well developed, however, the mite may cause symptoms immediately upon entering the skin and may be scratched out before burrowing begins.

Sites of predilection include interdigital webs, flexor surface of wrists, anterior axillary folds, penis, nipples, buttocks, and the sides of the feet. Except in infants, the head is usually spared. Two very characteristic findings are severe itching at bedtime and the presence of burrows: tortuous, raised, thread-like channels in the skin which curve or zigzag haphazardly in the areas of mite predilection. Papules, pustules, excoriations, and secondary bacterial infection also are seen.

A rare variant is called Norwegian scabies, in which thousands of organisms may cover a patient, who, for some reason, does not itch severely. Face, palms, and soles may be involved, and the inflammatory response includes extensive hyperkeratosis.

Scabies is acquired through intimate physical contact or may be transmitted via clothing, linens, or towels. The topical pesticides used for pediculosis are also effective for treatment of scabies. Medication should be left on the skin for twelve to twenty-four hours with each treatment.

REFERENCES

Ackerman, A. B.: "Crabs—The Resurgence of Phthirus Pubis," *N. Eng. J. Med.* **278:**950–951, April 1968.

Catalano, P. M.: "Broadening Spectrum of Herpesvirus Hominis (Herpes Simplex)," *Arch. Derm.* **101:**364–366, March 1970.

Conant, N. F. et al.: *Manual of Clinical Mycology,* W. B. Saunders Company, Philadelphia, 1971.

Dillon, H. C. Jr.: "Impetigo Contagiosa: Suppurative and Non-Suppurative Complications," *Am. J. Dis. Child.* **115:**530–541, May 1968.

Esterly, N. and M. Markowitz: "The Treatment of Pyoderma in Children,"
   JAMA **212:**1667–1670, June 1970.

Felber, T. D., E. B. Smith, J. M. Knox, C. Wallis, J. L. Melnick: "Photody-
   namic Inactivation of Herpes Simplex," *JAMA* **223:**289–292, January
   1973.

Keddie, F. "Clinical Signs in Tinea Versicolor," *Arch. Derm.* **87:**641–642,
   May 1963.

Lynch, P. J., and W. Minkin: "Molluscum Contagiosum of the Adult: Probable
   Venereal Transmission," *Arch. Derm.* **98:**141–143, August 1968.

Marples, M. J.: *The Ecology of the Human Skin.* Charles C Thomas, Publisher,
   Springfield, Ill., 1965.

Massing, A. M., W. L. Epstein: "Natural History of Warts. A two-year study,"
   Arch. Derm. **87:**306–310, March 1963.

Nobel, W. C.: "Streptococci, Nephritis, and the Skin," *Brit. J. Derm.*
   82:620–621, 1970.

Oriel, J. D.: "Natural History of Genital Warts," *Brit. J. Vener. Dis.* **47:**1–13,
   February 1971.

Orkin, M.: "Resurgence of Scabies," *JAMA,* **217:**593–597, August 1971.

Parnell, A. G.: "Facial Erysipelas," *Oral Surg.* **27:**166–168, February 1969.

Reiss, F.: "Present Status of Superficial Fungus Infections of the Skin, Hair,
   and Nails," *Med. Clin. N. Am.* **49:**725–736, May 1965.

Skin Bacteria and Their Role in Infection. Maibach, H. I., and G. Hildick-
   Smith, eds., McGraw-Hill Book Company, New York, 1965.

Wenner, H. A., and T. Y. Lou: "Virus Diseases Associated with Cutaneous
   Eruptions," *Progr. Med. Virol.* **5:**219–294, 1963.

Wheeler, C. E. Jr., and D. C. Abele: "Eczema Herpeticum, Primary and
   Recurrent," *Arch. Derm.* **93:**162–173, February 1966.

Marples, M. J.: "Life on the Human Skin," *Scientific American* 2 **30:**108,
   1969.

Kligman, A.: "The Bacteriology of Normal Skin" in *Skin Bacteria and Their
   Role in Infection,* Maibach, H. and G. Hildrick-Smith, eds., McGraw-Hill
   Book Company, New York, 1965, pp. 13–31.

Chapter 9

Disorders of Mucous Membranes

Common disorders affecting the oral cavity
Aphthous stomatitis
Venereal disease
  Syphilis
  Gonorrhea
  Chancroid
  Lymphogranuloma venereum (LGV)
  Granuloma inguinale

COMMON DISORDERS AFFECTING THE ORAL CAVITY

Oral mucosa represents an invagination of the skin. It is, like the skin, a stratified squamous epithelium. The lamina propria is the connective tissue counterpart of the dermis. In the epithelium of the oral cavity, the granular layer is usually absent and the stratum corneum is markedly reduced. The usual epidermal appendages are absent. Turnover time is much more rapid than that of normal skin. Many skin disorders affect mucous membranes; the presence of oral lesions and their morphology may give helpful diagnostic information (Figure 9-1).

Lichen planus (see Chapter 7). While the buccal mucosa is the most frequent site of oral involvement, lesions may occur on any mucous membrane. The usual presentation is that of nonindurated, white, minimally elevated papules, or lacy white reticulate lines (Wickham's striae) over variable amounts of erythema. Erosions occur less frequently and when

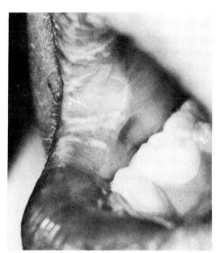
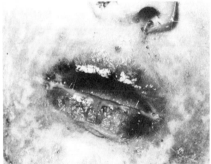
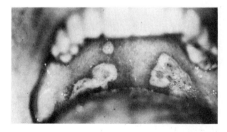

Figure 9-1 Mouth lesions. (*a*) Lichen planus; white streaks on reddened mucosa; (*b*) erythema multiforme; painful erosions of lips and intraoral mucosa; (*c*) aphthae; painful ulcer surrounded by erythema.

present are often surrounded by the more characteristic white striae. Lichen planus may be confined to the mouth.

Pemphigus vulgaris (see Chapter 12) is frequently accompanied by blisters in the mouth. The oral bullous lesions may precede skin lesions by several months. In the mouth the roofs of the blisters do not remain intact for long and the usual presentation is that of irregular, tender, bright red, denuded erosions with ragged shreds of necrotic epidermis remaining at their periphery. Lesions may extend beyond the vermillion border of the lip onto the skin. In contrast, the oral lesions of bullous pemphigoid are less common and less tender than in pemphigus and are less likely to precede skin lesions.

Erythema multiforme (see Chapters 5 and 12) frequently has oral involvement. Mucous membrane involvement may, in fact, be the most symptomatic aspect of erythema multiforme. Red macules or papules develop into vesicles which coalesce as they rupture, to leave irregular erosions or ulcers. The necrotic epidermis, exudates, and oral secretions may combine to form a gray-white pseudomembrane which leaves a bleeding raw base when removed. Lips may become crusted. Secondary infection is common, resulting in a foul smell. Eating may be painful; the patient may drool.

The mouth is frequently the site of *primary herpes simplex* infection (see Chapter 8), which can cause considerable discomfort. Grouped vesicles progress to confluent erosions. *Viral exanthems* (see Chapter 11) are often accompanied by erythema, petechiae, or vesicles within the oral cavity, especially on the posterior palate and posterior oropharynx. Oral lesions have been reported in more than one-fourth of patients with *lupus erythematosis*. The lesions are usually asymptomatic and morphology is varied.

Persistent, unexplained, white plaques on mucous membranes that are not easily removed should be biopsied. Such white plaques (*leukoplakia*) may be benign epidermal hyperplasia which occurs spontaneously or in response to repeated trauma. It could, however, be carcinoma *in situ* or invasive squamous cell carcinoma.

APHTHOUS STOMATITIS

Aphthous stomatitis (canker sores) is a recurrent painful mucosal erosion of the mouth and oropharynx. The cause is not known and aphthae may actually have several etiologies. A certain alpha streptococcus which can produce mouth erosions in animals is frequently isolated from the lesions. Since it has been shown that lymphocytes from patients with recurrent aphthous stomatitis can cause necrosis of mucosal epithelial cells, it seems reasonable to assume that cell-mediated immunity plays a role in the etiology of some lesions. Herpes simplex virus is not isolated from the recurrent aphthae.

Tingling and burning may precede the appearance of a lesion by twenty-four to forty-eight hours. The first objective change is a focal erythema which is accompanied by considerable pain. After another twelve to twenty-four hours a tiny superficial white or gray slough appears in the center of the erythema and gradually increases in size. The fully formed lesion appears as single or multiple small shallow erosions with sharp borders. The erosions may be covered by a gray, white, or yellow membrane, and are surrounded by a halo of intense erythema. Lesions heal without scarring after eight to ten days. Recurrences are the rule.

No treatment is uniformly effective, and none regularly prevents recurrences. Topical anesthetics help relieve pain and permit the patient to chew. Suspensions of tetracycline retained in the mouth for several minutes three to four times a day prevent or treat secondary bacterial infection and may shorten the duration of the lesions. Topical steroids sometimes reduce inflammation.

VENEREAL DISEASE (V.D.)

Although the origins, attributes, and myths of the Italian goddess Venus are obscure and often confused with those of Aphrodite, the name of Venus has come to be popularly associated with love and lovers. When man sought a euphemism for the genital sores of the active lover, he called them venereal diseases (Latin genitive of Venus is *veneris*). Venereal diseases are really a number of entirely different contagious diseases with little in common other than the fact that, at some stage, they have a genital location. Venereal diseases are usually acquired when the mucous membranes or skin of the genitals come in direct contact with infected mucous membranes or skin. This mode of spread is the only common bond of all the venereal diseases.

Venereal disease is divided into major and minor groups. This separation is actually based primarily on incidence. The major venereal diseases are *syphilis* and *gonorrhea* which together account for over 95 percent of the infectious venereal diseases. The "minor" venereal diseases are *chancroid, lymphogranuloma venereum,* and *granuloma inguinale,* which are much less common in North America. More common than any of these are the "paravenereal" diseases. These are infectious diseases which can be spread by sexual and nonsexual exposures (see Figure 9-2). Lesions of the genitalia caused by trauma, allergic contact dermatitis, and primary irritants are also very common.

V.D. symptoms, complaints, visible lesions, and complications vary

Disorders almost always acquired only by sexual contact

Disease	Common Name	Name of organism
Syphilis	"Syph" "Pox" Bad blood Chancre	*Treponema pallidum* (Spirochete)
Gonorrhea	Drip Dose Seed	*Neisseria gonorrhea* (Bacteria)
Chancroid	Soft chancre	*Hemophilus ducreyi* (Bacteria)
Lymphogranuloma venereum (LGV)	Bubo	(Possibly *bedsonia*) (Virus)
?Granuloma inguinale	Venereal ulcer, Venereal granuloma	*Donovania granulomatis* (Donovan bodies)

Disorders which may be acquired by sexual contact as well as by other person to person contacts

Disease	Common Name	Name of organism
Pediculosis pubis	Crabs	*Phthirus pubis* (louse)
Moniliasis	—	*Candida albicans* (yeast)
Herpes progenitalis	Fever blister	*Herpes simplex* (virus)
Condyloma accuminata	Venereal warts	*Papova*—DNA (virus)
Molluscum contagiosum	—	Pox virus (virus)
Scabies	"The itch"	*Sarcoptes scabiei* var. hominis (mite)
Trichomoniasis	"Trich"	*Trichomonas vaginalis* (flagellate protozoan)

Figure 9-2

considerably. A person infected with a venereal disease may have no symptoms and may be entirely unaware that he has V.D. He may or may not infect others and may or may not ever have any complications. Such silent V.D. may go away by itself or may last a lifetime.

Most people who have a major venereal disease know something is wrong. Discharge, visible lesions, pain, dysuria, or itching may occur. Symptomatic V.D. may eventually go away by itself. But it may not. The longer a person has V.D., the more likely he is to have complications. Complications range from simple scars to strictures to sterility and may lead to severe illness, insanity, or death.

V.D. may be serious business. But it need not be. V.D. is diagnosable and treatable.

Syphilis

Syphilis is an infectious disease caused by a spirochete, Treponema pallidum. It can be acquired *in utero,* by intimate contact with an infectious lesion or by blood transfusion. It is most frequently spread by sexual contacts. Although the most obvious manifestations at some stages may be localized, syphilis is a systemic disease from the onset. The course, signs, and symptoms are variable. Host defense mechanisms may lead to self-cure or the parasite may exist for a lifetime without clinical evidence of disease. On the other hand, serious sequelae which disable or kill may become manifest decades after infection. In its early stages, syphilis is treatable.

The microscopic spirochete can penetrate intact mucous membranes or abraded skin. Infection begins immediately after exposure, with spirochetes multiplying locally. Within hours, the organisms have entered the blood stream and lymphatics where they continue to divide and are carried to all organ systems where they reside, divide, and recirculate. There are no measurable signs that significant host defenses are mobilized against this early invasion by the spirochetes. No lesions, signs of inflammation, or signs of systemic toxicity occur during this early incubation stage. Tests for syphilis are negative.

As immunologic responses gradually reach measurable proportions, clinical manifestations begin to appear. Ten to ninety days (average twenty-one days) after infection has occurred, inflammatory responses begin. The first lesion to appear is at the site where the most spirochetes remain, the site of their original entry. This inflammation leads to the formation of the chancre; this stage of host-spirochete interaction is called primary syphilis.

The chancre is, characteristically, a painless, round, slightly raised lesion whose most obvious feature is a clean-based erosion (Figure 9-3). The induration may be striking, but the lesion is not bound down. It often

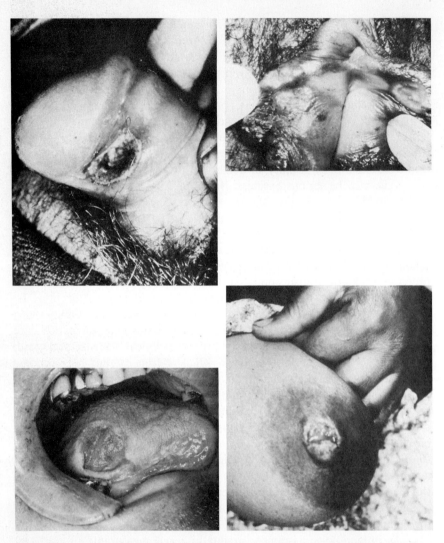

Figure 9-3 Chancre. Cleaned, based, painless ulcer surrounded by induration. (a) Penis; (b) vulva; (c) tongue; (d) nipple.

feels as though a coin were buried within the skin beneath the erosion or ulcer. This induration which extends beyond the erosion can be partially lifted or tugged with the examining fingers. The lesion is relatively non-tender. Lesions are usually single and are usually on the genitalia, but they may occur anywhere, depending upon where and how the original exposure occurred. Local, discrete, rubbery, painless adenopathy usually accompanies the appearance of the chancre. The untreated chancre usually heals in one to three months. The overt signs and symptoms may be self-limiting, despite the fact that the patient still has syphilis.

Spirochetes are present in the chancre and can be found microscopically by examining serum from the lesion. Therefore, the chancre is infectious, and it can spread syphilis by direct contact. Lesions suspected of being caused by venereal disease should be examined only with gloved hands.

Shortly after the appearance of the chancre (zero to three weeks), the serologic tests for syphilis may become positive. This simply means that by this time the immunologic reactions to the infection have reached a point at which antibodies are measurable in the blood. About six weeks after the appearance of the chancre, the continually developing immunologic responses of the host are ready for a total body reaction. The result is a generalized inflammatory response to the spirochetes which, since the beginning, have been traveling throughout the blood stream. This response has been termed secondary syphilis. If large numbers of spirochetes remain at the site of the original chancre, it may reappear at this time (chancre *redux*).

Secondary syphilis is characterized by generalized skin lesions which are nonconfluent, nonpruritic, and of uniform size and morphology. The lesions may appear on all skin surfaces, including palms, soles, and mucous membranes (Figure 9-4). The morphology may differ from one patient to another—the skin lesions of secondary syphilis may be macular, papular, papulosquamous (raised and scaling), or hyperpigmented—but on any one patient the lesions all appear the same, i.e., all macular, all papuosquamous, etc. Except in the newborn, lesions of secondary syphilis are never bullous. The size of each lesion remains relatively uniform on any one patient. The lesions remain discrete, becoming confluent only at the creases of the palms and soles or around the mouth. Secondary syphilis does not usually itch.

Internal reactions also occur during secondary syphilis. Fever, malaise, and adenopathy are common. Rarely, specific organs may be severely involved, resulting in hepatitis, nephritis, iritis, or signs of meningeal irritation. Arthritis may occur. Mucous membranes are also involved. Mucous patches are white plaques with a red base which occur in the mouth and if removed may leave denuded areas on the tongue. Moist, flat, flesh-colored papules called *condyloma lata* may group around the anogenital region or any moist area. These are sometimes mistakenly thought to be tumors or warts, and are removed surgically. Scalp involvement may lead to alopecia over the scattered skin lesions, leaving a temporary spotty, moth-eaten pattern of hair loss.

The serologic examination for antibodies is always positive by the

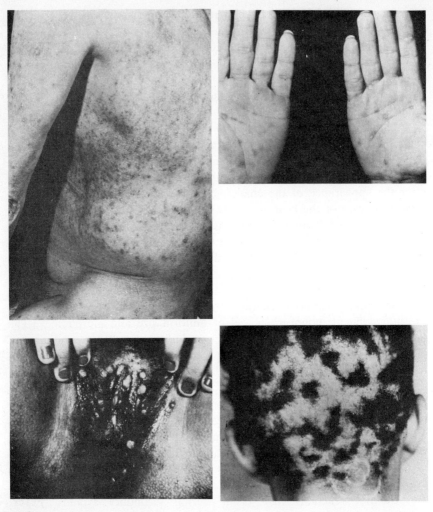

Figure 9-4 Secondary syphilis. (*a*) Generalized lesions; (*b*) palm involvement; (*c*) condyloma lata; (*d*) "moth-eaten" alopecia.

time lesions of secondary syphilis appear. The skin lesions contain viable spirochetes which may spread the infection to others. If untreated, the noticeable signs of secondary syphilis disappear over weeks to months to years. The patient may then enter a long period during which there is no evidence of infection (latent syphilis), except for the antibodies which are detectible in the blood (positive serology). He remains infected but does not appear sick. After two years he is no longer infectious to others but remains infected himself.

Primary and secondary syphilis and the first part of latent syphilis are collectively referred to as early syphilis. This is the period of infectivity. The symptoms outlined above are the classic and most common, but persons may have modified or absent symptoms during early syphilis. Early syphilis is also the time when therapy is curative.

In latent syphilis, there are no signs or symptoms. There is no way to determine infection, except by detecting antibodies. This is why routine serologies have traditionally been a part of the screening tests done on patients hospitalized for any reason. It is possible thereby to detect persons with latent syphilis. These persons should be treated.

Over many years, three things can happen to the host-spirochete balance in the chronically infected person with latent syphilis. In about one-third of such persons, the disease disappears. All clinical or serologic evidence of syphilis goes away. In another one-third, the serologic test always shows some evidence of antibodies but no clinical manifestations of disease ever occur during the remainder of that person's lifetime. In the remaining one-third of patients, late sequelae of syphilis eventually become obvious. Slowly, progressive, but severe, destructive, and scarring tissue reactions to remaining spirochetes cause permanent lesions ten to thirty years after the original infection. If such lesions are in skin, bone, or liver, no threat to life exists; but when such lesions occur in the brain, in the aorta, or in the vital centers, severe neurologic symptoms, insanity, heart disease, or death may occur.

The lesions of late syphilis are probably due to hypersensitivity to the spirochete. One or a few organisms can lead to extensive local tissue destruction. The characteristic focal lesion of late syphilis is called a gumma. In the skin, gummas may be indolent, indurated, arciform lesions that usually show signs of progression and healing at the same time. They may be psoriasiform, nodular, or noduloulcerative. The scarring and destruction are often marked and lead to perforations of palate or nose or erosion into bone. Once this state of hypersensitivity is reached, new spirochetes from another exposure may lead to gummas at the site of contact. Gummas can occur in any organ.

When syphilis involves the cardiovascular system, it usually involves the aorta, or one of its major branches. The spirochetes may lodge in the wall of the aorta during the early infectious stages of the disease; when the hyperimmune stage of host-spirochete relations is reached, scarring and destruction occur within the wall of the vessel. The aorta may become dilated, or an aneurysm may form in its ascending portion.

The destructive chronic inflammation of late syphilis may primarily affect the central nervous system. Since nerve tissue as well as blood vessels may be involved, almost any constellation of signs or symptoms may occur.

Two common symptom complexes which classically result from late syphilis of the nervous system have been named *paresis* and *tabes dorsalis*. Paresis occurs when the brain and small vessels are diffusely involved. Irritability, headache, poor memory, and character changes result. In the absence of treatment, progressive mental destruction may be followed by insanity and death. Tabes dorsalis is focal syphilitic meningitis of the posterior spinal roots and dorsal ganglia. As the nerve fibers degenerate, the patient experiences lightening pains and peripheral sensory abnormalities. Loss of sensation and position sense lead to ataxia, to joint changes, and foot ulcers secondary to repeated trauma to the insensitive extremities.

Spirochetes may be transferred via the placenta to the newborn, which may result in abortion, stillbirth, or congenital infection. Congenital syphilis may manifest itself shortly after birth with pneumonia, periostitis, rhinitis (snuffles), or a rash which may resemble that of secondary syphilis, including the appearance of condyloma lata. The only time that syphilis ever appears as bullous lesions is in the rash that occurs early in postuterine life in congenital syphilis.

As with acquired latent syphilis, the patient infected with *T. pallidum* at birth may have no signs of infection. The only evidence of his infection would be antibodies present in the serum. Late sequelae, which are comparable to the late reaction in acquired syphilis, may then appear. The manifestations of late congenital syphilis include interstitial keratitis, eighth nerve deafness, gummas, and bone and joint lesions.

Invasion of *T. pallidum* into a human host causes the development of many varieties of antibodies. The antibodies normally measured in hospital laboratories may not be those acting directly to produce or prevent clinical signs, but they do offer helpful diagnostic information. There are two basic types of antibodies:

1 Those antibodies resulting from antigens created by the complex spirochete-tissue reactions. These are called reagins and are measured in routine serology tests (also called nontreponemal tests or STS, serologic test for syphilis).
2 Those antibodies made against the organism itself. These are measured in the so-called treponemal tests.

Nontreponemal tests are *very sensitive* (very likely to detect syphilis). A high percentage of persons infected with syphilis for a long enough period will have these antibodies in measurable titer. But these tests are not completely *specific* for syphilis. That is, they may be positive in conditions other than syphilis. The treponemal tests are more *specific* for syphilis. They are too expensive and complicated to do for routine screening.

The nontreponemal tests are quick, easy, and inexpensive. If a patient has a positive nontreponemal test, a treponemal test can then be done to see if the specific antibodies against treponemes are present. The most widely accepted treponemal test is the FTA-ABS (fluorescent treponeonal antibody absorption).

When large groups of persons are screened with the nontreponemal serology test, most of them will have a negative test for syphilis. The small percentage of positive results can be explained by one of the following: (1) laboratory error, (2) syphilis, or (3) false positive (positive for some reason besides syphilis). Some of those in the last group, called biologic false positive (BFP), remain unexplained, but a high percentage of them have some explanation, as listed in Figure 9-5. Some healthy persons have reagins that give positive tests for serology. Immunizations and acute diseases listed in Figure 9-5 usually give transient, weakly positive reactions while the chronic diseases and noninfectious diseases may give strongly positive reactions that last for many years.

To determine whether the positive result was a laboratory error, the test is repeated. To determine the difference between syphilis and BFP, the more specific treponemal antibody test is performed. If the treponemal test is positive, the patient has syphilis. If it is negative, it is probably due to a BFP. The most common cause of a positive reagin test is syphilis.

Early syphilis is treatable. Early latent syphilis is treatable. Late syphilis may be treatable but scars and damaged organs cannot always be adequately repaired. The earlier syphilis is treated, the better the chance for the serology to return to negative and the lesser the chance of spreading the disease. Penicillin is the drug of choice, given in doses that maintain adequate blood levels for seven to ten days. Erythromycin or tetracycline can be given to those patients known to be allergic to penicillin.

Penicillin is adequate prophylaxis to those exposed, the amount of drug required depending upon how much time has elapsed between contact and treatment. Often contacts of infected people are treated with full courses of the drug as if they had the disease. This is done in order to avoid the theoretical possibility of lower doses masking an early infection and failing to prevent late sequelae of syphilis.

The time to treat all of the serious, crippling, family-destroying, expensive, and life-threatening late manifestations of syphilis is at the stage of the chancre. Penicillin kills spirochetes effectively only if administered to the infected patient. The biggest single challenge in treating syphilis is educating people to seek help before they have sequelae and before they pass the disease on to others. People feel encouraged to seek medical attention only if adequately informed about V.D. and if received and treated in a courteous, sympathetic, mature, and professional manner.

Infectious Diseases
  Bacterial
    Chancroid
    Leprosy
    Scarlet fever
    Pneumococcal pneumonia
    Subacute bacterial endocarditis
      (SBE)
    Tuberculosis

  Spirochetal
    Leptospirosis
    Relapsing fever
    Rat bite fever

  Viral
    Infectious hepatitis
    Infectious mononucleosis
    Measles
    Mumps
    Chicken pox
    Vaccinia
    Lymphogranuloma venereum
      (LGV)
    ?Common cold

  Other
    Malaria
    Typhus
    Trypanosomiasis
    PPLO (pleuropneumonia-like
      organisms)

Noninfectious Diseases
  Lupus erythematosus
  Scleroderma
  Rheumatoid arthritis
  Dermatomyositis
  Periarteritis nodosa
  Dysgammaglobulinemia
  Sarcoid

Pregnancy, Especially Early

Narcotic Addiction, Especially Opiates

Old Age

Figure 9–5 Causes of biologic false positive (BFP).

Gonorrhea

Gonorrhea is an infectious disease caused by the gonococcus, *Neisseria gonorrhoeae*. It is primarily a bacterial infection of mucous membranes, caused by an organism which quickly dries up and dies when removed from tissue and which therefore must be spread from person to person by direct contact from one mucous membrane to another. Dissemination is usually accomplished by sexual contact.

In males, the infection usually occurs in the anterior penile urethra with symptoms beginning two to five days (rarely much longer) after the infective exposure. Burning on urination, and a clear, white or yellow penile discharge are noted. Without treatment, these symptoms last several weeks and disappear or the infection may ascend to the posterior urethra or prostate gland. Proctitis and epididymitis may also occur.

In the female, acute gonorrhea symptoms usually do not exist. Mild and intermittent pain, tenderness, or vaginal discharge may occur but often there are no symptoms at all. The cervix is the usual site of initial infection. The postpubertal mucous membrane of the vagina seems relatively resistant to infection. The infection may persist unnoticed, it may gradually disappear, or it may ascend to infect the epithelial lining of the uterus or the fallopian tubes, or spill into the abdomen, causing acute symptomatic pelvic inflammatory disease. Proctitis can occur from direct anogenital contact or from exposure to infected vaginal discharge.

Untreated gonorrhea may lead to other complications besides those of direct mucous membrane extensions. Transient bacteremias may occur, which lead to any combination of transient arthralgias, purulent arthritis, tenosynovitis, or skin lesions. The skin lesions are characteristic. A countable number of lesions are located distally on the extremities. These begin as discrete, nonconfluent macules which progress from papules to vesicles to vesicopustules, and often further, to hemorrhagic vesicopustules surrounded by erythema.

The prepubertal vaginal mucosa itself is susceptible to the gonococcus so that bacterial vulvovaginitis can occur in young girls infected from contact with towels, clothing, or personal exposure. Newborns exposed to infected mucous membranes may acquire keratoconjunctivitis which may lead to blindness. Gonorrhea in postpubertal males and females is almost always acquired by sexual contact.

Diagnosis can be confirmed by finding the gram-negative diplococcus in a smear and by growing the organism in culture. The organism dies quickly when exposed to air. Smears must be rapidly planted on special media and immediately placed in optimum growing conditions.

The treatment of choice is penicillin. Whereas the goal of penicillin therapy of syphilis is to achieve prolonged modest blood levels, the goal

of treatment of gonorrhea is to reach high levels briefly. The clinical complications require higher and more prolonged dosages than simple male
urethritis, or the routinely discovered female carrier. The increase in relative penicillin resistance, as demonstrated in the laboratory, and the hazard
of penicillin allergy, make therapy with tetracycline or erythromycin a reasonable alternative. Contact tracing, routine screening for asymptomatic
carriers, patient education, and receptive attitudes are all equally important
parts of the therapy of gonorrhea.

Chancroid

Chancroid is an acute localized bacterial infection which is usually spread
by sexual contact. Two to five days after exposure, a vesicopustule noted
on the genitalia rapidly breaks down to form a painful purulent ulcer with
undermined edges. Other lesions may occur from accidental autoinoculation. Tender adenopathy may occur. The tender, foul-smelling, purulent,
deep, and undermined ulcer of chancroid contrasts with the clean-based,
nonpainful erosion of primary syphilis. Syphilis and chancroid may coexist,
however.

Chancroid is caused by *Hemophilus ducreyi*, a gram-negative bacillus
which can be seen in smear or grown with difficulty, using special culture
techniques. Sulfonamides are specific therapy. Tetracycline or streptomycin
are alternative drugs. Penicillin is not effective.

Lymphogranuloma Venereum

Lymphogranuloma venereum (LGV) is a viral disease primarily affecting
the lymphatic system. A transient, unimpressive, painless skin lesion, usually acquired by sexual exposure, is followed by regional lymphadenitis.
The serious long-term complications are the result of lymphatic obstruction.

Often the first manifestation noticed is the inguinal bubo. Firm, tender
adenopathy progresses to a larger mass formed by several nodes bound
to one another by inflammation about the nodes. The skin over the nodes
may break down and drain seropurulent fluid. The inguinal ligament may
pass through and indent the large mat of inguinal nodes causing the characteristic "groove sign." Late complications resulting from scarring and obstruction of lymph channels include elephantiasis of the genitalia, rectal
stricture, and protrusion of polypoid masses.

Diagnosis is based upon clinical features and diagnostic procedures,
which include a serum antibody test, skin test (Frei test), and skin biopsies.
The disease responds to wide spectrum antibiotics. The complications
caused by scarring may respond to surgery.

Granuloma Inguinale

Granuloma inguinale is a contagious, chronic, granulomatous process which usually occurs in the anogenital or inguinal region. It is caused by gram-negative, encapsulated, parasitic organisms called Donovan bodies which grow intracellularly. Its incubation period and mode of spread are not certain. Venereal spread is accepted as the most likely, but person to person transmissions are not often observed. Since there is some evidence that Donovan bodies may be a natural inhabitant of the bowel, it is possible that they secondarily invade other traumatic or infected lesions of the genital region.

The process starts with a small nodule on the genitalia which erodes and becomes filled with velvety red granulation. The lesions gradually spread to involve large areas of the inguinal region. The advancing border has a red, raised, rolled edge and the central lesion may be filled with beefy-red, granulation tissue or ulcers. Involvement around lymph nodes can simulate adenopathy. Scarring can lead to distortion of genitalia and to lymphedema.

Diagnosis is confirmed by finding the organism in tissue spread or from biopsy. Two weeks of tetracycline is specific therapy. Chloramphenicol, erythromycin, and streptomycin are also effective, but penicillin is ineffective.

REFERENCES

Abrams, A. J.: "Lymphogranuloma Venereum," *JAMA* **205**:199–202, July 1968.

Alergant, C. D.: "Chancroid," *Practitioner* **209**:624–627, November 1972.

Brown, W. J., et al.: *Syphilis and Other Venereal Diseases,* Harvard University Press, Boston, 1970.

Burket, L. W.: *Oral Medicine: Diagnosis and Treatment,* J. B. Lippincott Company, Philadelphia, 1971.

Cohen, L.: "Oral Candidiasis: Its Diagnosis and Treatement," *J. Oral. Med.* **27**:7–11, January–March 1972.

Davis, C. M.: "Granuloma Inguinale: A Clinical, Histological and Ultrastructural Study," *JAMA* **211**:632–636, January 1970.

Graykowski, E. A., M. F. Barile, and W. B. Lee: "Recurrent Aphthous Stomatitis," *JAMA* **196**:637–644, May 1966.

Johnson, R. L.: "Ulcerative Lesions of the Oral Cavity," *Otolaryngol Clin. North Amer.* **5**:231–247, June 1972.

Krull, E. A., A. C. Fellman, and L. A. Fabian: "White Lesions of the Mouth," *Clinical Symposia,* **25**(2): 1973.

McCarthy, P. L., and G. Shklar: *Diseases of the Oral Mucosa: Diagnosis, Management, Therapy,* McGraw-Hill Book Company, New York, 1964.

Rudolph, A. H.: "Control of Gonorrhea: Guidelines for Antibiotic Treatment," *JAMA* **220:**1587–1589, June 1972.

Ship, I., and D. A. Galili: "Systemic Significance of Mouth Ulcers," *Postgrad. Med.* **49:**67–72, January 1971.

Sim, S. K., et al.: "Chemotherapy of Gonorrhea: A Review of Current Status," *Can. Med. Ass. J.* **107:**986–992, November 1972.

Sparling, P. F.: "Diagnosis and Treatment of Syphilis," *N. Eng. J. Med.* **284:**642–653, March 1971.

Syphilis: A Synopsis, Public Health Service Publication #1660, U.S. Government Printing Office, Washington, D.C., 1968.

Tindall, J. P., and J. L. Callaway: "Hand-Foot-and-Mouth Diseases—It's More Common Than You Think," *Am. J. Dis. Child.* **124:**372–375, September 1972.

Chapter 10

Skin Cancer

Skin tumors
Etiology of skin cancer
Basal cell carcinoma
Squamous cell carcinoma
Malignant melanoma

SKIN TUMORS

The word tumor is used in many ways and, therefore, expresses general and nonspecific information. Tumor literally means swelling. Edema, one of the traditional signs of inflammation, is tumor. However, the term is most often used to describe a local excess of tissue, including malformations, as well as benign and malignant neoplasms. Some experts, however, restrict the use of the word tumor to neoplasms while others use it to refer specifically to malignant neoplasms.

The literal meaning of neoplasm is "new growth." This term is usually used to describe a group of cells which grow uncontrolled by the normal regulatory mechanisms of the organ system. Neoplasia differs from hyperplasia, in which an entire organ or parts of an organ increase in size in a regular, regulated, and harmonious fashion. The degree of maturity, differentiation, maturation, and cell size of neoplastic cells may be greater or less than that of normal cells. The major difference between neoplastic cells and normal cells is that the former do not work in harmony to serve the specific function of the organ and are not regulated by the normal growth-limiting factors.

Benign neoplasms may expand or compress surrounding tissues but they do not begin new growths elsewhere beyond their own tumor mass or outside the organ system. Malignant tumor cells are so defiant of the normal growth-regulatory mechanisms that the cells are able not only to grow at a higher than normal rate and to invade and destroy normal surrounding tissue, they are also able to survive and divide in new surroundings, either inside or outside the organ of origin. This distant growth is a metastasis.

In addition to this definitive sign of malignancy, other criteria are also used. Pathologists use histologic criteria based on number and form of mitoses, nuclear pattern and size, destruction or maintenance of normal architecture, and extension through tissue-limiting membranes. Clinicians may define a malignant tumor as one which kills the host. Cancer is the term often used to describe a malignant tumor, a growth consisting of cells which defy regulatory influences and can, therefore, metastasize. Carcinoma refers to a malignant neoplasm of epithelial cells. Malignant neoplasms of mesenchymal tissue (connective tissue, blood vessels, muscle, fibroblasts, bone, etc.) are called sarcomas.

In most instances the causes of malignant change are not known and are probably multiple. Somatic gene mutations may result in the acquisition of some biologic property which either supports malignancy of a cell or results in loss of ability to respond to control factors. Chemicals, x-irradiation, viruses, ultraviolet light, and hormones play permissive, supportive, or causative roles in some cancers. Cells that have been inactive since intrauterine development may persist and begin to grow in adult life. Actually, cells which no longer respond to normal regulating factors may arise more often than is recognized, but these cells may be altered in such a way that the immune system recognizes them as abnormal or "not self" and destroys them. If such is the case, cancers may result from a failure of this immune mechanism.

Some types of skin lesions, especially those induced by chronic sun exposure, seem to progress into cancer if left untreated. Such skin lesions are sometimes called "premalignant." Such a term cannot be accurately used to prognosticate about a particular lesion; it is a statistical statement suggesting that a high number of cancers do eventually arise from such "premalignant" lesions. The term also suggests that acquisition of malignant properties is not a sudden event that occurs in a single generation of cells but is the result of the addition of various biologic properties which are acquired serially over several cell generations. The skin happens to be the only organ in which these developments are easily available for continuous observation. When hyperplastic skin begins to have atypical cells and becomes slightly less regular and regulated in its growth, the corresponding morphologic changes may be grossly visible. Such lesions are noticed long before they have acquired the full status of biologic malignancy with ability to invade blood vessels or survive in sites other than skin. "Carcinoma *in situ*" refers to lesions which have the atypical cellular structure required to suggest malignant change to the pathologist, but which have remained completely confined to their site of origin without invading blood vessels or membrane barriers.

Actinic or solar keratoses are lesions which have cellular atypism and have lost the normal orderly arrangement of the epidermal cells (Figure 10-1*a*). Actinic comes from the Greek word for ray and suggests the relationship to radiation. Actinic keratoses have been shown—by epidemiology, by anatomic site of occurrence, and by accompanying "solar" or "actinic" dermal changes—to be related to sun exposure (see Chapter 5). An actinic keratosis is a premalignant lesion occurring on sun-exposed surfaces and presenting as a slightly elevated, dry, hyperkeratotic, scaly papule. The surface can be flat, rough, or verrucous. The scale is adherent and, characteristically, returns each time it is removed, the chronicity becoming an important factor in differentiating the lesion from more benign causes of keratotic papules. The hyperkeratosis may be excessive, creating a cutaneous horn (Figure 10-1*c*). Erythema and minimal induration may surround the lesion. Actinic keratoses are often multiple.

Treatment should be removal or destruction of lesions early in their development. Curettage, electrosurgery, cryosurgery, chemical caustics, or

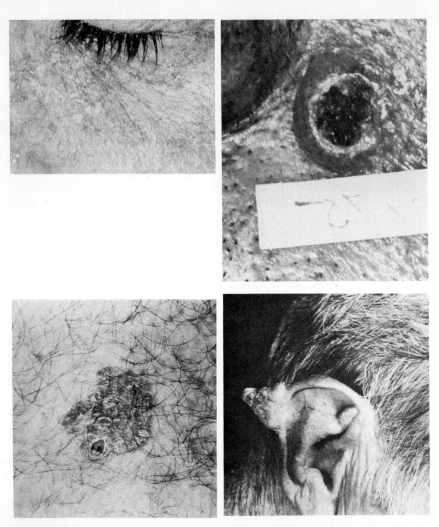

Figure 10-1 Skin tumors. (a) Actinic keratosis; telangiectasia, erytnema, crusting; (b) keratoacanthoma; a keratinous plug in a crater formed by rolled, elevated epidermis; (c) cutaneous horn; (d) Bowen's disease.

topical application of 5-fluorouracil, an antimetabolite, accomplishes this goal. Large, indurated, or recurrent lesions should be biopsied to rule out squamous cell carcinoma.

Bowen's disease is an intraepidermal carcinoma which represents carcinoma *in situ* (Figure 10-1*d*). The course is usually chronic and benign but invasion and metastasis can occur. Lesions are usually solitary and can occur on any exposed or unexposed site. A discrete, slightly erythematous brown plaque is covered by varying amounts of scale. Configuration is irregular with a polycyclic border and islands of normal skin scattered through the lesion. Nodules, erosions, crusting, and hyperpigmentation may occur irregularly over the slowly growing lesion.

Statistical studies suggest that patients with Bowen's disease have a higher than normal incidence of noncutaneous internal malignancies. This fact, along with the absence of a clear relationship to sun exposure and the occurrence of Bowen's disease in persons ingesting arsenicals, suggests that the development of Bowen's disease may be related to chemical carcinogens. Treatment of choice is surgical removal.

Most skin tumors are benign. Moles, lentigines, and nevi are malformations. Warts, skin tags, seborrheic keratoses, and molluscum contagiosum are benign neoplasms. The word keratosis used alone means any keratotic papule, horny growth, or cornification, including seborrheic keratoses, warts, calluses, and others. Therefore the term keratosis does not imply malignancy. Similarly, cutaneous horns are not all malignant but may be caused by benign epidermal hyperplasia, keratoacanthoma, or wart virus. Biopsy which includes tissue from the base of the lesion is the one sure way to determine the cause of a cutaneous horn.

Many different kinds of malformations and benign neoplasms may arise from the sweat glands and pilosebaceous units. Cells of the skin appendages and of the basal layer of the epidermis remain pluripotent; i.e., they remain capable of differentiating toward any of the epidermal specializations to look like and perform like manufacturers of hair, sebum, stratum corneum, sweat ducts, etc. Therefore, cell differentiation or morphology may not be directly related to the microanatomic site of origin of a tumor. Malignant neoplasms of appendage structures are rare.

When the term skin cancer is used, it most often refers to basal cell carcinoma or squamous cell carcinoma. These skin neoplasms, however, are difficult to classify in terms of biologic activity. The basal cell carcinoma does meet many of the pathologist's microscopic criteria for malignancy but rarely metastasizes or kills. The squamous cell carcinoma can be malignant by every criterion but is usually treatable and curable in its early stages.

It is true, however, that untreated skin cancer can lead to disfigurement, discomfort, and death. Such an occurrence is unfortunate because skin cancer is recognizable and treatable at early stages. To a large extent, many skin cancers are preventable. Malignant melanoma can metastasize and kill. Its early recognition can be life-saving.

ETIOLOGY OF SKIN CANCER

Epidemiologic and experimental evidence has shown that chronic systemic administration of arsenic may lead to premalignant keratosis, Bowen's disease, and carcinoma. Arsenical compounds have been used in medicines (Fowler's solution, Asiatic pills, Dover's powder), insecticides, and herbicides. Chronic ingestion may lead to keratoses of palms and soles, scattered macular hyper- and hypopigmentation, and increase in the incidence of various premalignant and malignant neoplasms of the skin and other organs. Carcinoma of the scrotum, found frequently in chimney sweeps, was found to be related to soot collected in the folds of the scrotal skin. Skin cancer is among the late complications of x-irradiation and radium exposure.

The most frequent, most preventable, and least disputed exogenous factor in the cause of skin cancer is chronic sun exposure. Persons with less pigment receive more ultraviolet penetration and have a higher incidence of skin cancer. Genetic factors also play a role. Celtic people not only have less pigment to block ultraviolet radiation, but they may also be more prone to development of skin cancer from the sun exposure which they absorb.

The role of ultraviolet light in causing skin cancer has been reinforced by studies of a rare recessive hereditary disorder called xeroderma pigmentosum which is characterized by a severe intolerance of the skin and eyes to light. Photophobia, persistent erythema, and pigmentation occur early in life. Premature wrinkling and early degeneration of the skin is followed by multiple skin cancers in childhood. Death may occur in early adult life as a complication of widespread cutaneous malignancies. It has been shown that these patients have an enzymatic defect which prevents them from being able to repair the usual damage which ultraviolet radiation causes to DNA.

BASAL CELL CARCINOMA

Basal cell carcinoma (basal cell epithelioma, rodent ulcer) is not only the most frequently encountered of the skin cancers, but probably the most common human malignancy (Color Plate III*A*, back endpaper). It is derived from pluripotent basal cells of the epidermis. The tumor is caused by a local change or defect in the basal cell which prevents the cell from maturing and keratinizing normally yet allows it to retain the property of cell replication. The cells do not become squamous cells (prickle cells) and stratum corneum and then fall off the surface; they remain as basal cells and as they continue to divide an enlarging mass results. Although it grows slowly, basal cell carcinoma can invade subcutaneous tissue, bone, or any other tissue. Because the tumor rarely metastasizes, some experts prefer the name basal cell epithelioma to that of basal cell carcinoma. Both terms are widely used and refer to the same lesion.

Sunlight is a major causative factor. Basal cell carcinomas are more frequent on sun-exposed areas, in fair-skinned Caucasians, in outdoor workers in southern sunny climates, and in older persons. Genetic diathesis, arsenicals, x-irradiation, scars, and some types of nevi may also predispose to basal cell carcinoma.

The most characteristic presentation is the noduloulcerative basal cell carcinoma. This lesion begins as a small, slowly enlarging papule. The borders of the lesion assume a semitranslucent, ground glass, or "pearly" appearance as the center begins to erode, ulcerate, and become depressed. The epidermis is stretched thin over the border, showing dilated capillaries (telangiectasia) and is missing in the center of larger lesions (rodent ulcer). The tumor smooths away skin markings and destroys other skin structures as it enlarges; it usually maintains its rolled "pearly" edge as it progresses. Pigment in varying amounts may be scattered throughout the lesion.

Basal cell epitheliomas may be deep and erosive, firm and morphea-like, or they may be superficial erythematous lesions with thin epidermis and fine semitranslucent borders. The most typical of lesions are characteristic enough to make clinical diagnosis possible. However, because of the destructive nature of treatment, because of the invasive potential, and because many atypical forms exist, the safest way to make the diagnosis is by histologic examination.

Basal cell carcinomas should be removed or destroyed. Conventional excisional surgery as well as chemosurgery, electrosurgery, and cryosurgery are used. Some lesions, especially those of the central face, are best treated with x-ray therapy. Success with each of these modalities is good with cure rates of well over 95 percent. Those that do recur are usually only local recurrences. Selection of treatment must be based on consideration of anatomic site of lesion, expected cosmetic results, patient's age, physician's expertise, and equipment at hand.

SQUAMOUS CELL CARCINOMA

Squamous cell carcinoma (epidermoid carcinoma) is a malignant tumor of the prickle (squamous) cell of the epidermis (Color Plate III*B*). Rate of growth is variable but invasion into dermis and surrounding tissue is unrelenting. If untreated, metastasis to regional nodes will eventually occur.

Squamous cell carcinoma may arise from what appears to be normal skin, but it frequently occurs in areas of chronic solar degeneration, scar, chronic irritation, and on skin damaged by thermal burn, x-irradiation, or chronic draining fistulae. It may arise from preexisting skin lesions such as discoid lupus erythematosis or tuberculosis of the skin, or more commonly from actinic or arsenical keratosis. The risk of metastatic squamous cell carcinoma arising from preexisting actinic keratosis is minimal. Those lesions arising from chronic scarred, irritated, or dermatitic skin or from normal skin are most likely to metastasize. Squamous cell carcinoma arising from lip, penis, vulva, and anus are dangerous lesions, prone to early and multiple metastasis.

Appearance is variable. Early lesions may look like arsenical or solar keratosis, Bowen's disease, or erythroplasia, except with slightly more in-

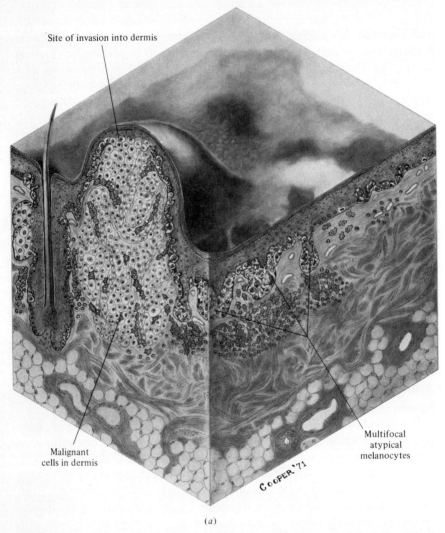

Site of invasion into dermis

Malignant
cells in dermis

Multifocal
atypical
melanocytes

COOPER '71

(*a*)

Figure 10-2 Diagram of types of malignant melanoma. (*a*) Melanoma type I (lentigo maligna melanoma); (*b*) melanoma type II (superficial spreading melanoma); (*c*) melanoma type III (nodular melanoma); (*d*) malignant melanoma. Levels of tumor invasion. (*Used with permission of Thomas B. Fitzpatrick, M.D. and Martin C. Mihm, Jr., M.D.*)

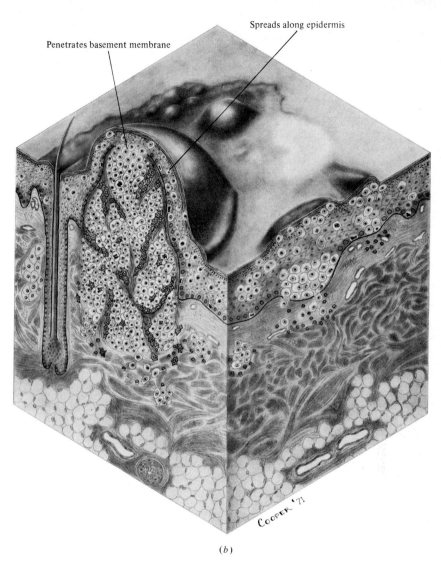

(b)

Figure 10-2 For legend see opposite page.

duration. Firm nodules with indistinct borders may be covered with scale or may ulcerate. As the lesion enlarges, firmness increases and the lesion becomes fixed to deeper tissue. Advancing rolled edges of relatively normal epidermis may leave behind a central ugly area of vegetation and ulceration, but, more commonly, abnormal keratinization results in the lesion being covered with scale or horn. Early surgical removal or complete destruction is the treatment choice. All skin cancer patients should be instructed in the use of sunscreens and should return for inspection of their skins at regular intervals.

Keratoacanthomas (KA) are rapidly growing crateriform skin tumors. Although they have a histologic similarity to invasive squamous cell carcinoma, most keratoacanthomas eventually regress or disappear. They occur on exposed hairy skin, grow rapidly to 1 to 3 centimeters in size, and slowly involute over several months. They are probably of multiple etiol-

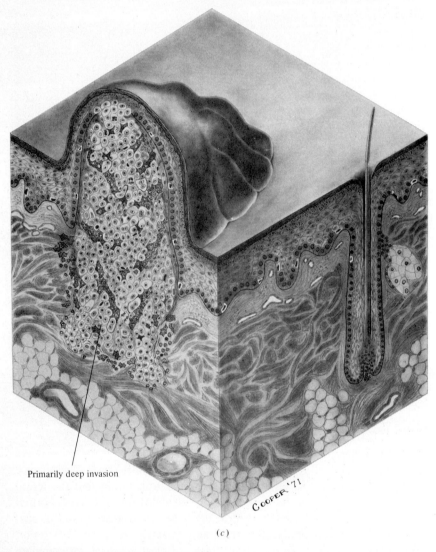

Primarily deep invasion

(c)

Figure 10-2 For legend see page 208.

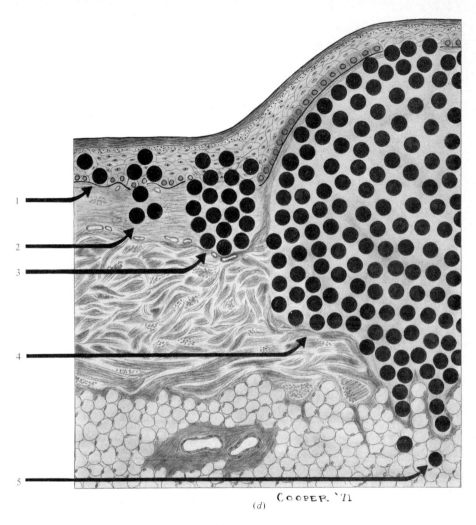

(d) COOPER. '71

Figure 10-2 For legend see page 208.

ogy. Keratoacanthomas have been produced experimentally in animals and accidentally in man by trauma, insect bite, viruses, and chemical carcinogens. Hereditary multiple keratoacanthomas occur.

A bud-shaped, dome-shaped lesion appears as a cup filled with a firm, granular keratin plug (Figure 10-1b). Although such lesions can be expected to regress, they are usually removed for cosmetic, practical, and diagnostic reasons. Spontaneous regression may leave a scar which is more unsightly than that caused by careful surgical removal.

MALIGNANT MELANOMA

Malignant melanoma is a neoplasm of melanocytes which is malignant and which has the potential for invasion, widespread metastasis, and subsequent death. The tumor is rare before puberty but can occur at any age. It occurs slightly more frequently in sun-exposed areas but may occur anywhere on the skin, the eye, or on mucous membranes. Patients with congenital pigmented hairy nevi and xeroderma pigmentosa are predisposed to the development of malignant melanoma.

Lentigo maligna is a hyperpigmented flat spot which occurs primarily on the faces of older persons (Color Plate IIIC). It begins as a tan freckle-like lesion but grows in size and changes in outline and color as it spreads. Reticulate areas of brown, black, and white appear. Lentigo maligna is a premalignant lesion. Biopsy shows atypical melanocytes. As many as one-third give rise to invasive malignant melanoma.

Even though 20 to 30 percent of malignant melanomas arise from the melanocytes of moles, moles (nevus cell nevus—see Chapter 3) should not be considered premalignant. Melanoma is more likely to occur in a mole than in adjacent normal skin, simply because there are more melanocytes in the mole. Each individual melanocyte within the mole is no more prone to malignant changes than are other melanocytes anywhere in the skin. Therefore, with the exception of the repeatedly irritated or traumatized mole, the only medical indication for removing a mole is the presence of features which suggest malignant melanoma.

Melanomas can be classified according to their major histologic mode of spread which correlates with their gross appearance and their malignant aggressiveness (Figure 10-2 and Color Plates IIID, E, F). Type I arises from lentigo maligna which already has widespread multifocal atypical collections of melanocytes. Malignant melanoma is considered to be present when this process breaks through the basement membrane into the dermis. Type II, also called superficial spreading melanoma, spreads primarily along the epidermis but penetrates the basement membrane and metastasizes. Type III, also called nodular melanoma, invades deeply from the beginning. A nodule of malignant melanocytes pushes up to make an elevated mass and down to invade dermis and subcutaneous tissues.

In all of these types of melanoma, the survival rate is correlated with depth of invasion. Treatment is complete, wide, and full-thickness surgical removal of the lesion, followed by skin grafting. The major life-saving step is early diagnosis and removal before metastasis occurs. There is no satisfactory treatment for metastatic malignant melanoma.

Malignant melanoma is a killer. Early diagnosis saves lives. Every person who examines, cares for, bathes, dresses, or attends the sick and injured patient should be trained to recognize early lesions. The signs of malignancy of a pigmented lesion are three:

1 *Variegated color, including red, white, and blue.* Lesions which are brown, tan, or black, especially if uniformly pigmented, are usually benign. The presence of red or white or blue shades within a pigmented lesion, especially when the colors are quite varied, is suggestive of malignancy.

2 *Irregular border.* A sizable notch in the border of a pigmented lesion is suggestive of malignant melanoma.

3 *Irregular surface.* Uneven elevations, loss of skin markings, and irregular topography suggest malignant melanoma.

Whenever questions arise, a skin biopsy is diagnostic.

REFERENCES

Advances in Biology of Skin, Vol. VII, Carcinogenesis, "Ultraviolet Radiation and Skin Cancer in Man," Montagna, W., and R. L. Dobson, eds, Pergamon Press, New York, 1966, pp. 195–214.

Belisario, J. C.: *Cancer of the Skin,* Butterworth and Co., (Publishers), Ltd., London, 1959.

Blum, H. F.: *Carcinogenesis by Ultraviolet Light,* Princeton University Press, Princeton, N.J., 1959.

Freeman, R. G., J. M. Knox, and C. L. Heaton: "The Treatment of Skin Cancer," *Cancer* **17:**535–538, April 1964.

McGovern, V. K., and M. M. Lane-Brown: *The Nature of Melanoma,* Charles C Thomas, Publisher, Springfield, Ill., 1969.

Mihm, M. C. Jr., T. B. Fitzpatrick, M. M. Lane-Brown, et al.: "Early Detection of Cutaneous Malignant Melanoma: A Color Atlas," *N. Eng. J. Med.* **289:**989–996, 1973.

Chapter 11

Cutaneous Signs of Systemic Disease

Skin signs of ill patients

Drug eruptions
Scarlet fever
Measles
German measles
Viral exanthems
Typhoid fever
Secondary syphilis
Erythema marginatum
Serum sickness

Chicken pox and Herpes zoster
Variola
Rocky Mountain spotted fever
Gonococcemia
Meningococcemia
Staphylococcemia
Pseudomonas septicemia
Subacute bacterial endocarditis

Skin signs of endocrine and metabolic disorders

Pituitary
Thyroid

Diabetes mellitus

Skin signs of diseases of connective tissue

Lupus erythematosis
Dermatomyositis

Scleroderma

Mastocytosis

Histiocytosis

Skin signs of diseases which affect the gastrointestinal tract

Peutz-Jegher syndrome
Hereditary hemorrhagic
telangiectasia

Pyoderma gangrenosum
Acrodermatitis enteropathica

Cancer, lymphoma, leukemia, and mycosis fungoides

Sarcoidosis

Miscellaneous conditions

Summary

SKIN SIGNS OF ILL PATIENTS (Fever and Rash)

The skin is one of the best indicators of general health. Young persons in good health have a certain glow, unwrinkled skin, and a wholesome complexion. However, we seldom notice skin for its normalcy, its absence of sun damage and skin disorders, or its reflection of good health. When health is impaired, the skin may provide important signs of the absence of health. Pallor connotes fewer red blood cells in the skin because of anemia, peripheral vasoconstriction, or central or dependent pooling of blood. The first sign of liver disease may be jaundice noted in the skin, or on mucous membranes. Fever may be noted by the warmth of the skin. Sweating may accompany a sudden fall in temperature or sympathetic nervous system discharges. Changes in skin turgor, moisture, pigmentation, and hair distribution give clues about electrolyte, endocrine, and nutritional status.

During illnesses patients often develop rashes. Since the rash of many diseases is relatively characteristic, special attention to skin changes may make diagnosis possible. In some illnesses, the *morphology, distribution,* and *arrangement* of skin lesions gives important clues to the etiology of the illness. It is important to note the *timing* of the rash (the temporal relationship of the rash to the other symptoms) and its *duration.* Additional information comes from noting the *evolution* of the rash—both the sequence in which various parts of the body are involved and the changes in individual lesions over the course of time.

Figure 11-1 lists some diseases in which a rash may accompany a febrile illness. On this chart, diseases are separated by the morphology of the skin lesions. Other characteristics will be discussed under each illness. Drug eruption and erythema multiforme which can have varied morphologies are listed in all three columns.

Drug Eruptions

When approaching the sick patient who has a rash, always consider drug eruptions as a possible cause for the skin eruption (Color Plate IV *A,* back endpaper). Drug eruptions may assume any morphology. They may exhibit macular, papular, urticarial, bullous, eczematous, or other expressions. Almost any drug can cause a drug eruption. Although in some cases drug eruptions are accompanied by involvement of other organ systems, most drug eruptions are manifested clinically entirely in the skin.

Allergic mechanisms appear to be the most likely explanation for drug eruptions, but this has been well demonstrated only with penicillin eruptions, insulin urticaria, and some photoallergic compounds. Urticarial eruptions which begin within hours after administration of a drug may be medi-

Diagnosis according to morphology of individual lesion*

Diseases Manifested by Macules or Papules	Diseases Manifested by Vesicles, Bullae, or Pustules	Diseases Manifested by Purpuric Macules, Purpuric Papules, or Purpuric Vesicles
Drug hypersensitivities	Drug hypersensitivities	Drug hypersensitivities
Scarlet fever	Dermatitis from	Bacteremia[2]:
Measles (rubeola)	plants (5)	Meningococcemia
German measles	Varicella (chicken	(acute or chronic)
(rubella)	pox)	Gonococcemia
Viral exanthems	Generalized herpes	Staphylococcemia
(ECHO, coxsackie,	zoster	Pseudomonas bacter-
adenovirus)	Disseminated herpes	emia
Typhoid fever	simplex[1]	Subacute bacterial
Secondary syphilis	Eczema herpeticum	endocarditis
Rocky Mountain spotted	(7)	Enterovirus infections
fever (early lesions)	Disseminated	(ECHO and coxsackie)
Pityriasis rosea	vaccinia[1] (7)	Rickettsial diseases:
Erythema multiforme	Eczema vaccinatum	Rocky Mountain
(5, 12)	(7)	spotted fever
Erythema marginatum	Variola[1]	"Allergic" vasculitis
Systemic lupus	Enterovirus infections	
erythematosus	(ECHO and cox-	
Dermatomyositis	sackie), including	
"Serum sickness"	hand-foot-mouth	
(manifested only as	disease	
wheals)	Toxic epidermal	
	necrolysis (12)	
	Erythema multiforme	
	bullosum (5, 12)	

* Modified from "Fundamentals of Dermatologic Diagnosis," by T. B. Fitzpatrick, D. P. Johnson, and M. Fisher in *Dermatology in General Medicine,* T. B. Fitzpatrick, K. A. Arndt, W. H. Clark, Jr., A. Z. Eisen, E. J. Van Scott, and J. G. Vaughn (eds.), McGraw-Hill Book Company, New York, 1971. Numbers in parentheses refer to chapters in the present text.

[1] The characteristic lesion of these exanthems is an umbilicated papule or vesicle on an erythematous base.

[2] Often presents as infarcts.

Figure 11–1   Rashes in the seriously ill patient.

ated by IgE or skin-sensitizing antibodies and may be a signal of anaphylaxis. The more typical appearance of a drug eruption is that of an erythematous, macular and papular, semiconfluent eruption which is generalized in distribution, is symmetrical, and is of relatively sudden onset. When this type of drug eruption is caused by penicillin, a measurable IgM and IgG antibody rise has been demonstrated (see Chapter 5).

Scarlet Fever (Scarlatina)

Scarlet fever (scarlatina) is caused by a streptococcal infection (Color Plate IV*B*). A painful tonsillopharyngitis with lymphadenopathy is followed by the appearance of a diffuse erythematous rash. A traumatic or surgical wound infected with streptococci may also lead to the rash. The vasodilation is caused by an erythrogenic toxin elaborated by some strains of group A streptococci. Redness usually appears on the neck first, then rapidly spreads to the trunk, and then to the extremities, sparing the palms and soles. Total involvement of the body is complete in about thirty-six hours. Superimposed on a diffuse bright red background, there are countless punctate papular lesions at the site of hair follicles. These papules give the skin the feel of rough sandpaper.

On the face, there are usually no discrete papules, but a marked flushing of the cheeks and forehead contrasts sharply with a characteristic absence of redness about the mouth (circumoral pallor). The rash is accentuated in the body folds, especially the antecubital fossae; the eruptions in these locations may become petechial (Pastia's sign). Purpuric macules or vesicles may be present on the palate and uvula. On the tongue, which is usually coated, there are enlarged red fungiform papillae, giving the appearance of a "strawberry tongue." Desquamation occurs in thin sheets as the eruption fades.

Measles (Rubeola; Morbilli)

Measles (rubeola; morbilli) is a contagious systemic viral disease (Color Plate IV*C*). The illness is characterized by a three to four day prodromal period of coryza, conjunctivitis with photophobia, a "barking" cough, and, finally, the appearance of blotchy macular erythema of the soft palate. Often appearing 1 to 2 days before the rash are the Koplik spots, characteristic tiny white lesions surrounded by an erythematous ring ("grains of sand"). Koplik's spots are usually found on the buccal mucosa opposite the second molars. They may last until the first or second day of the body rash.

The purplish-red rash appears first on the neck, behind the ears, and over the forehead and then spreads slowly to involve the entire body by the third day. The eruption extends over the shoulders and trunk and then distally over the upper and lower extremities. As new discrete macular lesions extend downward and distally, the erythema on the sites first involved becomes more and more confluent. The rash lasts a week or more, may take on a brownish hue, and finally fades away with mild desquamation.

German Measles (Rubella)

German measles (rubella) is a virus infection which is probably spread by respiratory transmission. It is most important because of the association of birth defects with *intrauterine* infection. A mild prodrome consists of fever and malaise and lymphadenopathy which involves the suboccipital, postauricular, and cervical nodes. After the appearance of the lymphadenopathy, the rash appears on the hairline and face and rapidly proceeds to involve the entire body within twenty-four to thirty-six hours. In contrast with the rash of measles, the rash of rubella disappears from each site as it spreads and is not associated with desquamation. It lasts only two to three days. Young adult and teenage females with rubella often have accompanying arthralgias. The infection can be documented by laboratory examination of antibody levels during acute and convalescent phases.

Viral Exanthems

Generalized infection with the enterovirus (coxsackie and ECHO) and adenovirus groups cause malaise, myalgias, a low grade temperature rise, and mild upper respiration symptoms. These symptoms may precede or accompany a generalized macular and papular semiconfluent erythematous eruption which is difficult to distinguish from a drug eruption. Bilaterally symmetrical urticarial eruptions, as well as macular, papular, and finely vesicular eruptions, may also occur. There may be a vesicular enanthem, especially on the palate or the posterior oropharynx. Hand-foot-and-mouth disease is an infectious disease caused by coxsackie virus which causes small tender linear blisters surrounded by erythema. The blisters are located on the hands and feet, and within the mouth.

Typhoid Fever (Enteric Fever)

Typhoid fever is an acute illness caused by the bacterium *Salmonella typhosa,* which is manifested by fever, headache, prostration, cough, leukopenia, and a rash. Seven to ten days after the appearance of the high temperature, characteristic "rose spots" appear on the upper abdomen, the lower anterior chest, and the mid-back. At a given time, they usually number 10 to 30, and appear as discrete 2 to 4 millimeter blanchable pink papules. Individual lesions last three to four days and may become brownish before they disappear. New crops continue to emerge over a two to three week period. Bacteria may be found in the skin lesions.

Secondary Syphilis

Although they can have a great variety of presentations on the skin, the classic lesions of secondary syphilis (see Chapter 9) are generalized, nonconfluent, erythematous, nonpruritic lesions of uniform size and morphology which often include palms, soles, and mucous membranes. Patients with secondary syphilis may feel ill and may often have a low grade temperature rise and generalized adenopathy.

Erythema Marginatum

Erythema marginatum is seen in about 10 percent of patients with acute rheumatic fever. The lesions begin as simple red papules or macules, but quickly enlarge to spread peripherally and clear centrally. Several red rings may join to form annular and gyrate lesions with borders which may be flat or raised. The outstanding feature of the eruption is the rapid movement of the ringed lesions (within hours to days) to form polycyclic, irregular, geographic lesions that seem to move over the trunk and proximal extremities. The rash usually comes after the joint involvement, and is often associated with carditis.

Serum Sickness

Serum sickness is an allergic reaction characterized by skin eruption, edema, fever, joint pain, lymphoadenopathy, and malaise. Erythema and intense pruritus may appear initially and most intensely at the site at which serum or a drug was administered. Urticarial lesions follow. The rash can progress further, to look like erythema multiforme or vasculitis. The most common skin manifestation is urticaria. Serum sickness is caused by circulating antigen-antibody complexes, and, therefore, its onset is several to ten days after initial exposure to the antigen, after the immune system has had time to produce antibodies. There may be renal involvement.

Chicken Pox and Herpes Zoster

Infection with the zoster-varicella virus may be asymptomatic. If symptoms are produced, one of two clinical entities develops, depending on the absence or presence of antibodies in the host. In the nonimmune host, there is a generalized, highly contagious, and usually self-limiting illness called *chicken pox* or *varicella*. In the partially immune host, a localized eruption called *herpes zoster* (shingles) develops in a band-like (dermatomal) distribution. The completely immune person exposed to zoster-varicella virus develops no disease. Microscopic examination of cells scraped from the bases of vesicles of chicken pox and herpes zoster show giant cells (see positive Tzanck test, Chapter 6) which distinguish the disease from other vesicobullous diseases except for herpes simplex.

Chicken Pox Chicken pox is an acute viral infection usually acquired by inhaling virus-laden air droplets. Children usually tolerate the disease very well. Adults may become severely ill and develop a viral pneumonia.

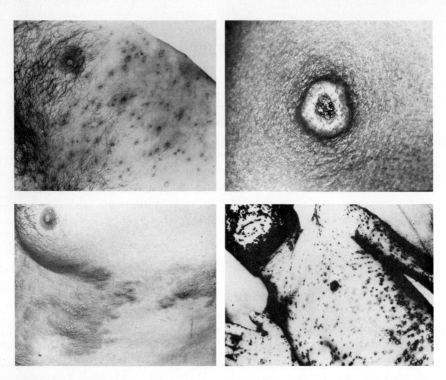

Figure 11-2 Cutaneous manifestations of systemic disease. (*a*) Chicken pox; papules, vesicles, and pustules in various stages of development; (*b*) chicken pox; close-up of umbilicated lesion; (*c*) herpes zoster; grouped vesicles in a bandlike distribution around the trunk; (*d*) smallpox; severely ill man covered with necrotic vesicles and pustules.

After an incubation period of two weeks, the disease begins abruptly with one to two days of malaise and fever, followed by the appearance of many erythematous macules and papules over the trunk (Figure 11-2*a* and *b*). These lesions rapidly progress to form 2 to 3 millimeter clear, tense, fragile vesicles which are surrounded by erythema. The vesicles eventually break and crust but some become umbilicated or filled with pus for three to four days before doing so. Several crops of new lesions appear over five to six days, so that lesions in all stages of development may be seen side by side. Itching may be severe and is often the most annoying symptom of the infection. The illness lasts seven to ten days, after which lesions heal and disappear. Scarring may occur.

Most persons with varicella require only symptomatic therapy. Topical drying lotions and systemic antihistamines may relieve pruritus in some patients. Infants and young children should have their nails cut short and may have to wear gloves to prevent severe excoriations. Patients who become severely ill with chicken pox may have to be hospitalized; they should be in a private room, separated from patients susceptible to infection.

Herpes Zoster (shingles, zoster)   Herpes zoster results from reexposure to virus or reactivation of latent virus in persons who already have some partial immunity. Shingles is unusual in infancy or childhood; two-thirds of patients are over 40 years old. Zoster occurs in a band or nerve segment (dermatome) which corresponds to the area of skin whose sensation is supplied by a single posterior spinal root or facial nerve. It usually occurs on the trunk and is almost always unilateral. The eruption usually begins posteriorly, progresses toward the anterior part of the body, and may be preceded by pain, itching, or burning. Red macules, papules, and plaques appear first and are rapidly followed by grouped vesicles (Figure 11-2c). Lesions crust and disappear over one to three weeks. As many as 10 to 20 vesicles may normally appear outside of the band of affected skin. In immune-suppressed patients, the lesions may become generalized and may be life threatening.

Occasionally, scarring may occur, especially if secondary bacterial infection is present. If zoster occurs on the face and the eye becomes involved, a scarring keratoconjunctivitis may occur. Pain sometimes accompanies zoster and may persist in the affected dermatome after the zoster skin lesions heal. The incidence of pain after shingles (postherpetic neuralgia) increases with advancing age. Rarely, muscle weakness occurs at the affected site.

Patients with serious underlying conditions, particularly diseases which alter immunologic competence, such as lymphoma or leukemia, are more prone to get herpes zoster. Shingles has been seen to occur at sites of prior radiation therapy or of a neoplastic lesion with higher frequency. The vast majority of persons with zoster are, however, otherwise normal, and the lesions heal without complications.

Variola

Smallpox (variola) is a serious virus infection which is now rare in this country because of the successful vaccination program that uses cowpox (vaccinia) virus to stimulate the production of antibodies which are active against the smallpox virus. The disease still exists in some countries, and epidemics do occur. Papules appear after several days of fever and prostration. The lesions become vesicular and pustular and then begin to umbilicate as they become deepseated and necrotic (Figure 11-2d). In contrast to chicken pox, the lesions are mostly distally located, with relative sparing of the trunk. Since a single crop of lesions is the rule, the lesions all appear to be in one stage of development.

Rocky Mountain Spotted Fever

Rickettsiae are microorganisms which have some of the characteristics of both bacteria and viruses. They are obligate intracellular parasites which are transmitted to man by arthropods. Rickettsial infections respond to certain broad spectrum antibiotics if administered early in the illness. Rocky Mountain spotted fever is the most serious of a group of infectious diseases caused by the rickettsiae occurring in this country. Delay in treatment of this disorder may lead to death.

Rocky Mountain spotted fever is caused by *Rickettsia rickettsii* which is transmitted by the tick bite. Rocky Mountain spotted fever occurs in many areas of the United States in addition to the Rocky Mountains, including Cape Cod and the Carolinas. Infection may be relatively asymptomatic or it can produce serious illness whose full blown classic picture carries a 50 percent mortality rate if untreated. This latter form of the disease is often accompanied by a rash. Recognition of the rash may lead to appropriate life-saving therapy long before any laboratory confirmation is available (Figure 11-3*b*).

Fever, headache, and severe myalgias precede the rash by two to four days. The eruption begins on the wrists, ankles, and forearms. The pink, blanchable, macular rash can be made more obvious by a rise in the patient's temperature, or by warm soaks. Within one day, the rash spreads distally to palms and soles, extending simultaneously to the trunk and face. Within another day, the rash becomes palpable and deeper red and petechiae begin to appear in the rash over the following days. By the fourth day of rash (seventh to eighth day of illness) the skin lesions no longer fade on pressure. The scrotum or vulva are often involved. Ulcers and gangrene may appear at the tips of the digits, nose, or earlobes.

The usual laboratory tests are not helpful. A special test (Weil-Felix), using certain proteus bacterial antigens, is positive in patients with rickettsial diseases. Skin biopsy shows a diffuse vasculitis; rickettsia may be seen within the endothelial cells of small vessels.

Both tetracycline and chloramphenicol are effective in treatment of Rocky Mountain spotted fever. Penicillin is not effective; sulfonamides may make the patient worse. Since Rocky Mountain spotted fever may be fatal, and laboratory results may require one to two days, it is wise to begin treatment if the clinical picture is suggestive. Tetracycline is a drug with few and nonserious side effects. Once extensive vasculitis occurs in the brain, heart, or kidney, the prognosis is not good and it may be too late for antibiotics.

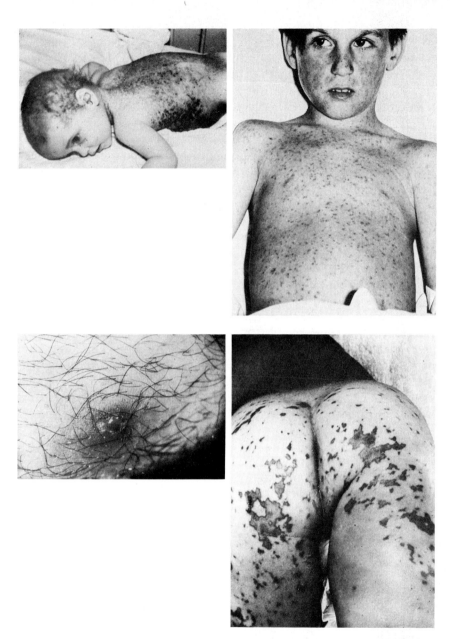

Figure 11-3 (a) Hand-Schüller-Christian disease; eczematous-appearing dermatitis with induration and purpura; (b) Rocky Mountain spotted fever; generalized purpuric lesions; (c) gonococcemia; hemorrhagic vesico-pustule; (d) meningococcemia; jagged, many-sided, flat, purple lesions with gun-metal gray centers.

Gonococcemia

Gonococcemia (see Chapter 9) results from bloodstream spread of gonorrhea. It is manifested by macules, purpuric papules, purpuric vesicles, or purpuric infarcts or pustules which may be surrounded by a narrow rim of purpura (Figure 11-3c). Migratory polyarthritis and tenosynovitis are usually present. The lesions are few in number, distal in location, often painful, and often occur around the joints. The most characteristic lesion is a hemorrhagic vesicopustule surrounded by erythema. The lesion may yield gonococci on smear or culture. A cervical or rectal swab from the patient with these lesions has a much higher percentage of positive cultures. All cultures may be negative. Diagnosis and treatment can be based solely on the morphology of the characteristic lesions, especially in patients with tenosynovitis, fever, and a history of exposure to gonorrhea.

Meningococcemia

In its acute form, meningococcemia is characterized by various, nonspecific lesions. Petechiae usually become scattered over the trunk and extremities early in the disease. As the petechiae enlarge, they may develop papules, vesicles, or pustules in their centers. Distribution is random and asymmetrical. As the lesions increase in number they begin to coalesce to form larger purpuric or ecchymotic areas. Large, fully developed lesions appear as purple, many-sided flat or slightly raised lesions with gun-metal gray centers and many straight edges at their borders (Figure 11-3d). Such lesions suggest advanced meningococcemia and the prognosis is guarded even in the face of maximum antibiosis.

Staphylococcemia

Staphylococcemia is manifested by pustules surrounded by an erythematous or purpuric halo. Petechiae may occur adjacent to the lesion. The lesion may remain as a large tender pustule or it may become infarctive. Distribution is random and lesions may be few or many. Gram's staining of the aspirated contents of the purulent center often reveals gram-positive cocci in clusters.

Pseudomonas Septicemia

Pseudomonas septicemia occurs usually in very sick hospitalized individuals who have underlying medical problems, or who are receiving significant doses of antibiotics, antitumor agents, or steroids. The patients are usually toxic and febrile. The lesions may be painful, but the patients are usually too sick to complain about them. Hemorrhagic bullae become necrotic and develop into round ulcers which are indurated and firm, are surrounded by considerable erythema, and have a central gray to black eschar. Such a lesion is called *ecthyma gangenosum*. Larger lesions begin to resemble decubitus ulcers. Scattered showers of generalized purpuric or erythematous macules and papules may occur, which usually signal a massive terminal sepsis and/or dangerous clotting derangements.

Subacute Bacterial Endocarditis

Subacute bacterial endocarditis (SBE) is an infection of the heart valves caused by viridans and Group-D streptococci. Painful urticaria-like nodules in the pulp of the fingers (Osler's nodes), purpuric macules of the acral areas (Janeway lesions), and subungual splinter hemorrhages occur.

SKIN SIGNS OF ENDOCRINE AND METABOLIC DISORDERS

Endocrine and metabolic abnormalities may result in quantitative alterations in the functions, reaction patterns, pigmentation, and composition of the skin. Hormones affect the electrolytes, fluids, and mucopolysaccharides of the skin, alter blood flow and heat regulation, and influence the metabolism of the cells. The rate of melanin production, the size of hairs, the excretion of sebum, and the secretion of sweat are dependent on hormones. The influence of the sex hormones has been discussed elsewhere (see Chapters 3 and 7).

Pituitary

Since it controls many endocrine glands, the pituitary has much indirect influence on the skin via target gland hormones. Its major direct effect is mediated by growth hormone, which affects the connective tissue. Collagen and mucopolysaccharides are increased by this hormone.

Increased levels of growth hormone can lead to thickening of the dermis which, in turn, stimulates hyperplasia of the epidermis and its appendages. Too much skin is present. The skin may feel thickened or doughy or may be thrown into folds with deep furrows and accentuation of normal wrinkle lines. Eyelids, lips, and tongue enlarge; hair and nails thicken. Excessive apocrine and eccrine sweating occurs and hyperpigmentation may be present. Overgrowth of fibrous tissue forms small pedunculated fibromas and skin tags. The connective tissue of bones is also increased and giantism may occur. If the epiphyses have already closed, the long bones cannot increase in length but the skull, hands, and feet can enlarge, leading to acromegaly (acro = extremity, megaly = great or huge).

Thyroid

The level of thyroid hormone (thyroxine) is an important determinant of the metabolic rate of the skin. This is probably the result of some direct effect on the skin cells as well as an indirect effect caused by the increased heat production of the body as a whole and the increased perfusion of the skin. The increased blood flow to the skin is accompanied by increased sweating.

In hyperthyroid states, the skin is warm and moist, and may be slightly erythematous. The epidermis is thin and the skin feels soft, smooth, and well hydrated. The increased cutaneous blood flow and increased sweating may account for most of these changes. Nails may become thin and curved upward at their free edge (Plummer's nails). Some patients with hyperthyroidism show hyperpigmentation while others become less pigmented. Vitiligo is seen with increased incidence in patients with overactive thyroid glands. There may be some diffuse alopecia in hyperthyroid patients.

Graves' disease is an intermittent, sometimes severe, overactive state of the thyroid gland of unknown etiology which may be accompanied by eye changes. Retraction of the upper lid, paralysis of the eye muscles, and proptosis (bulging of the eyeball, exophthalmos) occur. Those patients with eye abnormalities may also have a localized increase in mucopolysaccharides in the dermis which is histologically indistinguishable from myxedema (see below). Since the most usual site for this localized swelling in the dermis is over the anterior tibia, it is called *pretibial myxedema*. Flesh-colored, pink, or purple-brown nodules in the skin are at first covered by smooth, shiny epidermis but as the infiltrate becomes more extensive and confluent, the epidermis may become slightly thickened, resembling pigskin. Further hypertrophy of the dermis is accompanied by scaling and verrucous changes of the epidermis. Rarely, clubbing of the fingers and periosteal new bone formation occur in the extremities (*thyroid acropachy*).

Hypothyroidism is accompanied by pale to yellow, cold skin, and a dry, slightly hyperkeratotic epidermis with follicular plugging. Hair is coarse, dry, and brittle, and may be thin or absent. Loss of hair over the outer third of the eyebrows is frequent. Dermal accumulations of mucopolysaccharides in the skin cause a generalized nonpitting edema called myxedema. Broad nose, thick lips, large tongue, and distended, expressionless face in a sleepy, slow moving, slow talking patient suggests hypothyroidism.

Diabetes Mellitus

Diabetics have an increased incidence of infections (especially furuncles), superficial fungus infections, and yeast infections. They are more likely to develop xanthomas, benign aggregates of lipid-laden cells which present as white to yellow plaques in the skin. Persons with diabetes are also more likely to have increased amounts of carotene, an orange lipoid pigment derived from vegetables, which lend an orange-yellow hue to the skin. In addition, diabetics develop some fairly characteristic skin lesions which are probably related to abnormalities in the microcirculation of the skin. Even the capillaries and arterioles of clinically normal skin of diabetics may show abnormalities in the vessel walls and in the surrounding dermal supportive tissue. Two specific skin signs of diabetes are diabetic dermopathy and necrobiosis lipoidica diabeticorum. *Diabetic dermopathy* (shin spots, ladder spots) is manifested by small, atrophic, brown, slightly depressed lesions over the tibias, bilaterally. The border of each lesion is irregular and the overlying epidermis appears thin and smooth. *Necrobiosis lipoidica diabeticorum* (NLD) begins as small purple to red nodules or sharply circumscribed plaques which slowly enlarge and become atrophic, flat, and depressed, to form the characteristic lesion. The fully developed lesion of necrobiosis lipoidica diabeticorum is a yellow-brown depression covered with thin epidermis through which delicate vessels can be seen (Color Plate IV*D*). The border may remain elevated, with the morphology of the original red nodule or plaque, but an atrophic yellow center is left behind as it slowly progresses. Diabetic dermopathy is more common in men, whereas necrobiosis lipoidica diabeticorum is more common in females and may occur before chemical diabetes is apparent. Diabetes therapy with insulin can lead to local urticaria, erythema, and tenderness, or to a nonallergic atrophy or hypertrophy of subcutaneous fat (lipodystrophy).

SKIN SIGNS OF DISEASES OF CONNECTIVE TISSUE
(The "Collagen" Diseases)

The collagen or connective tissue diseases are a group of clinical syndromes which share the histologic features of widespread inflammatory damage in connective tissue and deposition of fibrinoid material in ground substance. Local changes in skin, joints, blood vessels, or internal organs may be accompanied by constitutional manifestations.

Lupus Erythematosis

Lupus erythematosis is a disease affecting the connective tissue of the skin, the vascular system, and the serous and synovial membranes. The clinical manifestations are varied; the course is one of exacerbations and remissions over a period of years. Many different kinds of abnormal serum proteins may be present. One of them causes the formation of the characteristic lupus erythematosis cell under certain laboratory conditions.

Discoid Lupus Erythematosis (DLE) Discoid lupus erythematosis is a skin disease characterized by well-demarcated, chronic, erythematous, raised lesions which have irregular outlines and may heal with scarring

(Figure 11-4a). Advanced lesions show telangiectasia, hyper- and hypopigmentation, atrophy, and dilated follicles. Scale is variable; when present, its under surface has "carpet tacks" of keratin that protrude down to fill the dilated hair follicles. Sun, cold, and trauma can induce a lesion in persons predisposed to have them.

Discoid lupus erythematosis is more common than systemic lupus erythematosis (SLE) and probably less than 1 percent of persons with chronic discoid lupus erythematosis go on to develop systemic lupus erythematosis. On the other hand, about 10 percent of SLE patients have discoid lupus erythematosis prior to the onset of systemic symptoms and diagnosis of SLE; about twice that many have discoid lupus erythematosis lesions sometime in the course of systemic lupus erythematosis.

Systemic Lupus Erythematosis (SLE)   Skin changes occur in more than three-fourths of patients with systemic lupus erythematosis. The "butterfly rash" has received the most attention but occurs in only about one-third of patients. It may initially look like sunburn on the cheeks and across the nose, but persists for weeks. A more generalized macular and papular semiconfluent rash which looks like a drug eruption also occurs. Discoid lupus erythematosis lesions, periungual erythema, ulcers of the mucous membranes, purpura, leg ulcers, and facial edema also occur. Vasculitis of small vessels may cause small ulcers of the distal digits. Diffuse and patchy alopecia may occur. Striking periungual telangiectasia is seen in systemic lupus erythematosis (Figure 11-6b) and sometimes in other collagen diseases but is very rare in normal people.

Dermatomyositis

Dermatomyositis is a connective tissue disease of unknown etiology characterized by edema, dermatitis, and inflammation in muscles. Muscle involvement causes progressive weakness of limb girdle muscles. When skin involvement is absent, the process is called polymyositis. Skin changes are variable. The most characteristic, almost diagnostic, skin changes are edema and a purplish-red discoloration about the upper eyelids (also called purple suffusion or heliotrope erythema). Two additional characteristic lesions include scaly, macular erythema over the knuckles and linear telangiectasia of the posterior nail fold. Butterfly rash may occur. A blotchy macular semiconfluent rash with scattered telangiectasia may be generalized or may be confined to light exposed areas. In children it may be a self-limited disease. In adults it is often associated with an internal malignancy.

Scleroderma

Scleroderma is a connective tissue disease of unknown etiology, characterized by leathery hardening of the skin. A localized form, *morphea,* is con-

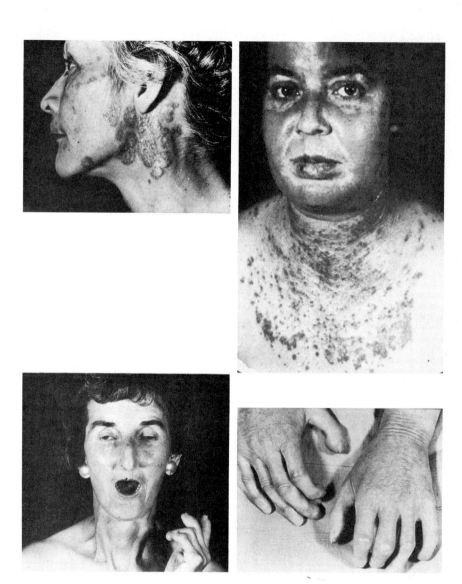

Figure 11-4 Cutaneous manifestation of collagen vascular disease. (*a*) Discoid lupus erythematosis; atrophy, telangiectasia, hyper- and hypopigmentation and scaling; (*b*) systemic lupus erythematosis; erythema, telangiectasia in sun-exposed areas; (*c*) scleroderma; "hide-bound" skin prevents wide opening of the mouth; (*d*) scleroderma; tightly bound skin and atrophy of ends of thumbs.

fined to the skin and a systemic form, *progressive systemic sclerosis* (PSS), is characterized by diffuse involvement of the connective tissue of the skin and certain internal organs (Figure 11-4*c* and *d*).

Morphea   Morphea begins as a slightly red, edematous plaque which evolves into a circumscribed, waxy, sclerotic, ivory-colored, shiny plaque. When the lesion is active and growing, it is surrounded by violaceous erythema. Oval, linear, and plaque types occur and involvement can be either a single lesion or generalized. Atrophy of dermis, subcutaneous tissue, and bone may occur beneath linear morphea. Progression to systemic involvement or progressive systemic sclerosis is rare and although, histologically, the two forms of scleroderma are often indistinguishable, their relationship is not clear. Morphea usually resolves gradually over months to years, sometimes with no residue but, more frequently, leaving some combination of atrophy and pigmentary change.

Progressive Systemic Sclerosis   Progressive systemic sclerosis is, like morphea, more common in women. The initial complaints may be chronic, nonpitting edema, or symptoms of Raynaud's phenomena (sequential pallor, erythema, and cyanosis of digits on cold exposure). Transient, mild edema usually begins with the fingers and hands, and extends centrally. The fingers may have a sausage-like appearance. In advanced stages, the skin becomes tense, smooth, hard, and firmly bound down to underlying structures. Painful ulcerations of the finger tips occur. The fingers may become stiff and develop flexion contractures. When these changes involve the skin of the face, a mask-like absence of expression occurs, accompanied by thinning of the lips and tightening of the skin over the nasal cartilage. Cutaneous calcifications may occur and telangiectasia may be prominent, especially on the face. Generalized hyperpigmentation can occur.

MASTOCYTOSIS

Mastocytosis is a disorder of unknown etiology characterized by the accumulation of mast cells in various body organs. When, as is most frequently the case, the mast cell proliferations are limited to the skin, the disorder is called *urticaria pigmentosa*. Urticaria pigmentosa usually presents as multiple red to yellow macules, papules, or nodules covered with variable amounts of pigment. Because the mast cells contain histamine, the lesions may become raised with surrounding flare when the skin is stroked firmly. This urticaria localized to the stroked lesion is diagnostic of urticaria pigmentosa (Darier's sign).

Patients with widespread urticaria pigmentosa may have systemic signs of histamine released from the mast cells of their skin lesions. Flushing, pruritus, tachycardia, hypotension, and gastrointestinal complaints may occur. Solitary papules composed of mast cells, called mastocytoma also occur. Rarely, skin involvement is diffuse and ubiquitous. The much less common *systemic mastocytosis* involves viscera, especially bone, liver, and the gastrointestinal tract, and may or may not involve skin.

HISTIOCYTOSIS

Histiocytosis (reticuloendotheliosis, histiocytosis X) is a disease of unknown cause, characterized histologically by a proliferation of histiocytes. The symptoms and seriousness of the disease depend on age of onset and on the site and rate of growth of the granulomatous collection of histiocytes. The three most common clinical forms have been given eponyms. When histiocytosis occurs during the first year of life, visceral involvement is widespread and often fatal (Letterer-Siwe disease). During early childhood, bone lesions, especially of the skull, are associated with skin lesions and less severe visceral involvement (Hand-Schüller-Christian disease; Figure 11-3*a*). If onset of histiocytosis is in later childhood and adult life, there may be one or several lesions confined to bone or skin (eosinophilic granuloma).

Whenever a rash of infancy or childhood, especially eczematous dermatitis, does not respond to treatment and becomes purpuric, histocytosis should be suspected and a biopsy should be performed. Cutaneous involvement in infancy may appear as scaling papules, petechiae and purpura, vesicles or bullae, or eroded areas of oozing and crusting which extend into body creases or into the perineum. Older children may also have yellow papules or well-demarcated plaques that can erode or ulcerate. Yellow papules with similar histiocytic histology may also occur in otherwise healthy children (juvenile xanthogranuloma) and are not of any but cosmetic concern.

SKIN SIGNS OF DISEASES WHICH AFFECT THE GASTROINTESTINAL TRACT

Peutz-Jeghers Syndrome

Peutz-Jeghers syndrome is a rare inherited trait (autosomal dominant) in which discrete, freckle-like, mucocutaneous pigmentation involving the lips, face, buccal mucosa, and hands is associated with polyps of the gastrointestinal tract, especially the jejunum and ileum. The 2 to 5 millimeters pigmented macules begin in infancy and early childhood. The multiple intestinal polyps are not necessarily premalignant but may cause bleeding, intussusception, or abdominal pain.

Hereditary Hemorrhagic Telangiectasia

Hereditary hemorrhagic telangiectasia (Osler-Rendu-Weber syndrome) is an autosomal dominant hereditary disorder of blood vessels characterized by delicate dilated vessels of the skin, mucous membranes, and viscera. Punctate red spots, spider-like angiomata, and linear and branched telangiectasiae appear on the skin and mucous membranes. Patients may note frequent episodes of nosebleed. Gastrointestinal bleeding may be occult, presenting as anemia, or may be more obvious and symptomatic.

Pyoderma Gangrenosum

Pyoderma gangrenosum is an ulcerative condition of the skin which is often associated with chronic ulcerative colitis. Minor trauma may initiate an ulcer which may be preceded by histologic signs of vasculitis. The lesion begins as an inflammatory nodule resembling a furuncle which breaks down, ulcerates, and gradually enlarges peripherally. Fully developed lesions are moderately deep, moist, red, granular, necrotic ulcers which partially undermine the surrounding skin. A border of violaceous edematous skin is present. In addition to ulcerative colitis, pyoderma gangrenosum is also seen in association with regional ileitis, rheumatoid arthritis, and dysproteinemia.

Acrodermatitis Enteropathica

Acrodermatitis enteropathica is an unusual, serious disease of children in which a vesicular or crusted dermatitis around body orifices and on distal extremities is associated with chronic diarrhea and alopecia. Onset is usually about the time of weaning. Superinfection with monilia is frequent. Although the etiology is not known, patients improve after ingestion of diiodohydroxyquinoline, an antimalarial.

CANCER, LYMPHOMA, LEUKEMIA, AND MYCOSIS FUNGOIDES

Cancer

Internal cancer can metastasize to the skin. The carcinomas most frequently associated with metastic lesions to the skin originate in the breast, stomach, lung, uterus, kidney, ovary, colon, and bladder. Usually when skin metastasis occurs, the prognosis is poor with life expectancy measured in months. Lesions may develop anywhere on the skin surface. A mass may develop in the subcutaneous tissue, within the dermis, or may fill the full thickness of the skin and may cause the epidermis to protrude but erosion or ulceration is unusual. The color may be pink, purple, or brown. Metastatic lesions are usually firm to stony hard.

Internal cancers may also release substances which act as hormones and cause skin changes which mimic certain endocrine disorders. Generalized pruritus, thrombophlebitis, dermatomyositis, blistering disorders, and coagulation defects have been related to the course of internal malignancies. Urticaria, erythema multiforme, gyrate erythemas, and other vascular reaction patterns may also occur. Exfoliative dermatitis and generalized acquired ichthyosis occur rarely.

Acanthosis Nigricans. Acanthosis nigricans, sometimes an indication of internal malignancy, is a thickening of the skin accompanied by hyperpigmentation. It chiefly affects the flexor areas of the skin, especially the neck, axillae, and groin. In its mildest form, it looks like dirty skin with slightly increased folds and skin markings. More extensive lesions are localized areas of verrucous or firmly papillomatous skin which is brown to black (Figure 11-5a). Acanthosis nigricans may also be independent of malignancy and associated with obesity or endocrine abnormalities.

Lymphoma

Skin manifestations may occur in as many as one half of patients with lymphomas. Papules, nodules, or plaques of varying size occur. They are firm, flesh-colored to red to purple, and may be deep or superficial. Pruritus and nonspecific erythemas also occur with lymphomas, especially Hodgkin's disease.

Leukemia

The most frequent cutaneous findings in leukemia are nonspecific skin changes related to anemia, infection, bleeding disorders, or rashes secondary to medications. Since most patients receive intensive chemotherapy, it is unusual to see patients with skin lesions caused by infiltration of the skin with leukemia cells (Figure 11-5b). Patients with chronic lymphocytic leukemia may eventually develop erythroderma, papules, nodules, or plaques filled with lymphocytes. Occasionally a patient with acute myeloblastic or monocytic leukemia will develop skin lesions that result from massive dermal infiltration with abnormal cells. The lesions, which are often hemorrhagic, do not have a characteristic appearance.

Mycosis Fungoides

Mycosis fungoides is an uncommon neoplastic disease of the lymphoreticular system of unknown cause. Lesions first appear in the skin which is the only site of involvement for weeks to decades, but lymph node or internal organ involvement often occurs eventually. The disease most often begins with chronic skin lesions that may originally be mistaken for eczema, psoriasis, or neurodermatitis. These lesions eventually become indurated,

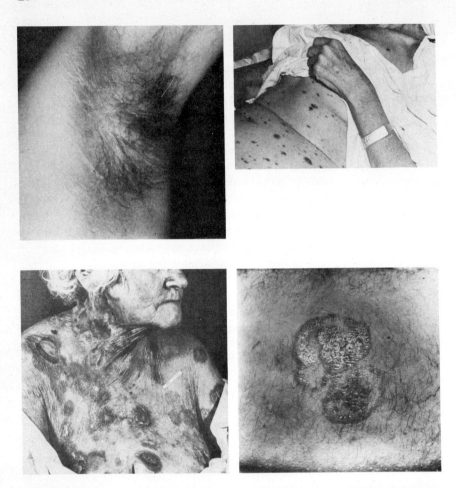

Figure 11-5 Cutaneous manifestations of malignancy. (a) Acanthosis nigricans; (b) leukemia cutis; (c) mycosis fungoides; (d) mycosis fungoides.

often respond poorly to treatment, or may show atypical dense dermal infiltrates on biopsy. Such changes should alert the clinician to the possibility of mycosis fungoides. Onset may also be with erythroderma, poikiloderma (atrophy, pigment change, and telangiectasia), or with a chronic, local, persistent, finely scaling, slightly hyperpigmented, and minimally erythematous plaque called *parapsoriasis en plaque*.

Eventually, indurated plaques, erosions, ulcers, and tumor masses appear in the skin (Figure 11-5c and d). Later, lymph nodes and internal organs become involved. Life expectancy after such occurrences is less than three years. Early stages can be treated with topical nitrogen mustard, steroids, superficial x-irradiation, electron beam, or ultraviolet light used with or without photoactive medications. Thick plaques or internal lesions require deep radiation therapy, systemic chemotherapy, or both.

SARCOIDOSIS

Sarcoidosis is a systemic granulomatous disease (or group of diseases) of unknown etiology which involves any organ or tissue. The process may be slowly progressive for many years or may undergo complete remission in its early stages. Approximately two-thirds of patients with sarcoidosis do not react to second strength tuberculin tests. Other forms of delayed hypersensitivity may also be diminished or absent (anergy).

Specific skin manifestations occur in almost one-fourth of patients with sarcoidosis. Plaques, flesh-colored papules, and nodules occur. They are often about the eyes or nose but may occur at any site. Previously flat scars from minor trauma or from surgery may become elevated and red to purplish in color. Biopsy of such scars shows granulomatous involvement of sarcoidosis. Erythema nodosum (see Chapter 5) is frequently associated with sarcoidosis.

MISCELLANEOUS CONDITIONS

There are skin signs associated with more uncommon systemic diseases. Erosions on the dorsa of the hands and facial hypertrichosis in older persons, especially those with compromised liver function, suggests *porphyria cutanea tarda*. Xanthomas may be seen in patients with elevated blood lipids secondary to *hyperlipoproteinemias*. Flat brown lesions (*café au lait*), axillary freckling, and soft tumors scattered over the skin are present in *von Recklinghausen's disease* (*neurofibromatosis*). Persons with *tuberous sclerosis* may have flat leaf-shaped areas of hypopigmentation present at birth. Most of these are chronic disorders and the patient is not acutely ill.

SUMMARY

When approaching the acutely ill patient with a rash it is important to remember several points:

1   Always consider drug eruption.
2   Palpable purpura is probably a vasculitis (Figure 11–6a).
3   Severe eczema in a child which does not respond to treatment or becomes purpuric may be histiocytosis X.
4   Purpuric lesions: Those on the palms may be Rocky Mountain spotted fever. Those with gun-metal gray centers and jagged, many-sided

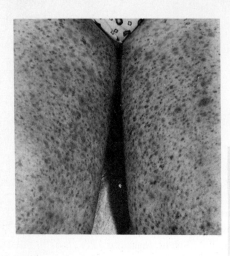

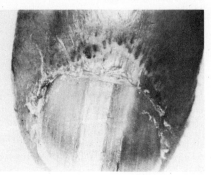

Figure 11-6 Cutaneous manifestations of systemic disease. (a) Palpable purpura is usually vasculitis; (b) paronychial telangiectasia is characteristic of collagen disease.

straight borders may be meningococcemia. Early diagnosis of either saves lives.

    5 Paronychial telangiectasia is highly suggestive of collagen disease (Figure 11–6b).

    6 Rashes which resemble secondray syphilis should be examined closely with gloved hands, as they are infective.

REFERENCES

Ashton, H., G. W. Beveridge, and C. J. Stevenson: "Management of Herpes Zoster," *Brit. J. Derm.* **81:**874–876, November 1969.

Binkley, G. W.: "Dermopathy in the Diabetic Syndrome," *Arch. Derm.* **92:**625–634, December 1965.

Bluefarb, S. M.: *Cutaneous Manifestations of the Malignant Lymphomas,* Charles C Thomas, Publisher, Springfield, Ill., 1959.

Braverman, I. M.: *Skin Signs of Systemic Disease,* W. B. Saunders Company, Philadelphia, 1970.

Brunell, P., H. Ross, L. H. Miller, et al.: "Prevention of Varicella by Zoster Immune Globulin," *N. Eng. J. Med.* **280:**1191–1194, May 1969.

Calabro, J. J., and J. M. Marchesano: "Rash Associated with Juvenile Rheumatoid Arthritis," *J. Pediat.* **72:**611–619, May 1968.

Caplan, R. M.: "Urticaria Pigmentosa and Mastocytosis," *JAMA* **194:**1077–1080, December 1965.

Castrow, F. F., and M. De Beukelaer: "Congenital Rubella Syndrome," *Arch. Derm.* **98:**260–262, September 1968.

Cherry, J. D.: "Newer Viral Exanthems," *Advances Pediat.* **16:**233–286, 1969.

Cooper, L. Z., and S. Krugman: "The Rubella Problem," *Disease-a-Month,* February 1969.

Cunliffe, W. J., R. Hall, D. J. Newell, et al.: "Vitiligo, Thyroid Disease and Autoimmunity," *Brit. J. Derm.* **80:**135–139, March 1968.

Curth, H. O.: "Pigmentary Changes of the Skin Associated with Internal Disease," *Postgrad. Med.* **41:**439–449, May 1967.

Eaglstein, W. H., R. Katz, and J. A. Brown: "The Effects of Early Corticosteroid Therapy on the Skin Eruption and Pain of Herpes Zoster," *JAMA* **221:**1681–1783, March 1970.

Gimlette, T. M. D.: "Thyroid Acropachy," *Lancet* **1:**22–24, January 1960.

Gordon, D. A., F. M. Hill, and C. Ezrin: "Acromegaly: A Review of 100 Cases," *Can. Med. Ass. J.* **87:**1106–1109, November 1962.

Hazard, G. W., R. N. Ganz, R. W. Nevin, et al.: "Rocky Mountain Spotted Fever in the Eastern United States," *New Eng. J. Med.* **280:**57–62, January 1969.

Hope-Simpson, R. E.: "The Nature of Herpes Zoster: A Long-Term Study and a New Hypothesis," *Proc. Roy. Soc. Med.* **58:**9–20, January 1965.

Juel-Jensen, B. E., and F. O. MacCullum: *Herpes Simplex Varicella and Zoster: Clinical Manifestations and Treatment,* J. B. Lippincott Company, Philadelphia, 1972.

Krugman, S., and R. Ward: *Infectious Diseases of Children,* The C. V. Mosby Company, St. Louis, 1968.

Lucaya, J.: "Histiocytosis X," *Am. J. Dis. Child.* **121:**289–295, April 1971.

Lupus Erythematosus, Dubois, E. L. ed., McGraw-Hill Book Company, New York, 1966.

The Thyroid, Werner, S. C., and S. H. Ingbar, eds; Wegelius, O.: "Skin and Connective Tissue," Harper & Row, Publishers, Incorporated, New York, 1971, pp. 522–535.

Chapter 12

Blisters, Ulcers, and Bedsores

Blisters
    Spongiosis
    Primary cell damage
    Acantholysis
    Dermoepidermal separation
Pemphigus
    Familial benign pemphigus
Pemphigoid
Erythema multiforme
Other dermatoses manifested by blisters,
        erosions, and ulcers
    Toxic epidermal necrolysis
    Dermatitis herpetiformis
    Mechanicobullous diseases
    Behçet's syndrome
Ulcers and erosions
Ischemia
Bedsores
Factitial ulcer

BLISTERS

Blisters are formed when an abnormal collection of fluid completely re-places preexisting skin architecture and the fluid is still capped by the epidermis or part of the epidermis. Such fluid accumulation results from damage to cells or fibers. Blisters may be microscopic, large enough to be grossly visible, or may cover large areas of skin. Vesicles are small, circumscribed, elevated blisters which range in size from barely visible to several millimeters. A blister larger than ½ centimeter is called a bulla. Blister walls may be so thin as to be translucent, so that the extracellular fluid, serum, blood, or pus within it can be seen.

Blisters can be classified on the basis of their *etiology*. Edema or fluid pressure may simply force the skin components apart. Fluid accumulation usually results from altered cells or fibers. Such alterations may result from infection, physical forces and chemical reactions, immunologic mechanisms, hereditary abnormalities, and abnormal cell metabolism. The cause for some blisters is not known. Blisters may also be categorized on the basis of their *location* or depth within the skin. Blisters can occur at many sites or levels within the skin. They may be just beneath the stratum corneum, in the middle of the epidermis, or just above the basal cell layer. The plane of cleavage may be at or below the dermoepidermal junction. Blisters may also be classified according to their *microscopic morphology* (Figure 12-1). If early lesions are biopsied, the histologic changes may suggest the mechanism of formation of the blisters. The histologic end result may be similar for blisters of quite different and unrelated causes.

Spongiosis

The most common first stage of blister formation is spongiosis, which is edema between the cells of the spongy layer (prickle layer) of the epidermis. The earliest histologic change is simply the presence of fluid which seems to push the cells apart from one another so that the intercellular bridges appear more prominent. This early change is followed by liquefaction and lysis of parts of the cells themselves which gradually increases the size of the fluid spaces. As many of these small multiloculated microvesicles coalesce, they form macroscopically visible lesions. The spongiotic blister remains intraepidermal (within the epidermis). Spongiosis is the hallmark of eczema; it is also seen in skin disorders which do not usually present with visible blisters. These include impetigo, superficial fungus infections, and pityriasis rosea.

Primary Cell Damage

If epidermal cells are damaged or killed, fluid may fill in the spaces vacated by the destroyed cells. Viruses which cause chicken pox, herpes zoster,

EPIDERMAL
  Spongiosis
    Atopic dermatitis
    Contact dermatitis
    Nummular eczema
    Dyshidrosis
  Primary Cell Damage
    Virus
    UV, x-ray
    Heat and cold
    Friction, suction
    Pressure, ischemia
  Acantholysis
    Pemphigus
    Bowen's disease, actinic keratosis
    Darier's disease
    Mild thermal damage

DERMOEPIDERMAL SEPARATION
    Erythema multiforme
    Pemphigoid
    Dermatitis herpetiformis
    Porphyria
    Epidermolysis bullosa
    Pressure, anoxia
    Heat
    Suction

Figure 12-1 Classification of blisters by their microscopic morphology and etiology.

herpes simplex, and smallpox cause vesicles in this way. Blisters may also result when cells are radiated by ultraviolet light or x-irradiation, or when they are damaged by excessive heat or cold. Physical force such as friction or suction may destroy cells and may lead to fluid accumulation and blisters. Pressure results in prolonged ischemia and may lead to blister formation.

Acantholysis

Blisters may result when the cells of the epidermis do not adhere well to each other. If the complicated cellular attachments and intercellular cementing substances are anatomically or chemically altered, the cells can slip past one another, and fluid can accumulate in spaces between the cells. This "dyshesion" of the cells in the epidermis is referred to as acantholysis. It may result from genetic alteration, thermal injury, virus infection, altered immunity, or from unknown causes. The classic example of acantholysis is pemphigus vulgaris, a blistering and erosive disease of unknown etiology which, if untreated, is frequently fatal.

Dermoepidermal Separation

Blisters may result from a separation of the epidermis from the dermis. In erythema multiforme, the primary site of injury to the skin and collection of fluid within the skin is on the dermal side of the dermoepidermal junction. In pemphigoid, there is alteration of the basement membrane which leads to dermal-epidermal separation. In some mechanicobullous dermatoses, uncommon hereditary disorders of the skin, separation occurs in this area with minor trauma or friction. Physical forces such as heat, marked friction, or tissue anoxia can cause separation of epidermis from dermis in the skin of normal persons.

PEMPHIGUS

Pemphigus vulgaris is an acquired blistering disease of unknown etiology, characterized histologically by acantholysis. Blisters occur within the epidermis just above the basal layer. In contrast to the many-sided, "prickly" appearance of normal epidermal cells viewed with the light microscope, the epidermal cells in the area of the blister and those floating in the blister cavity appear rounded and without prickles (see Tzanck test, Chapter 6). The cells do not hold together well. By placing the thumb firmly on the skin and exerting lateral sliding pressure, the upper epidermis can be dislodged, resulting in an erosion or blister (Nikolsky's sign).

Onset is usually in middle age. In more than one-half of patients, the first lesion appears in the mouth, and the oral mucosa is eventually involved in almost all patients. Intact blisters are rarely seen in the mouth because they break quickly, to become painful erosions. Mucosal lesions characteristically spill over the rims of the lips and onto the skin. Distribution of skin lesions is random except that pressure and friction lead to detachment of the epidermis and blisters often arise around the nostrils, mouth, and eyes. Lesions arise on normal-appearing skin. The blister roof often breaks and leaves denuded areas which slowly enlarge, maintaining a collar of thin, detached epidermis at the periphery. Lesions gradually progress with little tendency to heal but scarring is unusual. The denuded areas may be quite tender (Figure 12-2a and b).

The usual course of untreated pemphigus vulgaris is slow progression and discomfort. Mouth pain prevents adequate food intake, secondary bacterial infection of the skin leads to sepsis, and extensive denudations of the skin lead to fluid and electrolyte imbalance. Death results in most un-

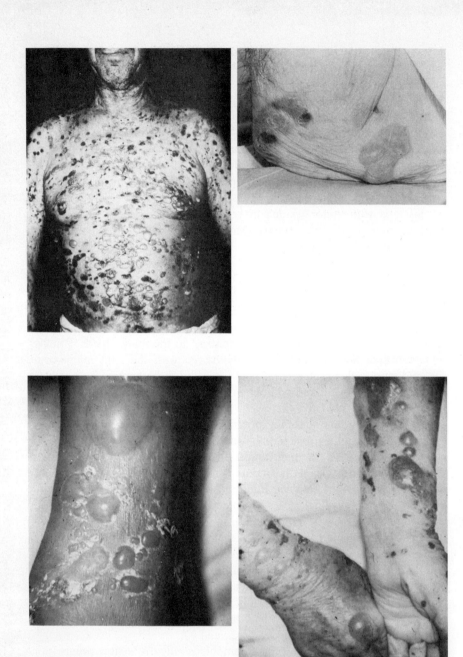

Figure 12-2 (a) Pemphigus vulgaris; (b) pemphigus vulgaris; (c) bullous pemphigoid; (d) bullous pemphigoid.

treated cases. High doses of systemic steroids over prolonged periods usu-ally result in control of the disease. Methotrexate or other antimetabolites are also useful in allowing the steriod dose to be lowered or may be used alone in maintainance therapy. Aggressive, persistent, and consistent nursing care is essential to the survival of the severely affected patient.

By immunofluorescent techniques, it is possible to demonstrate anti-bodies to the intercellular area of the epithelium or epidermis. Such anti-bodies are present in the serum and in the skin of patients with pemphigus. The direct relationship of these antibodies to the etiology of the blisters is not yet certain but many feel that pemphigus is a type of "autoimmune" disease.

There are four other diseases belonging to the pemphigus group (see Figure 12-3). *Pemphigus vegitans* is a variant of pemphigus vulgaris which heals with a hypertrophic, verrucous, "vegetative" surface, and carries the same serious prognosis. *Pemphigus foliaceous* is a less severe disease in which the acantholytic separation within the epidermis is in the upper por-tion of the prickle layer and often just beneath the stratum corneum. *Pemphigus erythematosis* may be a localized variant of pemphigus foliaceous. In Brazil, an acantholytic bullous disease called *fogo selvagem* (jungle fire) appears to be endemic and possibly even contagious. The histology is simi-lar to that of pemphigus foliaceous. The cause is unknown.

Familial Benign Pemphigus

Familial benign pemphigus (Hailey-Hailey disease) is an inherited dis-order, characterized histologically by suprabasal acantholysis. Groups of bullae arise on erythematous skin. The blister fluid becomes turbid and the lesions break easily. Spreading erosions often have vesicles and pustules at the border and a moist granular center. Lesions occur at the flexures of the neck and in intertriginous areas. Warm weather and superficial bac-terial infections can cause flares. Spontaneous exacerbations and remissions continue for years.

Familial benign pemphigus differs from other forms of pemphigus in its genetic pattern, absence of mouth lesions, benign course, and the ab-sence of intercellular antibodies in the serum. Some experts believe familial benign pemphigus is a vesicular variant of Darier's disease (see Chapter 7). Systemic steroids are effective in controlling the disease but continuous maintainance is not indicated for a benign and chronic disorder. Antibi-otics, both topical and systemic, often improve acute flares of the disease.

PEMPHIGOID

Bullous pemphigoid is a chronic disease of unknown etiology characterized clinically by large tense blisters and histologically by subepidermal accumu-

Name	Location of blister	Characteristic lesion	Mouth lesions	Other features	Laboratory findings
Pemphigus vulgaris	suprabasal	erosion	usual		
Pemphigus vegetans	suprabasal	verrucous hyperkeratotic ± pustules	usual		eosinophilia
Pemphigus foliaceous	subcorneal	superficial erosions	unusual	erythema, scaling, oozing, and crusting	
Pemphigus erythematosus (Senear-Usher syndrome)	subcorneal	superficial erosions	unusual	erythema, crusting, oozing, seborrheic dermatitis-like "butterfly rash"	some patients have laboratory findings suggestive of SLE

Figure 12-3 Diseases of the pemphigus group.

lations of fluid. It occurs predominantly in old age, lasts several months to several years, and usually ends with complete recovery and no scarring. Mouth lesions, which occur in one-third of patients, are usually not the first sign of disease and are usually few in number.

The blisters of pemphigoid may be more tense and break less easily than those of pemphigus. When they do break, the denuded area does not continue to increase in size, does not develop the collar of necrotic epidermis, and heals well. Blisters may arise on normal, erythematous, or slightly edematous skin. They are large, irregular in outline, and randomly distributed (Figure 12-2c and d). Occasionally, hemorrhagic bullae appear. Itching may be severe, moderate, or absent. Microscopic examination of early lesions shows that the blister forms beneath the basement membrane and lifts the entire epidermis, transforming it into the blister roof. No acantholytic cells are found.

In the serum of patients with bullous pemphigoid, fluorescent microscopic techniques demonstrate an antibody to the basement membrane zone. This suggests than an autoimmune mechanism may play some role in the disease. No intercellular antibodies, such as those in pemphigus, are seen. Systemic steroids, in doses considerably smaller than those needed for pemphigus, usually control the symptoms. Methotrexate may be used concomitantly, or as the only treatment. Good nursing care aids greatly in preventing secondary bacterial infections.

Benign mucosal pemphigoid (cicatricial pemphigoid) is a subepidermal blistering disease which differs from bullous pemphigoid in that it has a predilection for mucous membranes, especially the conjuctiva, it has a tendency to heal with scarring which may result in blindness, and its course is long, lasting years to decades.

ERYTHEMA MULTIFORME

Erythema multiforme (EM) is a clinical syndrome which is the morphologic expression of a vascular reaction pattern (Figure 12-4a and b). It most likely results from hypersensitivity. Among the known causative agents are herpes simplex, infectious mononucleosis, histoplasmosis, primary atypical pneumonia, sunlight, and antibiotics. Erythema multiforme is an acute disorder which runs a three to eight week course and may recur. It may be preceded by a prodrome of symptoms similar to a viral syndrome. The lesions on the skin result from vascular changes and from leakage of fluid and cells into the dermis (see Chapter 7). If the fluid is extensive enough, the epidermis may be lifted up, and a blister may appear. Variable amounts of necrosis of the epidermis occur, which may be the result of the release of some unidentified necrotizing agent.

As the name implies, the morphologic expression is multiforme or

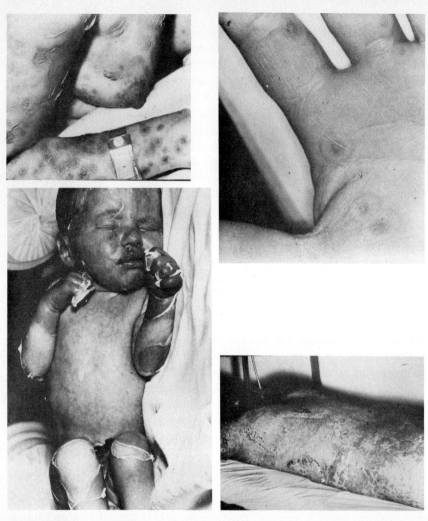

Figure 12-4 (*a*) Erythema multiforme; (*b*) erythema multiforme; (*c*) toxic epidermal necrolysis; (*d*) toxic epidermal necrolysis.

varied. Erthema, edema, urticaria, and blisters may occur. The characteristic lesion is made of concentric rings of the different morphologies (bull's eye or target lesion, Figure 5-5*b*). Distribution is bilateral and symmetrical and usually more impressive on the limbs than on the trunk. Individual lesions may last from several days up to two weeks; they heal with no scarring. Palms and soles are often involved. Mucous membranes may be involved, with blisters that quickly become erosions. While skin lesions are usually asymptomatic, extensive mouth lesions may lead to severe pain.

If erythema multiforme is severe and the mucous membranes are extensively involved, it is often referred to as Stevens-Johnson syndrome.

No specific laboratory test is abnormal or diagnostic. Antibodies to the basement membrane or intercellular space are not present. Treatment of this self-limited syndrome is symptomatic. It may be necessary to give systemic steroids to the severely ill patient. Most episodes are mild and require no therapy. Removal of the offending antigen is essential.

OTHER DERMATOSES MANIFESTED BY BLISTERS, EROSIONS, AND ULCERS

Toxic Epidermal Necrolysis

Toxic epidermal necrolysis (TEN, scalded skin syndrome) is a toxic erythema which has a time course similar to that of erythema multiforme (EM), i.e., it has a prodrome, a toxic phase with an eruption, recovery within a few weeks, and a possibility of recurrence. Occasionally a patient will have features of both toxic epidermal necrolysis and erythema multiforme. Histologically, there is extensive necrosis of the epidermis. Pain in the skin is followed by loss of epidermis and denudation. Clinically, the dead epidermis can be easily stripped away or made to slide off. Patients with extensive involvement look as if their skin has been scalded (Figure 12-4c and d).

Like erythema multiforme, toxic epidermal necrolysis is thought to be a reactive phenomenon, possibly initiated by a hypersensitivity. One-fourth of all cases and possibly most of the cases in adults are thought to be secondary to drugs. A distinct type of this syndrome occurs in children and infants and results from infection with a certain type of staphylococci which elaborate a substance toxic to the epidermal cells. This form of TEN has been called staphylococcal scalded skin syndrome (SSSS). The cause of many episodes of toxic epidermal necrolysis is never discovered. No laboratory abnormality is characteristic of toxic epidermal necrolysis.

Treatment is supportive. If the patient is severely ill, systemic steroids may be indicated. If staphylococci are playing some role, then systemic antibodies are needed. Fluids and electrolytes must be carefully managed and sound nursing care may be life-saving. The patients not only look like they have scalded skin, but in many respects must be treated like burn patients.

Dermatitis Herpetiformis

Dermatitis herpetiformis (DH) is a chronic, extremely pruritic, papular and vesicular eruption of unknown cause. It is seen most often in adult males, and is characterized by a "herpetiform" grouping of lesions and by a striking bilaterally symmetrical distribution. Lesions are most dense over the extensor surfaces of the limbs, on the buttocks, and on the scalp, but may occur anywhere. They heal with postinflammatory pigment changes, and may scar. Mucous membranes are usually spared. Erythema or urticaria may precede the grouped papules and vesicles or they may appear on previously normal skin.

The blisters occur below the basement membrane. Microscopic abscesses within the dermal papillae may precede the blisters. No laboratory tests are diagnostic. Some patients have an associated atrophy of the villae of the small bowel, which may or may not be accompanied by signs or findings of malabsorption.

Treatment is with systemic sulfapyridine or sulfones. The response is often dramatic and almost diagnostic. Patients with dermatitis herpetiformis are miserable because of the severe pruritus and some have been suicidal. The relief with medication is obvious and relapses may occur when treatment is discontinued.

Mechanicobullous Diseases

The mechanicobullous diseases (*epidermolysis bullosa*) are a group of inherited disorders in which blisters, erosions, or ulcers result from minor trauma to the skin. The clinical features and microscopic location of the blisters differ among the various rare disorders. Symptoms range from easily induced blistering, sloughing, scarring, secondary infections, and early death, to blisters which occur only after prolonged marching in boots. Heat and friction make these conditions worse. No specific therapy is available.

Behçet's Syndrome

Behçet's syndrome is a rare disorder usually affecting young adults. It is manifested by well-demarcated deep ulcers of the lips, cheeks, and genitalia. Inflammation of the eyes may lead to uveitis and blindness. Papulopustular lesions may occur at any site of minor trauma to the skin, such as venipuncture. Thrombophlebitis is common. Central nervous system involvement is unusual but may be serious when present. The cause is unknown. All treatments to date have been unsatisfactory. The course is prolonged but the symptoms may eventually cease.

ULCERS AND EROSIONS

When the epidermis is lost as a result of blistering, necrosis, or trauma, a circumscribed, slightly depressed, moist, denuded area appears. An *erosion* is an area of missing epidermis which extends no lower than the basal cell layer. An *ulcer* results when the entire epidermis is absent. Destruction of full-thickness epidermis and papillary dermis causes a superficial ulcer. Destruction down to the mid or lower dermis causes a deep ulcer. Erosions heal without scarring. Uncomplicated superficial ulcers may reepithelize if epidermal appendages remain intact or they may leave hyper- or hypopigmented scars. Deep ulcers heal with scarring.

Once the epidermis is missing, it may be difficult to determine the original cause of the insult. Diagnostic information can, however, be gained by noting the location and size of an ulcer or erosion and by examining other lesions which might be present. For example, nodules, plaques, varicose veins, or excoriations which are nearby may be related to the cause of the ulcer. An ulcer may have a characteristic border, configuration, base, or discharge. Ulcers are frequently related to vascular insufficiency. Examination of peripheral pulses, skin color, and hair distribution help to evaluate the blood circulation in the area.

Figure 12-5 lists frequent causes of simple ulceration of the skin. In addition to diseases with simple ulceration, there is a group of diseases characterized by nodules which ulcerate called noduloulcerative lesions. Malignant neoplasms, infectious diseases including cutaneous tuberculosis, syphilis, and bacterial, parasitic, and deep fungal infections may cause noduloulcerative lesions. In some skin disorders, depressed ulcers do not occur because the skin defect is filled with a densely adherent, dry, necrotic membrane called a sphacelus, which is firmly adherent to the floor of the ulcer. A sphacelus may be seen in decubitus ulcers as well as in defects caused by ischemia, x-irradiation, caustic chemicals, or diphtheria.

Excoriations may result in ulceration. The differential diagnosis for excoriations is the same as that for severe pruritus (Chapter 4). Accidental injury can scoop, cut, or scrape out sections of epidermis. Extreme heat or cold can destroy epidermis and dermis (Chapter 5), leaving ulcers.

Neurotrophic ulcers (anesthetic ulcer, mal perforans) occur in areas of skin which have lost their sensory innervation (Figure 12-6a). The skin is repeatedly injured, because pain, pressure, ischemia, or repeated trauma are not noted. Ulcers may result from such insults, or from prolonged pressure. Neurotrophic ulcers are seen in Hansen's disease (leprosy), tertiary syphilis, syringomyelia, peripheral nerve injury, congenital absence of pain, vascular diseases affecting the spinal tract, and diabetes mellitus.

Neurotrophic ulcers are painless, persistent, relatively noninflammatory, and usually appear over pressure points. Lesions on the bottoms of the feet are often surrounded by hyperkeratosis. Other common sites are the hands, as a result of burns and abrasions, and around the nose, as a result of "picking" with the fingernail.

I. Trauma

excoriations
mechanical, thermal, x-ray
neurotrophic
artifacta

II. Ischemia

arterial insufficiency
  arteriosclerosis
  hypertension

venous stasis
  stasis dermatitis
  postphlebitic syndrome

small vessel
  vasculitis
  ergotisms
  collagen diseases
  Arthus
  Raynaud's disease

occlusive
  embolus
  thrombus
  dysproteinemia
  sepsis

anemia
  sickle cell
  Cooley's

pressure
  acute—CNS compromise trapped victims
  chronic—decubitus ulcer

III. Specific disorders

infection—fungus, bacteria
pyoderma gangrenosum
Behçet's syndrome
primary blistering diseases (mechanicobullous dermatosis, occasionally EM)
chancroid, LGV, granuloma inguinale
malignancy (basal cell, squamous cell)
diabetes mellitus—NLD

Figure 12-5 Ulcers of the skin.

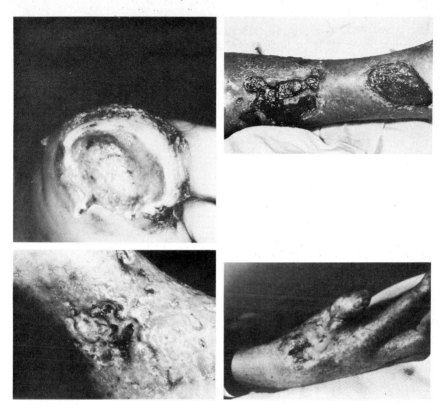

Figure 12-6 Ulcers. (a) Neurotrophic ulcer; (b) stasis ulcer; (c) arterial ulcer; (d) post-radiation ulcer.

Diabetes mellitus requires special consideration when discussing ulcers. Diabetics are more prone to develop ulcers because they are more susceptible to certain bacterial infections. Diabetics also have an increased incidence of arteriosclerosis which can lead to ischemic ulcers, and of neuropathy, which leads to neurotrophic ulcers. Lesions of necrobiosis lipoidica diabeticorum (NLD) may break down and lead to chronic ulcers.

ISCHEMIA

Arterial insufficiency may be related to organic arterial disease such as arteriosclerosis, to hypertension, or to any transient factors which cause vasoconstriction. The signs of arterial disease include hair loss, nail dystrophy, and dry, cool, pale, atrophic skin of an extremity. Leg ulcers of arteriosclerosis appear on heels, toes, or at the site of trauma. Ulcers are pale or white with slightly elevated rolled edges rimmed with several millimeters of purple-red, which contrasts with the pale skin of the surrounding area.

The base is covered with an adherent grey or yellow membrane or may be gangrenous. Little or no beefy red granulation tissue is present. These ulcers tend to heal poorly and may gradually increase in size (Figure 12-6c).

In patients with essential hypertension, ischemic ulcers appear on the lateral aspects of the ankle or foot. These lesions begin as a painful red plaque, which becomes cyanotic, then purpuric, and finally breaks down to form a tender superficial ulcer which fills with a thick adherent eschar (scab). Dressings which provide moderate pressure diminish the edema and venostasis and thereby allow better arterial flow. Such dressings may relieve the pain and allow healing.

Occlusive small artery and arteriolar diseases cause ulcers, especially on the legs. *Anemia* adds to the local tissue ischemia. Some abnormalities of red blood cells are exaggerated by the lower oxygen tension of the peripheral circulation which further exaggerates ischemia. Usually, arterial and small-vessel ulcers are more painful than venous ulcers. Elevation of the leg or cold exposure may increase the pain.

Venous insufficiency usually causes its most striking symptoms on the legs where dilated veins can often be seen grossly. Pitting edema gradually worsens during the day, because the body has been longer in an upright position. Pain or tenderness is made worse by a warm environment or prolonged standing. The skin is warm and red, red-purple, or cyanotic in color. Stasis dermatitis (Chapter 7), excoriations, delayed healing after minor trauma, and sluggish blood flow may eventually lead to ulceration of the skin (Figure 12-6b). Venous ulcers usually are on the medial leg, at or above the ankle, and usually do not involve the foot. The color is red and the base contains healthy granulation tissue. Crusting may occur. The ulcer is usually not deep or undermined. Pain is relieved by a cool environment or by elevation of the legs.

The first principle of treatment is rest. Bed rest is helpful but must be weighed against the hazards of staying in bed for prolonged periods of time (venous thrombosis, osteoporosis, loss of muscle tone, loss of motivation). A variety of dressings, topical medications, and relatively inert elements are commonly used to cover ulcers and each has its claims for assisting the healing process. Little scientific evidence exists to support most of these claims. Perhaps the major advantage of many of these compounds is simply that they are not harmful. Their application precludes the use of more irritating compounds and makes it necessary to put the extremities at rest for the applications. The water vehicle is beneficial and normal healing is allowed to procede.

To heal, an ulcer must have adequate blood supply, adequate drainage, and must be free of necrotic tissue, dirt, and significant numbers of pathogenic bacteria. When skin physiology returns to normal, healing follows. Measures such as elevation, wraps, modest pressure, rest, and diuretics, which help to reduce edema, promote healing. Heaped-up keratin, eschar, pus, and debris should be meticulously removed. Dressings should not be so occlusive that maceration occurs beneath them, and they should be changed frequently enough to prevent build-up of exudate or drainage.

Excessive pressure causes ischemia (local, temporary deficiency of blood) and resultant anoxia (reduction of oxygen). When tissues are compressed, blood is diverted from them; vessels are forcibly constricted, so that flow is inadequate. Cells get inadequate oxygen and are therefore impaired or killed. Tissue injury is proportional to the amount and duration of pressure. If pressure is great, cell damage can occur within minutes to hours. If pressure is slight it may take days to injure the tissue. Shock, vasodilator drugs, or other causes of inadequate perfusion both accelerate and exaggerate the damage.

BEDSORES

Bedsores are simply skin ulcerations resulting from prolonged pressure on discrete areas of skin (Figure 12-7a). Normally, muscle fatigue, position sense, minimal ischemia, pressure sensation, and pain provide conscious

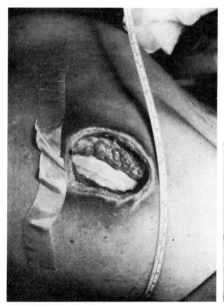
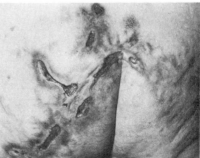

Figure 12-7 Ulcers. (a) Bedsore; deep ulcer showing fascia, muscle, and fat in base and rolled undermined edges; (b) factitial ulcer; linear- and fingernail-shaped ulcers.

and subconscious sensory input which keeps patients from maintaining pressure on one area of the skin for excessive periods of time. These sensory messages keep us shifting our weight during sitting, lying, and sleeping. Pressure injuries can, however, occur in persons who are unconscious and lie in one position or persons immobilized by accidents. Patients with neurologic defects may not perceive signs of pressure or may be unable to move parts of their bodies to shift pressure points. The earliest visible sign of pressure damage is simply erythema which may appear in minutes to hours at the site of pressure. If the pressure is sufficient, erythema is followed by some edema. In more severely injured tissues, bullae, with or without evidence of purpura, may form. Ulceration follows slough of the blister. Depending upon the amount and duration of pressure, this sequence may be reversed at any stage.

Chronic pressure occurs over bony prominences when patients are in bed for long periods of time. Decubitus ulcers, or pressure sores, are seen in debilitated persons or in patients with faulty sensory feedback. Prolonged pressure concentrated over a relatively small area of the body compresses the capillary circulation. The neurological patient not only has inadequate perception of pressure but is more likely to slip or fall. Blunt trauma may cause hematoma formation which causes further compression of tissue; sharp trauma interrupts the integrity of the skin. The resulting cell damage may result in full-thickness loss of skin. The devascularized margins of the ulcer may become undermined for a considerable distance. Variable amounts of granulation tissue gradually appear in the base of the ulcer. The necrotic tissue then provides an excellent environment for secondary bacterial infections. Cellulitis or abscess complicate the local broken-down skin site. Capillary and venous congestion further compromise blood supply and therefore make systemic antibiotic therapy less effective. Inadequate amounts of antibiotic reach the cells on the surface and the bacteria in the ischemic necrotic mesh are not affected.

General factors which make persons more likely to develop bedsores include diabetes, loss of skin sensation, marked increase or decrease in body movements, anemia, malnutrition, increased susceptibility to infection, compromised blood flow, and devitalization of deep tissues. Local factors such as infection, maceration, friction, or shearing force also make pressure ulcers more likely.

Prevention is the most essential therapeutic step. Since the cause of decubitus ulcer is prolonged concentration of body weight on a small area of soft tissue over a bony prominence, then any method which prevents prolonged pressure or distributes the weight over a larger area helps to prevent tissue ischemia. The single most important preventive measure is aggressive, constant, informed nursing care. Daily skin check should search for areas of erythema, superficial erosions, and minor trauma. Immobilized patients on standard flat beds should be turned every two hours. When handling patients, it is important to avoid sliding the skin across sheets or other surfaces. Patients should be lifted and replaced or turned and rolled. It takes three people to move a helpless patient properly. Excessive sedation should be avoided. Appropriate pads of foam rubber or other materials may relieve pressure. Alternating pressure mattresses, water beds, hamstring sitting boards, cushions, and electric beds help to redistribute pressure. Excessive moisture of the skin should be avoided because macerated skin is more easily injured and infected. Sheepskin can be used as a pad under the patient and directly against his skin. Incontinent patients must be kept clean.

At the first sign of tissue damage, the skin must be carefully cleansed and covered with a dry protective bandage. Constrictive rings, doughnut devices, or poorly placed pillows may reduce blood flow to the area and lead to further damage. Full-thickness ulcers require surgical debridement. Small lesions may be treated with silver nitrate wet dressings. Large lesions may require grafting.

FACTITIAL ULCERS

Self-inflicted injuries (dermatitis artifacta) may result in ulcers (Figure 12-7b). People inflict injury upon themselves to elicit sympathy, gain attention, avoid responsibility or unpleasant obligations, or for financial compensation (see Chapter 13). The patient then denies knowledge of the etiology of the lesions. Lesions appear relatively suddenly.

Ulcers may be produced by caustic chemicals, sharp objects, fingernails, cigarette burns, or injections of substances into the skin. Like other factitial lesions, the ulcers may be any shape and size. Bizarre configuration with straight edges and sharply demarcated borders are frequent. Whenever the site or morphology of an ulcer is not characteristic of any disease pattern, factitial dermatitis should be considered. It is, however, a diagnosis made only by excluding all other possibilities.

REFERENCES

Behçet's Disease, Monacelli, M., and P. Nazzaro, eds., S. Karger, New York, 1966.

Dermatology in General Medicine, Fitzpatrick, T. B., K. A. Arndt, et al., eds.; Pearson, R.: "The Mechanobullous Diseases," McGraw-Hill Book Company, New York, 1971, pp. 621–643.

Dermatology in General Medicine, Fitzpatrick, T. B., K. A. Arndt, et al., eds.; Stoughton, R. B.: "Mechanisms of Vesicle Formation and Classification," McGraw-Hill Book Company, New York, 1971, pp. 589–597.

Evans, C. D., and I. D. Fraser: "The Natural History of Dermatitis Herpetiformis," Trans. *St. John's Hosp. Derm. Soc.* **49:**108–114, 1963.

Lever, W. F.: *Pemphigus and Pemphigoid,* Charles C Thomas, Publisher, Springfield, Ill., 1965.

Melish, M. E., and L. A. Glasgow: "Staphylococcal Scalded Skin Syndrome: The Expanded Clinical Syndrome," *J. Pediat.* **78:**958–967, June 1971.

Newcomer, V. D., and J. W. Landau: "Recent Advances in the Diagnosis and Treatment of Pemphigus," *Calif. Med.* **114:**1–11, February 1971.

Samitz, M. H., and A. S. Dana Jr.: *Cutaneous Lesions of the Lower Extremities,* J. B. Lippincott Company, Philadelphia, 1971.

Shelley, W. B.: "Herpes Simplex Virus as a Cause of Erythema Multiforme," *JAMA* **201:**153–156, July 1967.

The Psychological Importance of Skin

Attitudes toward skin disease
  Prejudice
  Secondary gain
  Patient's perception
Attitude of the health care team
  Looking and touching
  Listening and talking
  Respect and concern
Psychosomatic factors and psychiatric delving
  The psychosomatic approach
  The focus of psychiatric inquiry
Emotions, skin changes, and skin disorders
  Physiologic responses of the skin to emotional stress
  Skin diseases which often have a primary psychological component
  Skin diseases with important emotional components
  Self-induced skin eruptions
  Cutaneous manifestation of psychosis or phobia
  Hypochondriasis
Emotional aspects of therapy
  Drug side effects
  Therapeutic side effects
  Hospitalization side effects
Dermatologic disease encountered in psychiatric patients

Although most persons do not spend much time contemplating the essential physiologic and protective roles of their integuments, they are concerned with the appearance of the skin. Skin is an important part of the self-image and of the image presented to others. The skin—especially the 5 percent which covers the face—is part of the way we relate to the world. Humans communicate by means of their skin. We register and reflect emotions by flushing (blushing), perspiring, and becoming pale. The skin glows, tingles, and glistens. We have goose bumps. We wrinkle our brows and scratch our chins.

People also communicate by the way in which they groom and style their epidermal appendages. Hair may be long or short, styled or unruly. Nails may be long, shapely, manicured, painted. The beard is allowed full growth by some men, shaped and trimmed by others, or completely removed each day. The cosmetic industry is one of the biggest in this country. Skin texture, tone, and color are exaggerated, modified, and changed. A generation ago, fair pale white skin was a sign of nobility, a flag signifying that the upper class did not have to work out in the sunny fields. Parasols, "makeup," and powders were essential to maintain this image. Now a tan is the symbol of leisure and wealth. Prolonged sunbathing, "makeup," and sunlamps are used to acquire pigmentation.

Finally, we communicate by touch. The first mode of sensory exchange between mother and unborn child is through cutaneous sensation. Experiments show that touch is one of the most sensitive of the seven senses. Man is able to distinguish minute changes in forces applied to his cutaneous surfaces. Studies in man and monkey emphasize the importance of "the tender touch" in the psychological development of the infant. Later in life, the caress becomes an integral part of sexual activity and emotional communication. The importance of being "touchable" is not just a myth of the advertising age, but strikes at basic communicative chords in man.

ATTITUDES TOWARD SKIN DISEASE

Prejudice

There exists a basic prejudice about skin disease. Even the well-informed view cutaneous disorders as more than a "blemish" of the skin. Skin disease marks a person as flawed in a more general way. Ancient writings equate skin disease with evil. The Bible tells of boils (furunculosis) as one of the plagues for Job. Lepers were considered "unclean" and were segregated from the rest of the population. Careful review of old descriptions suggests that many of these unfortunate outcasts merely had psoriasis or vitiligo.

The notion that skin disease is equated with being "unclean" is subtle and subconscious but ubiquitous. It is a prejudice that is not easily dispelled. It confuses the arbitrarily aesthetically unappealing with some ill-defined inherent character defect. Cutaneous physiological aberrations are equated with some type of basic inadequacy or evil. Skin disease becomes a manifestation of the spiritually and physically unclean. Such an assumption is an unfair value judgment.

Our basic attitudes toward skin disease have not changed greatly over the centuries. Although we know that common dermatoses are not contagious and are not the result of poor hygiene, persons with severe acne, psoriasis, birthmarks, or vitiligo may have trouble getting good jobs. Minor changes in cutaneous appearance alter an individual's social relationships and economic prospects. Patients with skin diseases must deal not only with these negative messages from their fellows, but also with their own guilt and feelings of inadequacy. They feel as if they are in some way worthless or incomplete.

A complicated mythology about skin adds to the prejudice about skin disease. Anxieties, fear of cancer, attitudes toward hygiene, and basic concepts of self-images and personal appearance may be expressed through thoughts about the skin. Skin disease may become symbolic of much more than a cosmetic flaw or an itch. Persons with skin disorders must be made to realize that they are in no way bad persons because they have abnormal skin and that they do not have bad skin as a result of being bad. This simple message begins therapy.

Secondary Gain

An illness can have positive as well as negative implications for an individual. The positive aspect of being sick is called secondary gain. The classic example of secondary gain is the child with a stomach ache who is allowed to stay home from the school session which he doesn't want to attend. In this case, the secondary gain of the illness (stomach ache) is staying home from school. Similarly, there may be secondary gain in dermatologic illnesses. For example, a hand dermatitis established as job related may permit an individual to gain transfer to a less demanding activity, and represents the secondary gain of that illness. In ascribing disease etiology and prescribing treatment, it is important to consider the impact of these decisions on the patient, his family, his employer, and society. Secondary gain may be entirely psychological and very indirect yet still play a major role in a patient's reaction to his dermatosis. More importantly, it affects the patient's thoroughness of self-treatment.

Patient's Perception

A given physical condition may result in very different levels of apprehension in different individuals. For example, many individuals are apparently willing to tolerate a few acne lesions, but others find the same number of blemishes a threat to their attractiveness and social interactions. The degree of concern about skin disease is in part determined by the general focus of an individual's concern with appearance, and this may vary with age. For example, the adolescent is extremely concerned with sexual and social functioning, and any skin changes that affect personal appearance in this period result in much anxiety.

Patients' concerns cannot be dismissed simply because they are "only of cosmetic importance" or because they will "eventually go away." Lesions that may seem insignificant to a busy nurse or doctor may be a major worry to the patient. The patient's perception of the problem should be taken into account.

ATTITUDE OF THE HEALTH CARE TEAM

Looking and Touching

The reactions of health care personnel, from receptionist to physician, can greatly influence a patient's anxiety about the "uncleanliness," disfigurement, or infectious capacity of his skin. Persons with skin disorders are very sensitive to glances of distaste or disapproval, or to any reluctance to touch them. An automatic and unintended transient expression of disgust can do harm that much verbal reassurance cannot undo. A person with hand eczema is used to people moving away from him at the lunch counter but he is not prepared for a look of instant disgust from a medical person.

Both verbal and nonverbal communication play important roles in information transmission between patient and health personnel. Initial contact is very important in setting the tenor of subsequent communication between patient and practitioner. Establishing communication with skin patients can be facilitated by making physical contact with them. Such contact may consist of a handshake or initially clasping the patient's hands to examine the palms, fingers, and nails. The latter approach both provides clinical data about areas often overlooked during the cutaneous examination and reassures the patient that he or she is touchable and not deformed or disgusting. In addition to clinical information about skin diseases, much can be learned from the initial hand contact. A patient's chronic or acute anxiety state may be reflected in sweaty palms or chewed fingernails. The willingness with which an individual will allow his hand to be clasped may reflect his style in interpersonal relationships, his degree of "leper" complex, or his trust.

In most circumstances, patients are fully undressed and gowned. While this facilitates complete examination, being without clothes is anxiety-provoking to many patients. It is essential to keep in mind the patient's vulnerability, respecting modesty and keeping exposures as brief and discrete as possible. For example, in outpatient facilities, it is often best to leave an examining room, and allow the patient to dress between examination and discussion of diagnosis and therapy. A clothed patient is not distracted by trying to maintain his modesty or dignity as is frequently the case for the individual whose only covering is a short gown. Inpatients should be allowed the maximum privacy consistent with hospital facilities and the amount of medical observation required.

Listening and Talking

The best clues to a patient's concerns are obtained by listening. Knowledge of people's concerns is essential to providing good care. For example, one individual with a seborrheic keratosis may be completely satisfied by the information that this growing dark papule is completely benign. Another patient of identical age and sex may find little comfort in the benign character of the seborrheic keratosis. For him, these "old age spots" represent loss of youth and are a significant cosmetic disability.

Clear two-directional verbal communication is essential for diagnosis and treatment. The patient should be given the opportunity to share his concerns about his disease and be given reassurance when needed. Not uncommonly, a patient who presents with what seems a minor complaint has a morbid fear that his skin lesion represents cancer. It is also important for the health care provider to anticipate the patient's fears about a skin disease, for the patient may be hesitant to share them with the physician. For example, the adolescent acne patient may not feel comfortable enough to ask about the relationship of his disease to masturbation or sexual activity. Optimal health care requires that the unasked question be anticipated. This means that the physician or nurse must frequently initiate discussions in the sensitive areas of skin disease such as possibility of malignancy, relationship to sexual activity, and emotional implications.

"Some people think that acne is made worse by chocolate, potato chips, masturbation, evil thoughts, or dirt. That is not true." Such a statement relieves many a teenager. "That is not the kind of skin lesion that becomes cancer." A few seconds spent covering some usual fears, even in the absence of direct questions, not only relieves anxiety but prevents later phone calls from patients, their families, and friends. "That is not a dangerous or contagious skin disorder, and it does not make you sick inside."

Educating the patient is too frequently neglected. Among the essential information that should be clearly conveyed during each iatrogenic encounter are the diagnosis, the etiology and degree of infectivity, the treatment, the rationale for treatment, and the expected result of the treatment.

Respect and Concern

The most important of the requirements for being an effective member of the health care team is to care. Caring is made up of equal parts of respect and concern. Respect for patients' right to life and health and maximum medical care is not enough. Each patient's individuality, modesty, psychic feelings, and self-esteem must be preserved. Medical personnel have their own opinions about "proper" life style, sexual behavior, work ethic, and class consciousness. These opinions should not, however, influence approach, treatment, and follow-up. Welfare patients, the chairman of the board, persons with V.D., and patients with acne are people with problems who deserve help without loss of dignity based on income or diagnosis.

Concern involves accepting the patient's problem as your problem. Concern is feeling uneasy unless the patient is improved or helped in some way.

PSYCHOSOMATIC FACTORS AND PSYCHIATRIC DELVING

The Psychosomatic Approach

The psychosomatic approach attempts to elucidate the interactions between emotional factors and disease. Psychosomatic research has shown that in certain diseases both somatic and psychic development play a role in the susceptibility to disease, the timing of the onset of disease, the course of the disease, and an individual's adaptation to a disease. Although susceptibility and response to a disease may be influenced by an individuals' emotional state, psychological factors are only one of multiple determinants of illness, and the relative importance of psychological, genetic, environmental, and infectious elements may vary greatly between individuals and diseases.

While the importance of psychological state in adjustment to a disease is evident, the relationship of emotional factors to the development of a disease is not always as clear. Some physiologic events can be clearly related to emotional states. Some mood alterations are readily reflected in the skin. For example, the sweating and blanching which occur with stress are the result of the action on the cutaneous vasculature and epidermal appendages of neuroactive substances released under stress. For most skin diseases, however, the relationship between emotion and skin response is not as clear as it is for blushing or blanching.

The Focus of Psychiatric Inquiry

In order to assess the role of emotion in a skin disease for a particular individual, certain information about the individual, his environment, and his disease is important. While the full psychiatric evaluation of a patient in most instances requires specially trained personnel, any health professional should be able to make certain observations and inquiries that will help to elucidate possible emotional components of an individual's illness.

Among the key information for such an assessment is knowledge about a patient's personality and its vulnerabilities. For example, one patient may feel more comfortable with maximum information about the psychiatric implications of his illness. Another may choose to minimize his knowledge about the etiology of his disease. In some cases, an individual's emotional state may be so precarious that he may not be able to deal with certain information about his illness and in these cases it is better not to attempt to force "insight" on the patient. Instead, support and referral for treatment of the underlying psychological disorder may be much more helpful. This may be especially true in dealing with severely disturbed individuals.

With any acute illness, it is helpful to look at the recent life situation and stresses faced by an individual. This is not only important for the assessment of the etiologic significance of this stress, but also for assessing to what extent therapy should be modified because of life situation. For example, hospitalization may be required for adequate treatment of a benign skin disease when an individual lacks anyone to care for him at home. Choice of therapy for itching may vary with the individual's need to be alert; it would be unwise to sedate someone who must drive a car.

Directly related to the question of life situation is the patient's mood and degree of tension. While it is a generally observed phenomenon, too often it is forgotten that the capacity of the individual to tolerate stress varies greatly. A situation easily handled by one individual can be overwhelming to another. Similarly, a stress easily tolerated at one time in an individual's life may be overwhelming at another. These variations in personality must also be kept in mind in treating the individual patient.

EMOTIONS, SKIN CHANGES, AND SKIN DISORDERS

Physiologic Responses of the Skin to Emotional Stress

Skin changes, both pathologic and physiologic, vary greatly in their emotional component or impact. Since skin responses are a continuum and a sufficiently vigorous "physiologic" reaction pattern is in some instances considered to represent pathologic change, the border between "physiologic" and "pathologic" change must often be arbitrarily drawn. Figure 13-1 lists skin disorders related to emotional states. The temporal relationship of skin disease and psychosocial stress, the reproducibility of disease with similar stress, and the meaning of the illness to the patient are all factors which should be carefully considered in deciding to what extent a skin condition is emotionally determined.

The skin can reveal much to the outside world about one's emotional state. Blushing is a transient erythema of the skin which is generally most prominent on the face, the most visible part of the body. This erythema is the result of increased blood flow to the "blush" areas. Neurochemical mediators regulate both total blood flow and local cutaneous vasomotor activity. Among the psychosocial events most clearly related to blushing

---

Skin Diseases which often have a primary *psychological component*
    Pruritus vulvae
    Pruritus ani
    Neurodermatitis (atopic dermatitis) (7)
    Dyshidrosis (7)
    Alopecia areata (2)

Skin diseases with important *emotional component (etiologic and/or resultant)*
    Acne (7)
    Psoriasis (7)
    Vitiligo (7)
    Seborrheic dermatitis (7)

Self-induced skin eruptions—psychopathology always present
    Trichotilomania
    Neurotic excoriations
    Factita
    Munchausen's syndrome (Syndrome in which a severely disturbed individual
        seeks repeated treatment for multiple self-induced signs and/or symptoms)
    Self-induced changes in an existing dermatoses

Skin disorders seen in marked psychic disturbances
    Delusions of Parasitosis
    Conversion reactions

Hypochondriacal disorders
    Cancerophobia
    Syphilophobia

Numbers in parenthesis refer to chapters in this book.

Figure 13-1 Skin disorders related to emotional states.

in everyday experience are embarrassment and excitement. The sexual nature of blushing is evidenced by the fact that sexual thoughts can lead to a blush reaction which is indistinguishable from the vasodilation which normally occurs during sexual excitement. Artificial "blushers" are used by many women to make themselves more attractive. Blanching and pilo-erection are two other physiologic alterations in the cutaneous surface which may be triggered by emotions (e.g., fear) or physiologic stimuli (e.g., cold).

Hyperhidrosis (excessive sweating) may be an accentuated physiologic response to emotions. The palms and soles are most affected. While occasional hyperhidrosis is normal, its constant presence may be very bothersome. Palms may literally drip onto the table top or floor. Maceration (softening, by wetting) of the feet can lead to offensive odors. Constant wetness can lead to the development of a variety of dermatoses. For example, fungi that result in tinea pedis grow best in a warm moist environment and the individual with hyperhidrosis can be troubled by persistent or recurrent tinea or candida infections. In addition, excessive sweating can lead to maceration of the skin which in turn can lead to pruritus. Psychologically induced hyperhidrosis is difficult to treat. Antianxiety medications (e.g., minor tranquilizers) have been very unsuccessful in the treatment of such hyperhidrosis even when they appear to calm the patient in other ways. This perhaps reflects the masking of anxiety rather than the removal of the events causing the psychological stress.

Skin Diseases Which Often Have a Primary Psychological Component

Pruritus vulvae is a disorder characterized by itching of the genital or vulvar area in the female. Pruritus in this area can be the result of a variety of stimuli including the common yeast, bacterial or parasitic infections, irritant and contact dermatitis, or a systemic cause of pruritus such as diabetes mellitus. Some women have intractable genital itching although careful examination and laboratory studies reveal no etiology for their pruritus. Within this "idiopathic" group, secondary effects of scratching such as lichenification, redness, or excoriations may be the only physical findings.

These women with pruritus vulvae can be any age, have any occupation, and be members of any class. Studies have shown that they frequently share common behavioral traits and psychological problems. They frequently report sexual and marital difficulties, marked frustration about their lives, as well as ambivalence about being women. Many such women complain of sexual dysfunction, and the skin complaints can provide a means for avoiding sexual activity. Among these individuals, scratching may have multiple functions ranging from pleasure to pain, and the possible erotic aspects of scratching in this area should be recognized. While individuals with this disorder often have very disturbed lives, both in terms of interpersonal difficulties and dissatisfactions, they are very seldom psychotic.

If the criteria for psychosomatic disease are applied to pruritus vulvae, it is apparent that many of the linkages between psychosocial forces and disease can be present in an affected individual. As in all psychosomatic disorders, an individual's genetic constitution is also important in determining which disorder may develop. Organic illness may precipitate pruritus in the genital area which will persist after the organic disease has been treated. *Pruritus ani* occurs in both sexes and may also have mixed organic, infectious, and psychic causes.

Emotional factors are often the key to flares of atopic dermatitis. In addition, this disease has important psychological effects. In infantile atopic eczema, the effect of skin disease on maternal-child interaction is especially important, for it is through the sensation of touching that the child receives much of its initial feeling of intimacy and self-assurance. The mother faced with excoriated, disfiguring rashes rather than "baby smooth" skin would find less positive reinforcement in touching her infant. The resultant loss of intimacy could result in disordered communication between mother and child and subsequently alter the child's psychological development.

It is characteristic for atopic individuals to note itching prior to the onset of any skin changes. Emotions play a significant role in the appearance of pruritus. Any type of emotional stress can act as a trigger factor, with pruritus and scratching occurring soon after such a stress. This is especially evident in the childhood atopics. These children, when frustrated or angry, will frequently begin to scratch their initially normal-appearing skin with the subsequent development of an eruption in the scratched area. The aggressive nature of scratching in such circumstances is apparent. The initial scratching not only gives an outlet for emotional tension, but also focuses the parent's attention on the child and his disease. Thus a child can express hostile, exhibitionistic, and masochistic feelings as well as signal for help and love through the single act of itching.

While individuals with atopic dermatitis have been characterized as sharing certain personality and behavioral traits, the extent to which these traits are constitutional, developmental, or the result of their disease experience is not well established. Among the traits mentioned for atopics are restlessness and irritability as a child, ambitiousness and a high-strung personality, combined with sensitivity and introversion. These individuals have often been characterized as perfectionists. However, no one personality type encompasses all who have this disorder.

The importance of emotional stress as a trigger factor in atopic eczema should be considered in making therapeutic decisions. Since scratching susceptible skin worsens the dermatitis, therapy aimed at reducing pruritus and scratching would appear logical. Among the treatments aimed at doing this are antihistamines and soothing and anti-inflammatory skin creams. When a child is experiencing itching, letting the child express himself in some way that does not involve scratching and the consequent itch-scratch cycle can be helpful. Efforts to avoid emotional stress which can trigger the itching may include psychotherapy, tranquillizers, and changing social situations. Unfortunately, these measures are not necessarily successful in reducing the pruritus. It is important to point out to the patient the role that stress may have in precipitating an attack.

While limiting scratching is a key therapeutic goal, restraining or even gloving of the young child should not be undertaken lightly, for such restraint is extremely frustrating to a child. Also, hospitalization of the infant or child can be a very disruptive and frightening experience. In a disease where condemned behavior by the child (i.e., scratching) plays a prominent role, hospitalization may be viewed by the child as punishment for his activities.

The majority of atopics can be managed by the individual responsible for skin care. In some situations, referral to a psychiatrist can become necessary. These situations include a patient who is part of a very disturbed family which is unable to accept advice or assurance. When the family is rejecting, or very resentful of the affected individual, counseling becomes crucial. In addition, if the atopic individual has a severe personality disorder, psychiatric referral is indicated. In infantile or childhood eczema, psychiatric treatment frequently involves the whole family and may consist of family therapy alone or in combination with individual therapy. It is important that realistic expectations be given to the individuals referred for psychiatric care, for this care is not likely to cure the atopic individual, and is intended to aid in adjustment to this disorder and to minimize the occurrence of emotional trigger factors.

Patients with atopic dermatitis can be very frustrating to treat, and psychiatric referral should not be used as "punishment" for a family or individual who does not cooperate in a physician's therapeutic efforts. Referral to a psychiatrist should not mark the end of the primary practitioner's involvement with the atopic individual. It should signal the beginning of a new team approach.

Alopecia areata is a sudden loss of hair in a circumscribed area. A frequent temporal relationship to emotional stress is most apparent in children in whom alopecia areata frequently occurs two to four weeks after the loss of someone important to them. While hair will often regrow spontaneously in these patients, the larger the area of the alopecia the worse the prognosis for regrowth, which is said to occur only with resolution of the precipitating emotional conflict. The relationship to emotional stress is suggestive. The cause of alopecia areata is unknown.

Skin Diseases with Important Emotional Components

Acne is a disorder of the sebaceous gland which occurs most frequently at puberty and can vary greatly in severity. Acne's impact on the individual is primarily a result of its deleterious effect on appearance which can be permanent because of postacne scarring. The psychological effects of disordered appearance in the affected adolescent age group can be especially severe, because it is during this period that social adaptation and acceptance is most important to the individual. The development of secondary sexual characteristics is in itself stressful and any other changes in appearance cannot help but add to the difficulty of adaptation to sudden maturation. Insecurity about sexuality, masturbation, and impulses is very widespread, and the folklore of acne helps add to the psychological burden of this disorder. Among the common myths about acne is that its development is related to masturbation, constipation, evil or sexual thoughts, or a diet containing "forbidden" items such as chocolates or sweets. With this conditioning, the teenager sees new acne lesions as punishment for the failure to contain impulses. Dispelling these myths about acne should be part of every initial encounter involving acne even if these issues are not directly raised by the patient.

The endocrine influences upon acne activity are illustrated by the frequently reported premenstrual flare of acne. Stress also seems to worsen acne, and this may be an endocrinologically mediated event, perhaps related to changed adrenal hormone levels. Whatever the mechanism, emotional tension, family and school pressures, sleep loss, and chronic anxiety make acne worse.

Emotional factors must be considered in implementing effective therapy for this disease. The affected individual must be sufficiently motivated to perform faithfully the required topical and systemic care. Yet it is important that the individual understand the limits of improvement which results from such care. Unexpected disappointment with the degree of improvement may further accentuate the patient's loss of self-esteem. An individual operating under the dictum, "If a little is good, more is better," may cause extensive irritation by the overly zealous applications of the drying and peeling agents routinely used in acne therapy.

Reassurance is important in the treatment of acne. It is not necessarily reassuring for the adolescent to be told that he or she will eventually "outgrow" acne. Current problems involving appearance and peer acceptance often dwarf concern about ultimate good prognosis. Acne's effect on the adolescent's psychosocial development can be great, and this potential should be considered in treating these patients. This is a prime example of a cutaneous condition whose importance lies not so much in its pathophysiologic consequences as in what it means to the affected individual, his self-image, and his relationship to peers.

Psoriasis is a common dermatosis and may have a wide range of clinical expression. It may appear as a few thickened plaques of skin or may be a life-threatening eruption as is the case with acute generalized pustular psoriasis. A disabling arthritis sometimes accompanies the disease. The "cause" of psoriasis is not known but a constitutional genetic predisposition is known to be an important factor. While the role of emotional factors in the development of psoriasis has not been clearly elucidated, the relationship between emotionally charged events and flares of psoriasis has been emphasized by a variety of investigators. Alcoholism, obesity, and worry seem to be correlated with worsening of psoriasis.

Whatever the etiologic role of stress in psoriasis, the tremendous psychosocial impact of this disorder is readily apparent to anyone connected with the care of skin disease. Psoriasis can have tremendous impact on appearance, and individuals with obvious plaques may have difficulty in employment or find themselves the subject of revulsion. Those close to them may be unwilling to touch them even if it is to apply medication. A spouse may refuse to sleep in the same bed because of scaling, and sexual relations may also be curtailed. When support at home is lacking, therapy is often neglected, and hospitalization may be necessary to clear the skin.

In fact, psoriasis is responsible for more admissions to inpatient dermatology services than any other disease. It is likely that the nurse or physician in the inpatient setting will have frequent contact with these patients, and it is important to realize that hospital admission may be the result of lack of a supportive therapeutic environment at home. Hospitalization can create financial or emotional burdens on the patient and his family.

As with other chronic disease, psoriasis can frequently result in personality changes. Many of these individuals seem angry or self-absorbed, worrying only about what will happen to them and frequently demanding special attention. In addition, they may develop a "why me?" martyred attitude or they may be depressed. If depression is persistent, a psychiatric evaluation for possible drug or supportive therapy is indicated. It may be useful for staff to help the individual share his feelings about his illness, especially patients who have required repeated hospitalization. Training of the family to help in the care of the individual may necessitate desensitizing them to the cosmetic liability of the disease. Visiting nurses can be employed in advising the patient and family and in reducing the need for hospitalization.

Self-induced Skin Eruptions

Neurotic excoriations are the most frequent of the self-induced dermatoses. They are the result of conscious manipulations of the skin. People use fingernails, hairpins, small tools, nails, needles, or knives to excavate small portions of normal or excoriated skin. Neurotic excoriations should be differentiated from factitial dermatitis which is manifested by self-induced lesions of the skin in which the individual denies having any role or knowledge in their formation. Patients with neurotic excoriations admit to "picking" at their skin. Their reasons for doing so vary greatly: itching, abnormal-appearing skin, habit, imagined skin diseases.

Neurotic excoriations can vary in severity and extent, and it is often difficult to distinguish such excoriations from self-aggravation of a preexisting dermatosis such as dry skin or stasis dermatitis. Patients with neurotic excoriations will often present with complaints of uncontrollable itching or will focus their attention on a bump or blemish in the skin which they proceed to remove mechanically with resulting self-induced injury. Altered sensation may play a role in this disease. Self-destructive manipulations are reported as frequently relieving tension and may involve ritualized behavior. In such cases, it is often possible to elucidate disturbed emotional relationships or psychological conflicts. A variety of character traits are said to be associated with self-destructive behavior. In approaching a patient with apparent self-induced excoriations, it is essential to be sure that there is no underlying organic cause of pruritus such as dermatitis herpetiformis or scabies.

In addition to neurotic excoriations, a variety of other skin changes can take place in more disturbed persons with repetitive or compulsive movements. Thumb-sucking can result in nail changes including paronychia and nail deformities. Biting and sucking of the lips or mucous membranes can lead to fissured or thickened membranes. Mental defectives and the demented frequently exhibit compulsive repetitive activity which results in skin changes. A visit to a home for the retarded will reveal many residents who incessantly rub or stroke their skin. Such repetitive activity can result in lichenification, hyperpigmentation, and sometimes even hypertrichosis.

Trichotillomania is mechanically induced hair loss resulting from an individual's manipulations (pulling, breaking, twisting the hair). The degree to which patients will admit to being conscious of their pulling of their hair may vary but admission of such manipulation usually is eventually obtained. The hair loss in these cases is patchy and diffuse with broken hairs prominent. It is generally greatest on the areas of the scalp most accessible to touching, the frontal and parietal areas. The underlying emotional disturbance may be relatively minor, in which case psychological support, sedation, and showing the connection between hair manipulation and hair loss may be sufficient to improve the disorder. In other cases, the pulling of the hair may be a manifestation of a severely disturbed psychic state. In children with trichotillomania, it is best not to confront them before their parents because the conflicts which have resulted in this behavior often involve parent-child interaction.

Dermatitis factitia (see factitial ulcer, Chapter 12) is the result of a self-induced injury to the skin. It is most clearly differentiated from neurotic excoriations by the fact that individuals with dermatitis factitia will not admit to any activity that could be responsible for the lesions. Individuals with such a dermatosis are generally severely disturbed and may be psychotic or schizophrenic. Their refusal to admit responsibility for the disorder reflects their lack of awareness of their reasons for self-destructive behavior.

Because major psychiatric illness is present, direct confrontation of a patient may be unwise. Rather, a psychiatric evaluation and appropriate psychiatric therapy should precede any direct confrontation. While the psychiatric diagnosis may vary with a particular factitial dermatosis, in general the more severe the self-inflicted injury, the more severe the psychological disturbance. While the self-inflicted dermatosis may represent self-punishment and serves to relieve tension, it may also represent an infantile attempt to obtain some secondary gain.

Cutaneous Manifestation of Psychosis or Phobia

Delusions of parasitosis is a striking, not uncommon disorder occurring in very disturbed individuals. These individuals are convinced they are infested by parasites. In addition to having multiple excoriations, they frequently present the clinician with a jar containing a variety of objects such as skin scabs, dirt, and threads that they claim are the infecting organisms. These are persistent individuals, and they frequently consult many dermatologists, and even come to the attention of entomologists.

Among individuals with delusions of parasitosis, some are phobic and may respond to reassurance or counseling. More frequently, psychotic illness underlies delusions of parasitosis and psychiatric improvement is the principal hope for alleviation of this complaint. Delusions of parasitosis may develop in an individual whose borderline psychological status is challenged by some exogenous stress such as the death of a spouse. It may occur when an individual's psychotrophic medications are altered. Clearly, individuals whose delusions of parasitosis persist after reassurance need full psychiatric evaluation.

Hypochondriasis

Exaggerated response to lesions or symptoms is common. The skin as a sensory and readily apparent organ can be the focus of inordinate concern on the part of a patient. The normal skin changes that may occur with aging or minor dermatoses may lead to multiple complaints. This may occur particularly in the narcissistic individual who feels that the slightest blemish will destroy his attractiveness and threaten his relationship to others. It may also result from discomfort about facing the inevitable physical and role changes that come with aging. The extent of such concerns can be so great that a patient may devote substantial money, time, and effort in attempts to correct what are the normal ravages of time. Extreme concern about minor blemishes may be appropriate in individuals such as actors or models whose livelihood or life styles are dependent on "perfect" skin.

In dealing with patients with pathologic concern about the appearance of their skin, two facts should be kept in mind. Confronting an individual with the "banality" of his or her complaint is not generally reassuring, and is seldom able to divert his attention from his complaint. Surgical manipulation to remove minor complaints can be an unrewarding effort because the individual may be as critical of any result as he was of the initial dermatosis.

Cancerophobia can often extend to skin lesions. Some patients seek advice about every bump and blemish. The more disturbed of these patients will question clinical diagnosis and may demand biopsy. Some individuals even when shown a negative biopsy report will still remain fearful, and occasionally these individuals clearly harbor pathologic fears about cancer that may require psychiatric help in addition to medical reassurance.

Syphilophobia. Faced with a well-advertised epidemic of V.D., it is not surprising that many individuals will seek testing or treatment for venereal disease. Some individuals have a pathologic preoccupation with venereal disease and will continue to focus on minor symptoms as evidence of their disease despite adequate treatment or reassurance. When such individuals do not respond to reassurance, this fear of venereal disease, sometimes called syphilophobia, can represent a significant impairment of psychological functioning which requires psychotherapy much more than penicillin. Guilt about sexual activity, especially extramarital, may be related to these symptoms.

EMOTIONAL ASPECTS OF THERAPY

In addition to the direct physiologic effects of dermatologic care, the modalities used in dermatologic intervention may have a variety of indirect positive and negative emotional effects.

Drug Side Effects

A variety of medications used in the care of skin diseases have central nervous system effects. Perhaps the most striking effect is seen with systemic steroids which occasionally produce mania in a formerly normal individual. The most frequently prescribed class of systemic medicine used in skin clinics, the antihistamines, have sedative effects on the central nervous system. These can result in a patient's developing activity changes that in some cases may be interpreted as signs of depression. Treating a patient with high doses of antihistamines may result in such drowsiness that new stresses result for the patient. For example, the overly sedated student may sleep in class and develop problems in his work.

Occasionally medications intended to sedate an individual will have a paradoxical effect and make him very agitated. This paradoxical reaction to medication occurs most frequently in the very young and very old. Benadryl and phenobarbital are among those drugs which may lead to paradoxical reactions.

Therapeutic Side Effects

In attempting to relieve dermatologic complaints, advice may be given that, if followed, would fundamentally alter a patient's activities and relationships. For example, having the young housewife avoid contact with any irritant soaps or washing may be virtually impossible if she must manage infants in diapers. A textile salesman irritated by the formaldehyde contained in synthetic materials may want to have clear hands, but he might be unable to avoid such contact and continue to earn his living. The effects of any therapy on an individual's work, responsibilities, and relationships to others should be consciously considered and discussed with the patient and family. At times, a social worker or family therapist may be able to provide information to the doctor or nurse which would aid them in making realistic therapeutic suggestions.

Hospitalization Side Effects

Not infrequently, skin disease does not respond to outpatient therapy. This frequently happens in patients with psoriasis and atopic eczema. Although they are not acutely ill, such patients may require hospitalization if they are to make significant improvement. While hospitalization permits more intensive care of the disease, an equally important effect is that it changes the emotional milieu which surrounds the patient, and may reduce stress.

Hospitalization also has negative effects. While it can mobilize support from the family, the opposite may occur if the family is sufficiently angry at the individual for being sick. Unfortunately, patients can use their hospitalization to manipulate their families or others close to them. Hospitalization may become a way of avoiding social or emotional problems rather than confronting them.

The hospitalization of children presents very special problems. The child carried from home to hospital is bound to be frightened by this new environment. In addition, the child may view its being hospitalized as punishment for being bad (sick). Relationships to parents may also be disturbed, especially when it is not possible for parents to be in constant attendance. The routine of the hospital is strange, the people and their dress are different, there is far more stimulation than the child has in his own environment, and much of the treatment may be painful or uncomfortable. With skin diseases, these tensions add to the fact that the skin eruption may have already interfered with nonverbal communication between parent and child.

Parents of the hospitalized child are also strained by this event, and this cannot but affect their relationship to the child. One potential impact of hospitalization on parents that is often at least partially a result of hospital personnel's actions is that the parent feels his failure is in part responsible for the child's requiring hospitalization. Such guilt is unlikely to ensure greater cooperation in the future, and may lead to the parents' further abdication of responsibility for the child's care.

DERMATOLOGIC DISEASE ENCOUNTERED IN PSYCHIATRIC PATIENTS

The psychiatric patient is at least as prone as is the average individual to develop dermatologic disease. As has been discussed, the individual under stress may be more apt to develop certain dermatoses that can be related to stress. In addition, there are skin eruptions resulting from self-manipulation such as neurotic excoriations, factita, and self-induced changes from compulsive movements.

Medications commonly employed in psychiatric practice can have a variety of effects on the skin. In addition to the well-known semiconfluent generalized macular and papular allergic eruptions that can occur with any medication, phenothiazine tranquillizers such as thorazine can precipitate photosensitive skin reactions with extensive eruptions occurring in sun-exposed areas. If medication must be maintained, these individuals sometimes can be treated by being kept out of the sun. Pigmentary changes may be seen in individuals who receive high doses of phenothiazines.

The institutionalized patient presents special dermatologic problems. Approximately 400,000 individuals are hospitalized in public psychiatric institutions. The quality of care and hygiene varies greatly among institutions and with the type of patient. In any group living situation, communicable diseases are frequently a problem. Lack of adequate personal hygiene compounds this problem, and psychiatric patients and staff can be plagued with virtual epidemics of parasitic infections such as scabies and body lice. These infestations may lead to intense pruritus, the cause of which is not treated because the constant scratching may be attributed to a patient's psychiatric condition. The incontinent patient is also prone to develop intertrigo and the bedridden patient may develop ulcers.

REFERENCES

Eller, J. J., and S. Silver: "Psychosomatic Diseases of the Skin," *Behav. Neuropsychiat.* **1**:25–36, February–March 1970.

Friedman, D., and S. T. Selesnick: "Clinical Notes on the Management of Asthma and Eczema," *Clin. Pediat.* **4**:735–738, December 1965.

Kraus, S. J.: "Stress, Acne and Skin Surface Free Fatty Acids," *Psychosomatic Med.* **32**(5):503–508, September–October 1970.

Lodin, A., and O. Stigell: "Cutaneous Self-Mutilation and Potential Self-Destruction in a Schizoid Psychopath," *Acta Dermatovener.* **46**:224–227, 1966.

Mitchell, J. C.: "Dermatologic Aspects of Displacement Activity," *Can. Med. Ass. J.* **98**:962–964, May 1968.

Montagu, A.: *Touching: The Human Significance of Skin,* Columbia University Press, New York, 1971.

Musaph, H.: "Aggression and Symptom Formation in Dermatology," *J. of Psychosomatic Research* **13**:257–264, September 1969.

Musaph, H.: *Itching and Scratching: Psychodynamics in Dermatology,* S. Karger, New York, 1964.

Obermayer, E.: *Psychocutaneous Medicine,* Charles C Thomas, Publisher, Springfield, Ill., 1955.

Preston, K.: "Depression and Skin Diseases," *Med. J. of Australia* **1**:326–329, February 1969.

Recent Developments in Psychosomatic Medicine, Wittkower, E., and Cleghorn, eds.; Seitz, P. F. D.: "Psychological Aspects of Skin Disease," J. B. Lippincott Company, Philadelphia, 1954, pp. 245–266.

Schrut, A. M., and W. G. Waldron: "Psychiatric and Entomological Aspects of Delusory Parasitosis," *JAMA* **186**:429–430, October 1963.

Waisman, M.: "Pickers, Pluckers, and Impostors: A Panorama of Self-Mutilation," *Postgrad. Med.* **38**:620–630, December 1965.

Wittkower, E., and B. Russell: *Emotional Factors in Skin Disease,* Paul B. Hoeber, Inc., New York, 1953.

Zaidens, S. H.: "Self-Induced Dermatoses: Psychodynamics and Treatment," *Skin* **3**:135–143, May 1964.

Chapter 14

Principles of Dermatologic Therapy

Goals
  Relief of symptoms
  Protection
  Removal of debris
  Alteration of cell metabolism
Infectivity
Soaks and baths
Dressings
Topical medications
  Vehicles (bases)
  Specific agents
Systemic therapy
  Antihistamines
  Corticosteroids

GOALS

1 If it is dry, wet it; if it is wet, dry it.
2 If it is acute, rest it; if it is chronic, stimulate it.

These two old, overused, and oversimplified adages are still sometimes useful general principles of empirical dermatologic therapy. Comprehensive dermatologic treatment is, however, much more complicated. Recent advances in knowledge of cutaneous physiology, the mechanism of skin diseases, and reaction patterns have made it possible to have a more logical and specific approach to the care of skin and treatment of skin disorders. The general principles of treatment of skin disease are not different from those of any medical specialty. The goals are: to define and remove the cause of the disorder, to restore the structural and functional integrity of the organ, and to relieve symptoms.

Discovering the cause of disease is the first step toward cure or prevention. Removing the specific antigen, contact irritant, insect, trauma, or microorganism can do what months of vigorous topical or systemic therapy cannot. In obtaining a history from the patient, in examining the lesion, and in performing diagnostic tests there is no substitute for thoroughness. Careful, slow, deliberate consideration of different potential causes is essential; a specific diagnosis cannot be made if it isn't considered.

In many skin disorders the etiology is not known. Some skin diseases are inherited. In other disorders, even though some of the pathologic mechanisms are observable and measurable, it is not possible to eliminate all the trigger factors. Finally, symptoms and inflammatory reactions may persist long after specific etiologic agents have been removed. Removing the cause is an important step in therapy, but not the only one.

Relief of Symptoms

One of the goals of therapy must be simply to make the patient feel better. Whenever possible, it is best to relieve symptoms by directing definitive therapy to the specific skin disorder. When this is not possible or practical, symptomatic relief of itching, dryness, or scratching is often possible. Pruritus is a disturbing symptom, and scratching and rubbing can worsen and perpetuate skin diseases. Pruritus can be eliminated by treating the underlying dermatoses, or it may be lessened by many less specific measures (see Chapter 4) which include topical treatments as well as oral medications such as antihistamines and oral tranquilizers.

Dry skin is subjectively bothersome to some people. Diseased skin loses water more readily. Dryness may lower the itch threshold, and also lead to painful cracking and fissuring. Lubricants and simple measures which help to rehydrate the skin (see Chapter 3) relieve these symptoms. Some skin lesions, such as leg ulcers (see Chapter 12), cause pain. Soaks and supportive measures which promote healing gradually lessen such discomfort.

One of the major complaints related to any skin disorder is the patient's perception of the resulting cosmetic disfigurement. Such perceptions may not seem realistic to medical personnel, but they must still be dealt with; improving the patient's self-image is a reasonable goal.

Protection

Damaged or diseased skin needs protection. The skin cannot be put to rest as can an injured bone or muscle because its barrier function is a constant necessity. The skin can be partially put to rest by protecting it from unnecessary challenges and by assuming some of the barrier function with dressings. It is possible to limit the number of environmental insults and challenges which the skin must meet. Rubbing with the fingers, scratching, and the abrasive action of clothing can be minimized. The purposeful avoidance of soap and water, chemicals, and extremes of temperature is protective. Dressings can protect against exposures to irritants, dirt, and mechanical trauma. Wet dressings protect against the drying effect of air. Occlusive dressings increase the penetration of certain topical medications while they keep the patients from scratching.

Not only does diseased or damaged skin itself need protection, but the whole patient may need special protective or compensatory attention because of the loss of the outer barrier. Persons with atopic eczema should not be vaccinated for smallpox and should be kept away from persons recently vaccinated or persons with active herpes simplex. Patients with extensive vesicular, bullous, or erosive skin disorders, including burn patients, must be kept away from potential sources of secondary infection. If such patients with large areas of denuded skin do become infected, systemic antibiotics are needed to keep them from being overwhelmed by sepsis. Burn patients and some patients with bullous diseases often need fluid replacement because massive amounts of fluids escape through the skin.

Removal of Debris

Not only must the cause of skin disorders be removed, but other substances must be removed as well. Excessive scale can prevent penetration of medicine, retard healing, or be unsightly. In psoriasis, for instance, at the same time that treatments are directed toward decreased scale production by slowing skin metabolism; the scale can also be mechanically removed. Soaks macerate the scale, and make it more easily removed; brushing vigorously can scrub them away. Baths soak, macerate, and float off scales. Keratotic follicular plugs may be lifted out when certain primary irritants stimulate follicular and perifollicular epidermis to proliferate faster. Hyperkeratotic areas can also be softened, and thereafter more easily worn away, when chemicals such as salicylic acid or propylene glycol are applied under occlusion. Such chemicals alter the pH, which may permit increased hydration of skin from endogenous water.

Dirt, debris, and crust must also be removed. When skin continuity is interrupted, serum proteins coagulate, dehydrate, and form fibers and gel, and red blood cells and white blood cells become trapped in the tangled mesh. The crust is an essential step in early hemostasis and water barrier function. It is the temporary barrier under which the new epidermis forms. However, as time goes by, this crust is an unnecessary graveyard of white cells and bacteria. It retards healing, and provides food for bacteria. Sudden mechanical removal of crusts may cause pain and bleeding but gradual debridement of the useless elevated portions of scab is a useful process. This can be done by soaks and dressings. Excessive numbers of bacteria which do not normally colonize skin must also be removed. Soaks, frequent dressing changes, and attention to hygiene help to reduce the number of bacteria. A more specific approach involves topical and systemic antibiotics (see Chapter 7). The best way to protect the underlying tissue against bacteria is to restore the dry intact stratum corneum.

Alteration of Cell Metabolism

Topical medications, dressings, and treatments can alter skin temperature and blood flow and thereby affect the metabolism of the skin. The rate of delivery to and use of oxygen by the tissues can be changed. The rate at which toxins and mediators are absorbed can be modified. The speed, efficiency, and thoroughness of the inflammatory reaction may be altered.

Warm soaks and heat lamps cause local vasodilation and increased blood flow. Insulation of the skin alone will increase local temperature by several degrees. Besides bringing increased heat, increase in circulation of blood to the skin brings nutrients and metabolites to the cells which are dividing and manufacturing new proteins and also removes wastes and toxins at a faster rate. On the other hand, the cooling and vasoconstriction caused by wet dressings may help reverse the symptomatic hypermetabolic state of the eczematous or psoriatic epidermis and may reduce itching.

At times the inflammatory process appears excessive for the amount of protection it provides the host (see Chapter 5), so that the process itself is the major source of discomfort and disability. Topical glucocorticosteroids cause vasoconstriction and reduce blood flow to the skin. This vasoconstriction leads to a reduction in redness, heat, and itching. Steroids also reduce inflammation by other mechanisms which are not well understood. They appear to have a suppressive effect at each stage of the immune response. They interfere with certain cells and mediators of inflammation and may suppress hypersensitivity reactions.

Methotrexate causes a decrease in the mitotic rate, lengthens the turnover time, and slows the formation of stratum corneum or scale. Medications containing primary irritants stimulate the skin, and shorten turnover time. Ultraviolet light causes an initial decrease in the production of DNA and in cell replication which is followed by a rebound increase in these parameters. Since faster production of keratin leads to faster sloughing, such medications are often referred to as having "keratolytic" properties. It is imagined that the excess sloughing of keratin mechanically cleanses pores or that more keratin is lost than is made, but convincing evidence for these events is hard to accumulate.

Substances which evaporate rapidly, lower the surface temperature of the skin. Any measure that prevents rubbing or scratching stops the trauma that causes the release of mediators which lead to more irritation and to itching and scratching.

INFECTIVITY

Most of the common skin disorders are not contagious. It is safe to touch most skin patients to reassure them, provide nursing care, and apply medication. Topical creams and ointments are usually best applied with the hand, which permits delivery of an accurate amount of medication with little or no waste. Applicators absorb medication, leading to waste and making it more difficult to apply a uniform layer. Abnormalities in skin texture and surface characteristics can best be appreciated during application with an ungloved hand. Finally, direct application with the hand is more acceptable to the patient. However in bullous diseases, burns, or extensive skin ulcers, great care must be taken not to carry infection to the patient's skin.

There are only a few commonly encountered skin disorders that are markedly contagious. Persons caring for the ill should be able to recognize them and should always have a high index of suspicion. If in doubt, wear gloves. Acne, psoriasis, vitiligo, eczema, and seborrheic dermatitis are not contagious.

Bacterial infections (see Chapter 8). Impetigo and staphylococcal pyodermas should be treated with gloved hands. Dressings should be carefully discarded and hands washed thoroughly before treating other patients. Any dermatitis which is secondarily infected with bacteria should be considered possibly infectious to others.

Syphilis (see Chapter 9). Primary chancre and secondary syphilis lesions are contagious. Erosive lesions on the genitalia should be examined with gloved hands. Nonconfluent, generalized eruptions which involve palms and soles should not be touched until syphilis has been ruled out.

Scabies and pediculosis (see Chapter 8). These disorders are contagious through close contact with skin, bed clothes, or clothing. Patients complaining of severe pruritus which is worse at night and which leads to excoriations, should be examined closely for signs of parasites.

Others. Ringworm of the scalp is particularly contagious among children but is much less common since the introduction of griseofulvin. Fungus infections of the rest of the body are contagious but individual susceptibility plays a large role and the organisms are so ubiquitous that scrupulous sterile techniques are more ritual than protection. Warts can be spread from person to person but usually a scratch or implantation of the virus must occur and even then it is not easily transferred even under ideal experimental conditions.

Eczema patients, or any patients with extensive areas of denuded skin, should be protected from persons with active herpes simplex lesions, or from recent smallpox vaccinations. Herpes zoster lesions contain virus capable of causing chicken pox.

SOAKS AND BATHS

Soaks and baths provide comfort. They are soothing and antipruritic. They also provide irrigation to remove debris, contaminants, exudates, and devitalized tissue. They help rehydrate the wound. The rate of healing of surface epithelium is decreased if it is allowed to dry. Scale and crust which is macerated by soaking in water is more easily removed.

A tub bath may be better tolerated by tender skin than the rubbing of a sponge bath in bed. A tub bath also gently cleans within flexures and body folds better than soaks. With widespread skin disorders, medicated baths can evenly distribute soothing antipruritic, anti-inflammatory agents. Starch (soluble cornstarch), oatmeal, and soybean complex are commercially available in forms used for adding to tub baths. They frequently have a soothing effect. It is felt that the layer of solute left in the skin can provide protection and can decrease the oozing of acute dermatitis, but there is no evidence for this phenomenon. Symptom relief may be from some other mechanism, or may be psychological. Potassium permanganate, which is sometimes used for generalized weeping and bullous dermatoses, has deodorizing properties. Tar preparations added to baths are antipruritic to some patients. Bath oils are thought to prevent postbath drying by forming a thin film on the skin. They are especially useful in elderly patients or in patients with ichthyosis or chronic eczema. The tub becomes extremely slippery when bath oils are used. Patients should use caution, and move slowly and carefully to avoid falling. Elderly patients should be assisted.

The tub should be about half full and the duration of soaking no longer than one-half hour. Warm baths cause vasodilation. Cool baths cause vasoconstriction which may decrease itching. Weak and debilitated patients should have an attendant available throughout the bath. All patients should be warned about the slippery quality of most medicated baths. After a bath the skin should usually be patted dry. The best time to apply lubricants is immediately after the bath. This helps hold water in the recently hydrated skin and does not make a slippery tub.

DRESSINGS

Wet dressings. Liquids and solutions can be applied to the skin with dressings thoroughly soaked in the fluid. Wet dressings are modified soaks, and may have an antipruritic, soothing effect. They may be used to deliver medication or to macerate scale and crust to facilitate their removal. Pus and exudate goes up into the dressing and is removed from the diseased skin. There are two types of wet dressing, the open, or unoccluded method, and the closed or occluded method.

The *open wet dressing* is simpler, most commonly used, and is usually preferable. It consists of simply applying the saturated cloth or gauze directly on the skin and leaving the dressing exposed to the air. The fluid is allowed to evaporate, and thereby provides a cooling effect on the diseased skin. The natural vasoconstrictive response to cooling decreases the redness and decreases local blood flow of the inflammatory reaction. Wet dressings cleanse away exudate and crust and help maintain drainage. Such technique is especially useful in acutely inflamed, vesicular, or oozing dermatitis. For continued effect the dressing must be removed as it dries, remoistened, and reapplied.

Although various solutes and medications are added to wet dressings, the most important ingredient is the water. Solutions for wet dressings include saline (0.9 percent sodium chloride solution), aluminum acetate (Burow's U.S.P.), and potassium permanganate ($KMNO_4$). Silver nitrate ($AgNO_3$) has antiseptic and coagulant properties. Claims of inherent permissive, supportive, or even stimulating roles in reepithelization are difficult to confirm. Upon exposure to air, silver nitrate stains the skin a dark brown. Boric acid is readily available, is inexpensive, and is often used in wet dressings. Significant systemic absorption may take place if large areas of acutely eczematous, raw, oozing skin are treated. Possibilities of toxicity may outweigh definitive therapeutic benefits.

The dressing materials generally used are Kerlix gauze rolls for the extremities, light cotton toweling for the trunk, and gauze sponges without a layer of absorbent cotton for the face, neck, and flexural areas. The bed linens should be protected with plastic sheeting which is covered with an absorbent cotton blanket. If additional blankets are needed for comfort, a bed cradle should be used. Home treatments can be done with clean pillow cases, sheets, handkerchiefs, or white shirts torn into 2-inch to 4-inch strips. Clean material should be used but sterile technique is not necessary.

Application. Soak each dressing in a basin containing the prescribed solution and wring out excess moisture before applying; a single layer must be in contact with the surface of the affected area. The gauze sponges should be spread out to cover the specific areas, but some wrinkling or crumpling of the gauze is better than smooth adherence to the skin surface. Two to five layers of gauze may be necessary to prevent rapid drying of the dressing. Remoistening every ten to fifteen minutes provides maximum cooling effect. Wetting solutions can be kept in an intravenous bottle and the tubing positioned so that a continuous drip lands on the dressing. The same dressing material may be used, with repeated rewettings and reapplications, for a twelve-hour period except when drainage is excessive or if the prescribed solution has a cumulative effect, e.g., silver nitrate solution. Each toe or finger should be wrapped separately. When compressing more than one-third of the body with wet soaks, be especially careful that the room is warm enough and that the patient is not chilled. A bed cradle with a lamp may be necessary to provide heat so that evaporation does not lower body temperature below normal. Overmaceration should be avoided by having intermittent drying periods between soaks.

The *closed wet dressing* is one in which the wet fabric is applied to the skin as above and is then covered. Coverings can be occlusive to prevent evaporation of water or insulative to prevent escape of heat or they may be both. If a dressing is occluded with plastic, oil cloth, waxed paper, saran wrap, or some other nonpermeable layer, evaporation and epidermal maceration are increased. If occlusion is maintained uninterrupted for periods in excess of several hours, maceration may be excessive. Towels, incontinence pads, blankets, and other insulating materials which prevent heat loss temporarily elevate the skin temperture and blood flow to the skin is increased. This method is useful in treating cellulitis or erysipelas where increased blood flow may be helpful and where cooling, drying, and relief of itching are not essential. Prolonged occlusion may also encourage overgrowth of bacteria, both because of increased water and warmth.

Wet-to-dry dressings are simply wet dressings that are allowed to dry in place before they are removed. When this happens membranous exudate, debris, or eschar sticks into the mesh of the dressing and can be gently pealed away when the dressing is removed. Initially, wet-to-dry soaks are soothing and cooling and, finally, provide gentle debridement. In order to permit complete drying in a reasonably short period of time, the dressing should not be too thick.

Dry dressings protect the skin, hold medications against the skin, keep clothing or sheets from rubbing the skin, and keep dirt and air away. They also prevent infectious exudate from coming in contact with others. Dressings may also prevent patients from scratching or from rubbing. In the case of neurodermatitis or stasis dermatitis, they are often left in place for days. Soft casts or cast-like boots can serve the same purpose. Mesh gauze or other materials which permit passage of air, water, and heat are usually used. Totally occlusive dry dressings which prevent evaporation of endogenous cutaneous water could end up being wet dressings, and causing maceration.

TOPICAL MEDICATIONS

Vehicles (Bases)

Powders promote dryness by increasing the effective area for evaporation. They can be used to reduce moisture, maceration, and friction in intertriginous areas. Some powders may absorb moisture. Powders may be simple inert chemicals or they may contain medications. *Lotions* are suspensions of insoluble powders in water. When powder is present in excess, it settles to the bottom and the lotion must be vigorously shaken to resuspend the particles (shake lotion). As the water on the skin surface evaporates, it cools and creates the feeling of dryness. It also leaves a uniform film of powder on the surface. The addition of alcohol increases the cooling effect. *Creams* are emulsions of oil and water. They "vanish" into the skin because the water evaporates and the residual oil, which has a high melting point, is not noticed on the skin. They are cosmetically acceptable and are used as the base for the majority of topical medications. *Ointments* consist of oils with variable smaller amounts of water added in suspension. Some ointments are miscible with water, others are not. Ointments have a pleasant lubricating effect on dry or diseased skin but may also lead to an undesirable greasy feeling on skin and clothing. They prevent or retard water loss through evaporation and therefore allow endogenous hydration of stratum corneum. Ointments retain heat and may increase percutaneous absorption of some medications. The more occlusive ointments should not be used on oozing or infected areas because the resulting occlusion and warmth may increase bacterial growth. *Pastes* are mixtures of powder and ointment.

Specific Agents

Antibacterial agents. Some of the most effective and frequently used systemic antibiotics such as penicillin or streptomycin are not used topically because they have a high potential for causing allergic contact dermatitis. Most topical antibiotic medications include one or more of the minimally absorbable antibiotics: bacitracin, gramicidin, polymyxin, or neomycin. Arguments used to justify a combination approach include the difficulty of quick identification of the pathogenic organism, the frequent presence of more than one pathogen, and the fact that these agents are safe when used topically. They should be used after the skin is cleansed and crusts and debris have been removed. They should not be used with occlusion. *Bacitracin,* an antibiotic elaborated by a bacterium, is effective against many gram-positive organisms. *Neomycin* and *gentamycin* are effective against staphylococci and against most gram-negative organisms. They act by interfering with bacterial protein synthesis. *Polymyxin B* is also effective against gram-negative organisms and acts by altering the bacterial cell membrane.

Organic iodides slowly liberate iodine into the surrounding tissue. Because the resulting antiseptic action is effective against a wide range of bacteria, fungi (including yeasts), viruses, and protozoa, such preparations are sometimes used to prepare the skin for a surgical procedure or to cleanse it before applying dressings. Alcohol, which evaporates rapidly and has bactericidal activity that may be equally effective, is more widely used.

Antibiotic powders may prevent or reduce infection when sprinkled into ulcers, wounds, or denuded skin. Topical antibiotics are used as preventive and curative treatments. They should not be a substitute for vigorous cleansing, debridement, and supportive care. If extensive primary or secondary bacterial infection exists or if adenopathy or fever are present, systemic antibiotics are indicated.

Topical steroids. The most potent local anti-inflammatory medications are the topical corticosteroids. They are effective in treating most inflammations and pruritic cutaneous disorders. They are easy to compound, stable in many bases, and mix well with other medications. They are useful in a wide variety of common eruptions. The onset of action is rapid. Frequent topical use causes no pain, no tolerance to their action develops, the feel and smell is acceptable, and they do not stain.

The exact mechanism of the anti-inflammatory activity of topical steroids is not known. They cause vasoconstriction which reduces blood flow and that alone may reduce erythema and itching and may nonspecifically reduce the degree of inflammation. The mitotic rate in fibroblasts and epidermal cells is slowed. Enzyme activities within cells may be diminished by stabilization of various membranes. Steroids can interfere with the migration of cells, impede phagocytosis, and suppress hypersensitivity. Atopic eczema, seborrheic dermatitis, lichen simplex chronicus, and psoriasis respond to topical steroids.

Hundreds of compounds are available. Minor changes in molecular structure affect both potency and percutaneous absorption. Cortisone has no anti-inflammatory action when applied topically to the skin, but hydrocortisone is moderately effective, and fluorinated corticosteroids are extremely potent. Occlusion increases the efficacy of most of the topical steroid preparations. The increased state of hydration of the stratum corneum which occurs with occlusion appears to induce a reservoir of corticosteroid in the stratum corneum which may persist for days. Enough percutaneous absorption occurs so that, if large areas of severely compromised skin are treated with occlusion, transient adrenal suppression occurs. Careful studies of the pituitary adrenal axis document such suppression but clinically significant adrenal insufficiency is unlikely. Steroids are also injected into cutaneous lesions to provide a higher concentration or a prolonged depot. The side effects of topical steroids include telangiectasia (especially on the face), skin atrophy, and striae (especially in body folds). Topical hydrocortisone in 1 percent concentration does not appear to cause telangiectasia or striae and is perfectly adequate for many inflammatory skin disorders. The likelihood of side effects increases with increased potency of the steroid preparation used, and with occlusion, injection, and duration of therapy. Intermittent use for significant disease usually is justified when considering the risk-benefit ratio.

Tars. The distillation of certain organic substances yields tars. Four groups of substances are used as a source of tars for dermatologic use: wood, coal, bitumen (pitch), and crude petroleum. The commercially available mixtures vary and are very impure, containing many different hydrocarbon fractions and other chemicals. Crude coal tar is often applied directly to the body to treat psoriasis. Tars seem to increase the effectiveness of long-wave ultraviolet light and to reduce the mitotic rate in psoriasis. They are mixed into many topical medications and shampoos. Tars seem to be anti-inflammatory, antipruritic, and soothing. There is some evidence that they oxidize or change epidermal constituents.

SYSTEMIC THERAPY

Antihistamines

Antihistamines antagonize or block most of the pharmacologic actions of histamine. Since histamine is a major mediator of inflammation, especially of certain allergic reactions, antihistamines are useful in controlling these reactions. They are most helpful in controlling the symptoms of urticaria, angioedema, drug reactions, and other allergic cutaneous reactions. Antihistamines are only moderately effective in treating other (nonallergic) forms of pruritus, and are often not helpful in relieving the itching of eczema.

Antihistamines are rapidly absorbed after parental or oral administration. They also have antipruritic activity when used topically, but may produce allergic contact dermatitis when used in this manner. The most frequent side effect is sedation and patients driving cars or working around machinery should be warned of this. Patients on antihistamines are more sensitive to the central nervous system effects of alcohol or barbiturates. The different chemical classes of antihistamines have only minor variations in their properties but individuals may react differently to each of the compound's therapeutic and side effects. It may be necessary to try several different compounds before optimum relief of itching is found.

Corticosteroids

Systemic corticosteroids have a striking anti-inflammatory action and bring about improvement of many dermatologic disorders. However: (1) prolonged administration leads to serious medical and orthopedic disabilities, adrenal suppression, and susceptibility to infection. (2) Many diseases, such as psoriasis, alopecia areata, and atopic dermatitis, may rebound after steroids are withdrawn. (3) Safer and simpler therapy is available for many common dermatoses.

The decision to use systemic corticosteroids is therefore not based only on the likelihood of therapeutic response, but also on a careful consideration of the benefits versus the sizable number of risks. This limits the use to several types of dermatologic conditions.

A Short course. (It is known that duration of therapy will be short.)
  1 Burst therapy. Short-term (days to weeks) therapy to suppress an acute and severe allergic or inflammatory reaction with a known short, defined time course. Even in moderately high doses, short-term courses of steroids carry little risk for healthy people. Severe contact dermatitis, such as severe poison ivy dermatitis, extensive sunburn, acute generalized urticaria of known cause, and severe drug eruption can be "covered" with such burst therapy, starting with high doses and diminishing over a few days to two to three weeks.
  2 Life-threatening hypersensitivity or immunologic reactions may require steroid therapy. The long-term effects are a lesser consideration when life is in danger. Severe anaphylactic reactions, severe erythema multiforme, and acute exfoliative erythroderma may require systematic steroids.

B Prolonged Treatment. Disease is so severe (or alternate therapy is not as effective as, or is even more dangerous than, steroids) as to outweigh risks involved.

   1 Severe systemic effects of collagen disease such as systemic lupus erythematosus or dermatomyositis, or immunologic types of vasculitis.

   2 Chronic bullous diseases such as pemphigus, pemphigoid, epidermolysis bullosa.

   3 All other therapy fails and the patient is constantly symptomatic, as in exfoliative erythroderma and chronic severe eczema.

REFERENCES

Arndt, K.: *Manual of Dermatologic Therapeutics,* Little, Brown and Company, Boston, 1974.

Blank, I. H.: "Action of Emollient Creams and Their Additives," *JAMA* **164:**412–415, May 1957.

Burack, R.: *The New Handbook of Prescription Drugs,* Pantheon Books, Inc., New York, 1970.

Current Dermatologic Management, Maddin, W. S., and T. H. Brown, eds.. The C. V. Mosby Company, St. Louis, 1970.

Frazier, C. N., and I. H. Blank: *A Formulary for External Therapy of the Skin,* Charles C Thomas, Publisher, Springfield, Ill., 1954.

Handbook of Non-Prescription Drugs, Griffenhagen, G. B., ed., American Pharmaceutical Association, Washington, D.C., 1967.

Lerner, M. R., and A. B. Lerner: *Dermatologic Medications,* Second Edition, Year Book Medical Publishers, Chicago, 1960.

The Pharmacological Basis of Therapeutics, Fourth Edition, Goodman, L. S., and A. Gilman, eds., The MacMillan Company, New York, 1970.

Quinones, C. A., and R. K. Winkelmann: "Changes in Skin Temperature with Wet Dressing Therapy," *Arch. Derm.* **96:**708–711, December 1967.

Steigleder, G. K., and W. P. Raab: "Skin Protection Afforded by Ointments," *J. Invest. Derm.* **38:**129–131, March 1962.

Wilkinson, D. S.: "Dermatological Dressings," *Practitioner* **202:**27–36, January 1969.

Index

Abscesses, described, 150
Acantholysis, blister formation resulting from, 240, 241
Acanthosis nigricans, 233, 234
Acids causing alopecia, 21
Acne rosacea, 117–119
Acne vulgaris, 112–117
  adolescent, 43
  causes of, 23, 25
  characteristic lesions of, 112–114
  distribution of, 65
  external factors worsening, 115
  psychological component of, 264, 268–269
  therapy for, 107, 108, 115–117
Acquired skin disorders, defined, 65
Acrochordons (cutaneous tags, fibroepithelial polyps), 46, 49, 106
Acrodermatitis enteropathica, cutaneous signs of, 232
Actinic (solar) keratosis, 203, 204
  blister formation and, 240
  squamous cell carcinoma and, 207–209
Active immunity, defined, 84–85
Acute pressure, ulcers caused by, 250
Adipose layer (subcutaneous tissue, panniculus adiposus), 6, 15
Adolescent skin, 43–44
Aged, the:
  alopecia among, 20
  skin of, 48–50
Agents of medications, types of, 284
Alkalis causing alopecia, 21
Allergic contact dermatitis, 93–96
Allergic cutaneous dermatitis, 96
Allergic vasculitis, 216
Allergies, 83–91
  to drugs, 89–91, 215, 216
  erythema multiforme as, 87, 88, 91
    (See also Erythema mutiforme)
  to insect bites, 86
  as skin reactions, 83–85
  therapy for, 286–287
  urticaria as, 87, 90, 91, 227
    (See also Urticaria)
Alopecia (loss of hair, baldness):
  causes of, 20–22
  male pattern baldness, 21
    androgens and, 26
    in menopausal women, 48
    typical distribution of, 20
  secondary syphilis and, 191, 192
  thyroid disorders and, 226

Alopecia areata:
  described, 20–21
  psychological component of, 264, 267–268
  treatment of, 287
Alopecia totalis, 21
Alopecia universalis, 21
Amelanosis, defined, 56
Anaesthetic ulcers (neurotrophic ulcers, mal perforant), 249, 251
Anagen phase of hair follicles, 18–19
Anaphylaxis, described, 85
Anatomy, 6–31
  of apocrine glands, 23–24
  of dermis, 12–15
  of eccrine sweat glands, 26–28
  of epidermis, 8–12
  of hair, 17–22
  of melanocytes, 29–31
  of nails, 28–29
  of oil glands, 22–23
  of skin, 6–14
Androgens:
  function of, in adolescence, 43
  male pattern baldness and, 26
  sebaceous and apocrine glands responsive to, 23, 25, 34
  terminal hairs affected by, 20
Anemia, ulcers caused by, 250, 252
Angular stomatitis (cheilitis, perleche), 161, 162
Anhidrosis:
  causes of, 137
  defined, 28
Antibacterial agents, defined, 285
Antigens, defined, 84
Antihistamines, 286–287
Aphthous stomatitis (canker sores), 186–187
Apocrine glands:
  adolescent, 43
  of the aged, 49
  anatomy and physiology of, 23–24
  cerumen glands as modified, 24, 25
  embryological formation of, 17
  PEG and, 16
Apocrine nevi, 38
Arterial insufficiency, ischemia and, 250–252
Arterial ulcers, 251
Arteriolar diseases, ischemia and, 250, 252
Arteriosclerosis, ulcers and, 250
Arthus, ulcers and, 250
Atopic dermatitis, 127–131
  blisters in, 240

Atopic dermatitis:
  causes of, 95
  characteristics of, 127–128, 130
  infections and, 131
  pruritus in, 128–129
  psychological components of, 264, 266–267
  therapy for, 96, 132–133, 267, 286, 287
Atrophy of skin, 61
Autoeczematization as cause of eczema, 93

Bacitracin, 285
Bacterial folliculitis, 151
Bacterial infections, 151–159
  alopecia and, 21
  bacterial folliculitis as, 154
  carbuncles as, 156–157
  causes of, 151
  cellulitis as, 157
  ecthyma, 154
  eczema and, 131
  erysipelas as, 157–158
  erythrasma as, 151–152
  furunculosis as, 154–156
  hidradenitis suppurativa as, 158, 159
  impetigo as, 150–154, 280
    characteristics and treatment of,
      152–154
    crusts of, 61
    in newborns, 35
    spongiosis in, 239
  responsbile for BFP, 196
  therapy for, 280
  ulcers caused by, 250
Balanitis, 176
Baldness (see Alopecia)
Basal cell carcinoma (basal cell epithelioma,
    rodent ulcer), 206–207
  curettage of, 105
  ulcers and, 250
Basal cells:
  defined, 8
  kinetics of, 10
Bathing suit nevi, 38
Baths, 281–282
Bedsonia, 188
Bedsores, 253–255
Behcet's syndrome, ulcers and, 250
Benign malformations, 37–43
  dermal melanocytosis as, 41–42
  hemangiomas as, 37–41
  lentigo and freckles as, 42–43
  moles as, 38, 39, 41
    alopecia and, 21
    basal cell carcinoma and, 207
    as benign tumors, 205
    as premalignant neoplasms, 212
    sebaceous, 38
Benign mucosal pemphigoid (cicatricial
    pemphigoid), 245
Benign tumors, 45–47, 202
BFP (biologic false positive), 195, 196
Biliary diseases as cause of pruritus, 67
Biologic false positive (BFP), 195, 196

Biopsy, 104–105
  for cutaneous horn, 205
  for malignant melanomas, 213
Birthmarks (see Hemangiomas; Moles)
Blackheads (comedones), 112–113
Blepharitis, 119–120
  acne rosacea and, 117
Blisters, 239–247
  causes of, 239–241
  in erythema multiforme, 245–247
  fever, 178
  in pemphigoid, 242, 243, 245
  in pemphigus group, 240–244
    acantholytic cells of, 102
    characteristics of, 241–243
    microscopic examination of, 103
    therapy for, 243, 288
Blue nevi (dermal melanocytoma), 42
Blushing as physiologic response, 264–265
Body heat regulation, function of eccrine
    glands in, 26, 27
Body lice infestation (see Pediculosis)
Body odor, causes of, 24, 25
Body ringworm (tinea corporis), 164–165
Bowen's disease, 204–206
  blister formation in, 240
  causes of, 205–206
  squamous cell carcinoma and, 209
Bullae:
  defined, 57
  systemic diseases manifested by, 216
Bullous pemphigoid, 243, 245
Burns (see Thermal injuries)
Burst corticosteroid therapy, 287
Butterfly rash, 119, 120, 228, 244

Café au lait lesions, described, 235
Callus, described, 75
Cancer, cutaneous signs of, 232–233
  (See also Skin cancer)
Cancerophobia, 264, 272
Candida albicans, 160, 161, 163
Candidiasis (see Moniliasis)
Canker sores (aphthous stomatitis), 186–187
Capillary hemangiomas (strawberry mark,
    nevus vasculosus), 39–40
Carbuncles, 156–157
Carcinoma in situ:
  Bowen's disease as, 204, 205
  defined, 203
Cavernous hemangiomas, described, 41
Cell metabolism, effects of therapy on, 279–280
Cellulitis, bedsores and, 254
Cerumen glands as modified apocrine glands,
    24, 25
Cervicitis, herpes simplex and, 176
Chancre, syphilitic, 189–190
Chancroid, 196, 198
  acquired by sexual contact, 188
  as minor venereal disease, 187
Chapping, conditions causing, 12
Cheilitis (angular stomatitis, perleche),
    161–162

Cherry angiomas, 49
Chicken pox (varicella):
 cutaneous signs of, 216, 219, 220
 primary cell damage in, 239
 pruritus in, 67
Chloasma (melasma, pregnancy mask), 139–140
Chronic eczema, 92, 108, 281
Chronic hand eczema, 128
Chronic pressure, ulcers caused by, 250
Cicatricial pemphigoid (benign mucosal pemphigoid), 245
Circumscribed neurodermatitis (LSC, lichen simplex chronicus), 95, 135–136, 286
Classification of blisters, 239–240
Clavus (corns), 75
Closed wet dressings, 283
Coin-shaped eczema (see Nummular eczema)
Cold:
 blisters caused by, 240
 common, as cause of BFP, 196
Collagen:
 of the aged, 48, 49
 described, 13
Collagen diseases (connective tissue diseases):
 cutaneous signs of, 227–230
 paronychial telangiectasia and, 236
 therapy for, 288
 ulcers caused by, 250
Comedo nevi, 38
Comedones (blackheads), 112–113
Common cold as cause of BFP, 196
Common warts (verruca vulgaris), 171, 172
Compound melanocytoma (Spitz juvenile melanoma), 42
Condyloma accuminata (venereal warts), 171, 172, 188
Condyloma lata, 191, 192, 194
Configuration (arrangement) of lesions, defined, 64
Conjunctivitis:
 acne rosacea and, 117
 herpetic keratoconjunctivitis, 176
 seborrheic dermatitis and, 119
 sunlamps and, 76–77
Connective tissue diseases (see Collagen diseases)
Connective tissue nevi, 38
Contact dermatitis:
 allergic, 93–96
 atopic dermatitis and, 131
 blisters in, 240
 described, 96
 therapy for, 94–95, 287
Conversion reactions, 264
Cooley's anemia, ulcers and, 250
Corns (clavus), 75
Corticosteroids, 287–288
Corynebacterium acnes:
 inhibiting growth of, 116
 role of, 114–115
 in skin ecology, 148
Corynebacterium minitissimum, 151

Coxsackie (virus), 216, 218
Creams, 284
Crusts, 61–63
Cryosurgery, 107
 for actinic keratoses, 203
 for basal cell carcinoma, 207
 for hemangiomas, 40
 for molluscum contagiosum, 174–175
 for warts, 173
Curettage, 105–106, 203
Curly hair, 22
Cutaneous dermatitis, 96
Cutaneous horn, 204, 205
Cutaneous signs, 214–237
 of cancer, lymphoma, leukemia, and mycosis fungoides, 232–235
 of connective tissue diseases, 227–230
 of gastrointestinal tract diseases, 231–232
 of mastocytosis, 230–231
 of metabolic and endocrine disorders, 225–227
 of psychosis or phobia, 264, 271
 of systemic diseases, 214–225
Cutaneous tags (acrochordons, fibroepithelial polyps), 46, 49, 106
Cystic acne, 109
Cysts, 57–61
 described, 59–61
 surgery for, 47

Darier's disease (keratosis follicularis), 126, 127, 230
 blisters in, 240
 familial benign pemphigus and, 243
Decubitus ulcers (pressure sores), 254
Delayed hypersensitivity, defined, 85
Demodex folliculorum, 117
Dennie's line, 128, 130
Dermal atrophy, 61
Dermal melanocytoma (blue nevus), 42
Dermal melanocytosis, 41–42
Dermal nevi, 38
Dermatitis (see specific forms of dermatitis, for example: Allergic contact dematitis; Atopic dermatitis; Contact dermatitis)
Dermatitis artifacta (self-inflicted injuries), 255
Dermatitis factita (factitial ulcers), 253, 255, 264, 271
Dermatitis herpetiformis (DH), 240, 247- 248
Dermato fibromas, 47
Dermatomyositis:
 as cause of BFP, 196
 cutaneous signs of, 228
 as manifestation of cancer, 233
 therapy for, 168, 288
Dermatophytes, 164–168
 (See also Fungus infections)
Dermis:
 of the aged, 49
 anatomy and physiology of, 12–15
 described, 6
 thickness of, 8, 13

Dermoepidermal junction, 14
Dermoepidermal separation, blister formation caused by, 240, 241
Desquamation (scaling):
  in blepharitis, 120
  in cases of sunburn, 77
  in chronic eczema, 92
  in measles and scarlet fever, 217
  of newborn skin, 34
  in pemphigus diseases, 244
DH (dermatitis herpetiformis), 240, 247–248
Diabetes mellitus:
  bedsores and, 254
  as cause of pruritus, 67, 68
  cutaneous manifestations of, 226–227
  furuncles and, 155
  ulcers and, 250, 251
Diabetic dermopathy, described, 227
Diagnostic tests, 103–105
Diaper dermatitis (napkin rash), 35–37
Diascopy, 100–101
Differentiation compartment of epidermis, 11
  cells made by, 12
Diffuse capillary hemangiomas (nevus flammeus, plane nevus, telangiectatic nevus), 39, 40
Discoid lupus erythematosis (DLE), 227–229
Diseases (see specific diseases, for example: Liver diseases; Skin diseases; Systemic diseases)
Disseminated herpes simplex, 216
Disseminated vaccinia, 216
DLE (discoid lupus erythematosis), 227–229
Donovania granulomatis, 188
Dressings, 282–284
Drug addiction responsible for BFP, 196
Drug eruptions, 89–91, 93, 215–216, 287
Drug side effects, 273
  alopecia as, 21, 22
  eczema as, 95
  pruritus as, 67
Dry dressings, 284
Dry skin:
  of the aged, 49–50
  atopic dermatitis and, 128
  pruritus and, 67, 68
  relieving, 44–45, 277–278
Dysgammaglobulinemia as cause of BFP, 196
Dyshidrosis:
  blisters in, 240
  psychological component of, 264
Dyshidrotic eczema (pompholyx), 93, 133, 134
Dysproteinemia, ulcers and, 250

Early syphilis, 189–193
Ecchymoses, defined, 60
Eccrine sweat glands:
  adolescent, 43
  of the aged, 49
  anatomy and physiology of, 26–28
  at birth, 34
  as cause of benign neoplasms, 205
  occlusion of, 137–139

ECHO (virus), 216, 218
Echthyma, 150, 151, 154
Ecthyma gangenosum, 225
Eczema:
  of the aged, 49
  alopecia and, 21
  chronic, 281
  chronic hand, 128
  clinical manifestations of, in groin area, 167
  dyshidrotic, 133, 134
  hallmark of, 239
  hypopigmentation and, 56
  mycosis fungoides and, 233
  as skin reaction, 91–96
  stress and, 44
  therapy for, 96, 108, 287, 288
Eczema herpeticum, 176, 216
Eczema vaccinatum, 216
Eczematous dermatitis, 44, 127–136
  atopic dermatitis as, 127–131
    blisters in, 240
    causes of, 95
    characteristics of, 127–128, 130
    infections and, 131
    pruritus in, 128–129
    psychological components of, 264, 266–267
    therapy for, 96, 132–133, 267, 286, 287
  circumscribed neurodermatitis as, 95, 135, 136, 286
  hand eczema as, 134–135
    chronic, 128
  nummular eczema as, 93, 95
    atopy in, 128
    blisters in, 240
    characteristics of, 133, 134
    vesicular, 96
Eczematous pityriasis rosea, 93
Eczematous polymorphous eruptions, causes of, 93
Edema, defined, 56
Elastin fibers, described, 13
Electrocoagulation, described, 106
Electrodessication, described, 106
Electrolysis, basis of, 17
Electrosurgery, 106–107
  for actinic keratoses, 203
  for basal cell carcinoma, 207
EM (see Erythema multiforme)
Embolism, ulcers and, 250
Emotions:
  effects of therapy on, 272, 273
  skin disorders and, 263–271
  (See also Stress)
Endocrine disorders:
  acne and, 115
  alopecia and, 21, 226
  cutaneous signs of, 225–227
  pruritis and, 67
Endogenous causes of eczema, 93, 95
Enteric fever (typhoid fever), 216, 218
Enterovirus infections, 216

Eosinophilic granuloma, 231
Ephelides (freckles), 42–43
Epidermal appendages, 15–17
 (*See also* Hair; Hair follicles; Nails)
Epidermal nevi (epithelial nevi), 38
Epidermal proliferation, disorders of, 121–127
 (*See also* Darier's disease; Ichthyosis; Psoriasis; Reiter's syndrome)
Epidermis, 8–12
 anatomy of, 8–12
 composition of, 6
 dermis providing structural support for, 13
 junction between dermis and, 14
Epidermoid carcinoma (squamous cell carcinoma), 207–211, 250
Epidermolysis bullosa, 240, 288
Epithelial nevi (epidermal nevi), 38
Erector pili, junction of, 17
Ergotisms, ulcers and, 250
Erosion:
 defined, 62–63
 dermatoses manifested by, 247–248
 ulcers and, 248–249
Erysipelas, 157–158
Erythema marginatum, cutaneous signs of, 216, 219
Erythema multiforme (EM, Stevens-Johnson syndrome), 88, 185, 186
 as allergy, 87, 88, 91
 blister formation in, 240, 245–247
 characteristics of, 245–247
 as manifestation of cancer, 233
 therapy for, 88, 247, 287
 ulcers caused by, 250
Erythema multiforme bullosum, 216
Erythema neonatorum (toxic erythema, urticaria neonatorum, erythema neonatorum allergicum), 35
Erythema nodosum, 87
 from drug hypersensitivity, 91
 sarcoidosis and, 235
Erythemas:
 in acne rosacea, 118
 in actinic keratosis, 204
 causes of, 227
 chronic eczema and, 92
 defined, 53
 DH and, 248
 in echthyma, 150
 in moniliasis, 166
 in pemphigus, 244
 of pityriasis rosea, 143
Erythrasma, 102, 151–152
Eschar (scab), 81
Estrogens, role of, in aging of skin, 48
Evolution of lesions:
 defined, 65
 etiology of systemic diseases and, 215
Excoriations, 64–65
 in eczema, 129
 ischemia and, 250, 252
 neurotic, 264, 270

Excretion of apocrine glands, described, 24
Exfoliative erythroderma:
 effects of, 21
 therapy for, 287, 288
Exogenous causes of eczema, 93–94

Factitial ulcers (dermatitis factita), 253, 255, 264, 271
Familial benign pemphigus (Hailey-Hailey disease), 243
Feet ringworm (tinea pedis), 165, 166, 265
Female hormones, estrogens as, 48
Fever, cutaneous signs of, 215
Fever blisters, 178
Fibroblasts, function of, in dermis, 13
Fibroepithelial polyps (acrochordons, cutaneous tags), 46, 49, 106
Filiform warts (verruca filiformis), 171, 172
First-degree burns, 82, 83
Flat warts (verruca plana), 171, 172
Fogo selvagem (jungle fire), 243
Folliculitis:
 bacterial, 151
 described, 43
Foreign body granuloma, defined, 74
Freckles (ephelides), 42–43
Frei test, 198
Friction:
 blisters caused by, 240
 as cause of alopecia, 21
Frostbite as cause of alopecia, 21
FTA-ABS (treponemal test), 195
Fungus infections, 159–170
 alopecia and, 21
 as cause of eczema, 93
 dermatophytes as, 164–168
 diabetes mellitus and, 226
 of hyphae, 102
 infectivity of, 281
 moniliasis as, 160–163
  (*See also* Moniliasis)
 nail disorders and, 28, 29
 superficial, 95
 tinea versicolor as, 168–170
 ulcers caused by, 250
Furunculosis, 154–156, 226

Gastrointestinal tract diseases, cutaneous signs of, 231–232
Generalized pruritus without lesions, causes of, 67
Gentamycin, 285
German measles (rubella), 216–218
Germinative compartment (reproductive compartment) of epidermis, 11
Giemsa's stain, 103
Gingivostomatitis, 176
Glands (*see* Apocrine glands; Eccrine sweat glands; Melanocytes; Pilosebaceous apocrine unit; Sebaceous glands)

Globulins, defined, 84
Gonococcemia, cutaneous signs of, 216,
    223, 224
Gonorrhea, 197–198
    acquired by sexual contact, 188
    as major venereal disease, 187
Granular cells, described, 9
Granulation tissue, 81
Granuloma inguinale, 199
    acquired by sexual contact, 188
    as minor venereal disease, 187
    ulcers and, 250
Granulomas:
    defined, 74
    eosinophilic, 231
Groin ringworm (jock itch; tinea cruris),
    164–167
Ground substance, defined, 13
Gummata, described, 193

Hailey-Hailey disease (familial benign
    pemphigus), 243
Hair:
    anatomy and physiology of, 17–22
    hyphae of, 102, 103
    loss of (see Alopecia)
Hair-follicle nevi, 38
Hair follicles:
    anagen phase of, 18–19
    destruction of, 17
    embryological formation of, 17
    sebaceous glands as outgrowths of, 22
Hair growth:
    anagen and telogen phases of, 18–19
    changes in rate of, 19–20
Hair size, changes in, 20
Hand eczema:
    characterics of, 134–135
    chronic, 128
Hand-foot-and-mouth disease, cutaneous
    signs of, 216, 218
Hand-Schuller-Christian disease, cutaneous
    signs of, 223
Harlequin color change in newborns,
    described, 35
Hay fever, 128
Healed congenital ectodermal defects as
    cause of alopecia, 21
Health, skin as indicator of, 2
Health care personnel, attitudes of, toward
    skin disorders, 260–262
Heat, blisters caused by, 240
Heat rash (miliaria rubra), 137–139
Hemangiomas (vascular nevi), 37–41
Hematomas, defined, 60
Hemophilus ducreyi, 188, 198
Hereditary hemorrhagic telangiectasia
    (Osler-Rendu-Weber syndrome), 232
Herpes hominis, 175, 178
Herpes progenitalis, 177, 178
    acquired by sexual contact, 188
Herpes simplex, 175–179
    disseminated, 216
    eczema and, 131

Herpes simplex:
    infectivity of, 281
    multinucleate cells of, 102
    primary, 186
    primary cell damage in, 240
Herpes simplex (virus), 188
Herpes zoster (shingles):
    cutaneous signs of, 216, 219–221
    infectivity of, 281
    primary cell damage in, 239
Herpetic keratoconjunctivitis, 176
Herpetic whitlow, 176
Hidradenitis suppurativa, 109, 158–159
Hirsutism, 20, 48
Histiocytosis (reticuloendotheliosis,
    histiocytosis X), 231
Hives (see Urticaria)
Holocrine glands, sebaceous glands as, 23
Hookworm infestations as cause of pruritus,
    67
Hormones (see Androgens; Estrogens)
Hospitalization, side effects of, 273–274
Hyperhidrosis:
    defined, 28
    as physiologic response to emotions, 265
Hyperkeratosis, 60–61, 75
Hyperlipoproteinemias, cutaneous signs of,
    235
Hyperpigmentation, defined, 53
Hypersensitivity (see Allergies)
Hypertension, ulcers and, 250
Hypertrichosis, defined, 20
Hyphae of hair, 102, 103
Hypochondriasis, 264, 272
Hypopigmentation, defined, 53–56

Ichthyosis, 125–127
    causes of, 44
    soaks and baths for, 281
    turnover time in, 73
Ichthyosis vulgaris, 126, 127
Immediate hypersensitivity, defined, 85
Immunoglobulins, defined, 84
Immunity as skin reaction, 83–85
Impetigo, 150–154, 280
    characteristics and treatment of, 152–154
    crusts of, 61
    in newborns, 35
    spongiosis in, 239
Infections:
    atopic dermatitis and, 131
    enteroviral, 216, 218
    microscopic examinations for, 102–103
    responsible for BFP, 196
    ulcers caused by, 250
    (See also Bacterial infections; Fungus
        infections; Spirochetal infections;
        Viral infections)
Infectious hepatitis as cause of BFP, 196
Infectious mononucleosis as cause of
    BFP, 196
Infectivity, precautions against, 280–281
Infestations, 179–182
    pruritus caused by, 67, 181, 275

Inflammation:
  as basic reaction, 83–84
  causes and purpose of, 73–75
  sunburn as, 75
Infrared radiation (UV-B, middle ultraviolet radiation):
  effects of, 78–80
  melasma and, 140
Insect bites, 86
Inspection of skin, 100–103
Intertrigo, described, 35
Ischemia, 250–253
  blister formation caused by, 240
Itching (*see* Pruritus)

Janeway lesions, described, 225
Jock itch (groin ringworm, tinea cruris), 164–167
Jungle fire (*fogo selvagem*), 243
Juvenile xanthogranuloma, 231

KA (keratoacanthomas), 210–211
Keratin, 12
  (*See also* Hair; Hair follicles; Nails)
Keratinization, defined, 12
Keratitis, acne rosacea and, 117
Keratoacanthomas (KA), 210–211
Keratoconjunctivitis, herpetic, 176
Keratoses:
  actinic, 203, 204
    blister formation and, 240
    squamous cell carcinoma and, 207–209
  premalignant, 205–206
  seborrheic, 45–46
    of the aged, 49
    as benign tumor, 205
    crumbling away of, 106
  therapy for, 105, 106
Keratosis follicularis (*see* Darier's disease)
Keratosis pilaris, 125–126

Late syphilis, 193–194
Lentigines as benign tumors, 205
Lentigo, 42–43, 49
Lentigo maligna, 208, 212
Leprosy as cause of BFP, 196
Leptospirosis as cause of BFP, 196
Lesions:
  café au lait, 235
  configuration and morphology of, defined, 64
  etiology of systemic diseases and, 215
  evolution and distribution of, defined, 65
  generalized pruritus without, 67
  of pemphigus diseases, 244
  types of, in systemic diseases, 216
  (*See also specific kinds of lesions, for example:* Papules; Macules; *and specific diseases in which lesions appear, for example:* Skin cancer; Ulcers)

Letterer-Siwe disease, 231
Leukemia:
  as cause of pruritus, 67
  cutaneous signs of, 233, 234
Leukoplakia, 186
LGV (lymphogranuloma venerium), 187, 188
Lichen planus, 143–144, 185
  alopecia and, 21–22
Lichen simplex chronicus (circumscribed neurodermatitis, LSC), 93, 95, 135–136, 286
Lichenification, 60, 92, 130
Lipodystrophy, defined, 227
Lipomas, 47
Liver diseases, pruritus caused by, 68
Liver spots (senile lentigo), 42
Long ultraviolet radiation (UV-A):
  melasma and, 140
  primary cell damage from, 240
  vitiligo and, 142
  wavelengths of, 76–80
Loss of hair (*see* Alopecia)
Lotions, 284
LSC (lichen simplex chronicus, circumscribed neurodermatitis), 95, 135–136, 286
Lupus erythematosus:
  as cause of alopecia, 21, 22
  as cause of BFP, 196
  cutaneous signs of, 227–229
  in oral cavity, 186
Lymphangiomas, 38
Lymphogranuloma venerium (LGV), 187, 188, 198
Lymphomas:
  as cause of pruritus, 67
  cutaneous signs of, 233

Macules, 54
  described, 52
  systemic diseases manifested by, 216
Mal perforant (anaesthetic ulcers, neurotrophic ulcers), 249, 251
Malaria as cause of BFP, 196
Malassezia furfur, 169
Male hormones (*see* Androgens)
Male pattern baldness, 21
  androgens and, 26
  in menopausal women, 48
  typical distribution of, 20
Malignant melanomas, 208–213
Malignant tumors, 202–203
Mammary glands as apocrine glands, 25
Mastocytosis, cutaneous signs of, 230–231
Measles (rubeola, morbilli), 67, 216, 217
Mechanicobullous dermatosis, 250
Mechanicobullous diseases (epidermolysis bullosa), 248
Melanin, 29–31
  ultraviolet light absorbed by, 78
Melanocyte-like cells in nevi, 38
Melanocytes, anatomy and physiology of, 29–31

Melanomas, malignant, 208–213
Melasma (chloasma, mask of pregnancy), 139, 140
Meningococcemia, cutaneous signs of, 216, 223, 224
Meningoencephalitis, herpes simplex as cause of, 176
Metabolic disorders:
  causing pruritus, 67
  cutaneous signs of, 225–227
Microscopic tests, rapid, 102, 103
Middle ultraviolet radiation (*see* Infrared radiation)
Milia:
  described, 34
  scooping out of, 105–106
  size of, 47
  transient nature of, 37
Miliaria:
  defined, 28, 34
  diaper dermatitis and, 36
  types of, 137–139
Miliaria crystallina (sudamina), 137, 138
Miliaria profunda, 137, 138
Miliaria pustulosa, 137, 138
Miliaria rubra (heat rash, prickly heat), 137–139
Mitosis during anagen phase of hair growth, 19–20
Moles (nevus cell nevi), 38, 39, 41
  alopecia and, 21
  basal cell carcinoma and, 207
  as benign tumors, 205
  as premalignant neoplasms, 212
  sebaceous, 38
Molluscum contagiosum, 174, 175
  acquired by sexual contact, 188
  as benign neoplasms, 205
  scooping out of, 105–106
Mongolian spot, described, 42
Monilial intertrigo, 161–163
Monilial vaginitis, 116
Moniliasis (candidiasis), 160–163, 166
  acquired by sexual contact, 188
  as cause of pruritus, 68
  clinical manifestations of, in groin area, 167
Morbilli (measles, rubeola), 67, 216, 217
Morphea, cutaneous signs of, 228, 230
Morphology of lesions:
  defined, 64
  etiology of systemic diseases and, 215
Mosaic pattern of growth of hair follicles, 18
Mucous membrane diseases:
  aphthous stomatitis, 186–187
  common, 185–186
  venereal disease as (*see* Venereal disease)
  viral infections and, 176
Munchausen's syndrome, psychological component of, 264
Mycosis fungoides, cutaneous signs of, 233–235

Nails:
  anatomy and physiology of, 28–29
  psoriasis on, 122
Napkin rash (diaper dermatitis), 35–37
Narcotic addiction responsible for BFP, 196
Necrobiosis lipoidica diabeticorum (NLD), 227, 250
Neisseria gonorrhea, 188, 197
Neomycin, 285
Neonatal alopecia, 21
Neoplasms:
  benign, 205
  as cause of alopecia, 21, 22
  defined, 202
  premalignant, 212
  pruritus caused by, 67
  (*See also specific kinds of neoplasms, for example:* Moles; Skin cancer)
Neurodermatitis, 93
  causes of, 95
  mycosis fungoides and, 233
  psychological component of, 264
Neurofibromatosis (von Recklinghausen's disease), 235
Neurotic excoraitions as self-induced, 264, 270
Neurotrophic ulcers (anaesthetic ulcers, mal perforant), 249, 251
Nevus cell nevi (*see* Moles)
Nevus flammeus (diffuse capillary hemangioma, plane nevus, telangiectatic nevus), 39, 40
Nevus lipomatosus, 38
Nevus vasculosus (strawberry mark, capillary hemangioma), 39, 40
Newborn skin, 34–37
  diaper dermatitis on, 35–37
  general characteristics of, 34–35
Nits, 179, 180
NLD (necrobiosis lipoidica diabeticorum), 227, 250
Nodular melanomas, 208, 212
Nodules, 53, 54
Noninfectious diseases responsible for BFP, 196
Nonscarring alopecia, 20–22
Nontreponemal tests, 194–195
Normal epidermis, cross section of, 9
Normal skin, cross section of, 7
Nummular eczema (coin-shaped eczema), 93, 95
  atopy in, 128
  blisters in, 240
  characteristics of, 133, 134

Occlusive diseases, ulcers and, 250, 252
Oil glands (*see* Sebaceous glands)
Ointments, 284
Old age, responsible for BFP, 196
Onchocerciasis infestations as cause of pruritus, 67
Onychomycosis, 166
Open wet dressings, 282–283

Opium derivates, pruritus caused by, 67
Oral cavity, common disorders affecting, 185–186
Osler-Rendu-Weber syndrome (hereditary hemorrhagic telangiectasia), 232
Osler's nodes, described, 225

Palm ringworm (tinea manum), 166
Panniculus adiposus (adipose layer, subcutaneous tissue), 6, 15
Panugo hairs (vellus hairs), 18
Papillae, described, 14
Papillary dermis, described, 13
Papova, 188
Papules, 54
    of acne rosacea, 118
    of acne vulgaris, 113
    defined, 52
    systemic diseases manifested by, 216, 220
Parapsoriasis en plaques, described, 234
Parasitic infestations, 67, 179–182
Parasitosis, delusions of, 264, 271
    as cause of pruritus, 67
Paresis, described, 194
Paronychia, 163
Paronychial telangiectasia, collagen diseases and, 236
Passive immunity, defined, 85
Pastes, 284
Patch tests, 94, 104
Pathogenicity, defined, 151
Pediculosis, 179–181
    infectivity of, 281
    among psychiatric patients, 275
Pediculosis humanus, 179–180
Pediculosis pubis acquired by sexual contact, 188
PEG (see Primary epithelial germ)
Pemphigoid, 240, 242, 243, 245, 288
Pemphigus diseases, 240–244
    acantholytic cells of, 102
    characteristics of, 241–243
    microscopic examination of, 103
    therapy for, 243, 288
Pemphigus erythematosis (Senear-Usher syndrome), 243, 244
Pemphigus foliaceous, 243, 244
Pemphigus vegitans, 243, 244
Pemphigus vulgaris, 57, 186, 241–244
Periarteritis nodosa as cause of BFP, 196
Perleche (cheilitis, angular stomatitis), 161–162
Petechiae, defined, 60
Peutz-Jeghers syndrome, cutaneous signs of, 231
Pharyngitis, herpes simplex and, 176
Phobia, cutaneous signs of, 264, 271
Photosensitivity, defined, 77
Phthirus pubis, 179–181, 188
Physiology, 6–31
    of apocrine glands, 23–24
    of dermis, 12–15
    of eccrine sweat glands, 26–28
    of hair, 17–22

Physiology:
    of melanocytes, 29–31
    of nails, 28–29
    of oil glands, 22–23
    of skin, 6–14
Pigmentation, disorders of, 139–142
Pilosebaceous apocrine unit:
    as cause of benign neoplasms, 205
    function of, 25–26
    (See also Apocrine glands; Sebaceous glands)
Pituitary disorders, cutaneous signs of, 225
Pityriasis alba, 129
Pityriasis rosea, 93, 129, 142, 143
Plane nevus (nevus flammeus, diffuse capillary hemangioma, telangiectatic nevus), 39, 40
Plantar warts (verruca plantaris), 171, 172
Plaques, 53, 54
Pneumococcal pneumonia as cause of BFP, 196
Poison ivy dermatitis, 287
Polymorphonuclear leukocytes (polys), inflammation and, 74
Polymyxin B, 285
Pompholyx (dyshidrotic eczema), 93, 133–134
Porphyria, 102, 240
Porphyria cutanea tarda, cutaneous signs of, 235
Port wine stain, 39, 40
Post partum alopecia, 21
Post-radiation ulcers, 251
Postphlebitic syndrome, ulcers and, 250
Powders, 284
Pox virus, 188
Prausnitz-Küstner reaction, 128
Pregnancy mask (chloasma, melasma), 139, 140
Pregnancy responsible for BFP, 196
Premalignant keratoses, causes of, 205–206
Premalignant tumors, 203–204
Pressure, ischemia caused by, 250, 253
Pressure sores (decubitus ulcers), 254
Pretibial myxedema, 226
Prickle-cells, defined, 9
Prickly heat (heat rash, miliaria rubra), 137–139
Primary cell damage, blisters and, 239–240
Primary epithelial germ (PEG):
    epidermal appendage formation and, 16–17
    in formation of apocrine glands, 16, 23
    in formation of sebaceous glands, 16
    pilosebaceous apocrine unit developed from, 25
Primary herpes simplex in oral cavity, 186
Primary irritant dermatitis, described, 96–97
Primary syphilis, 189–191
Progressive systemic sclerosis (PSS), 230
Prolonged corticosteroid therapy, effects of, 288
Protective compartment of epidermis, 11
Prurigo nodularis as cause of eczema, 93

Pruritus (itching), 44, 65–69
  of the aged, 49–50
  in atopic dermatitis, 128–129
  causes of, 67–68
  in chicken pox, 220
  in dyshidrotic eczema, 133–134
  in hand eczema, 135
  hyperhidrosis and, 265
  in impetigo, 152
  in infestations, 67, 181, 275
  in lichen planus, 144
  liver diseases and, 68
  in LSC, 135
  as manifestation of cancer, 233
  in monilial intertrigo, 163
  in neurotic excoriations, 270
  in nummular eczema, 133
  in pityriasis rosea, 142
  in primary irritant dermatitis, 96–97
  in pruritus vulvae, 265
  in psoriasis, 121
  therapy for, 69, 277, 287
  in thrush, 161
  in urticaria, 57, 85
Pruritus ani, psychological components of, 264, 266
Pruritus vulvae, psychological components of, 264–266
Pseudomonas, 102–103
Pseudomonas septicemia, cutaneous signs of, 216, 224–225
Psoriasis, 60, 121–125
  characteristics of, 121–123
  mycosis fungoides and, 233
  nail disorders and, 28
  psychological components of, 264, 269
  stress and, 44
  treatment of, 107–108, 124–125, 286, 287
  turnover time in, 73
PSS (progressive systemic sclerosis), 230
Psychiatric approach to skin disorders, 262–263
Psychiatric patients, skin diseases in, 274–275
Psychogenic factors in pruritus, 67
Psychosis, cutaneous signs of, 264, 271
Psychosomatic approach to skin disorders, 262–263
Punch biopsy, 104–105
Purpura, 89
Purpuric macules, systemic diseases manifested by, 216
Purpuric papules, systemic diseases manifested by, 216
Purpuric vesicles, systemic diseases manifested by, 216
Pustules:
  of acne rosacea, 118
  of acne vulgaris, 113
  defined, 57
  systemic diseases manifested by, 216, 220, 223
Pyoderma gangrenosum:
  cutaneous signs of, 232
  ulcers and, 250
Pyodermas (*see* Bacterial infections)

Rapid microscopic tests, 102–103
Rat bite fever as cause of BFP, 196
Raynaud's disease, ulcers caused by, 250
Recurrent herpes simplex, 176–177
Regeneration of skin, 75
Rehydration of skin, 44–45
Reiter's syndrome, 127
Relapsing fever as cause of BFP, 196
Renal insufficiency, pruritus caused by, 68
Reproductive compartment (germinative compartment) of epidermis, 11
Reticular dermis, described, 13–14
Reticuloendotheliosis (histiocytosis, histiocytosis X), 231
Reticulum fibers, described, 13
Rheumatoid arthritis as cause of BFP, 196
Rhinitis, viral infections and, 176
Rhinophyma, 117, 118
Rickettsia rickettsii, 222
Rickettsial diseases, 216
Rocky Mountain spotted fever, cutaneous signs of, 216, 222, 223
Rodent ulcers (*see* Basal cell carcinoma)
Rubella (German measles), 216–218
Rubeola (measles, morbilli), 67, 216, 217

Salmon patch, 39
Salmonella typhosa, 218
Sarcoid as cause of BFP, 196
Sarcoidosis:
  alopecia and, 21, 22
  cutaneous signs of, 235
Sarcoptes scabiei, 181, 188
Scab (eschar), 81
Scabies, 181, 182
  acquired by sexual contact, 188
  infectivity of, 281
  pruritus and, 68
  among psychiatric patients, 275
Scalded skin syndrome (TEN, toxic epidermal necrolysis), 216, 247
Scales, 61, 62
Scaling (*see* Desquamation)
Scalp hair, at birth, 34
Scalp ringworm (tinea capitis), 109, 164, 165, 281
Scarlet fever (scarlatina):
  as cause of BFP, 196
  cutaneous signs of, 216, 217
Scarring alopecia, 20–22
Scleroderma:
  as cause of BFP, 196
  cutaneous signs of, 228–230
Sclerosis:
  defined, 61–62
  tuberous: cutaneous signs of, 235
    under Wood's light, 103
Scratching (*see* Excoriations; Pruritus)
Sebaceous glands (oil glands):
  adolescent, 43
  of the aged, 49
  anatomy and physiology of, 22–23
  disorders related to, 112–121

Sebaceous glands (oil glands):
  embryological formation of, 16–17
  as vestigial, 25
Sebaceous nevi, 38
Seborrheic dermatitis, 93, 119–121
  adolescent, 43
  causes of, 95
  described, 23
  psychological aspects of, 264
  treatment of, 120–121, 286
Seborrheic keratoses, 45–46
  of the aged, 49
  as benign tumors, 205
  crumbling away of, 106
Sebum, characteristics of, 23
Second-degree burns, 82, 83
Secondary gains of skin diseases, 259
Secondary syphilis:
  cutaneous signs of, 216, 218–219
  effects of, 21, 191–192
Secretion of apocrine glands, 24
Self-induced skin eruptions, 264, 270–271
Self-inflicted injuries (dermatitis artifacta), 255
Senear-Usher syndrome (pemphigus erythematosis), 243, 244
Senile lentigo (liver spots), 42
Sepsis, ulcers and, 250
Serum sickness, cutaneous signs of, 216, 219
Sexual contact, venereal diseases acquired by, 188
Shingles (see Herpes zoster)
Short corticosteroid therapy, 287
Short ultraviolet radiation (UV-C), 76, 108
Sickle cell anemia, ulcers and, 250
Skin:
  functions of, 1, 5–6
  as indicator of health, 2
Skin cancer, 201–213
  among the aged, 49
  basal cell carcinoma as, 206–207
    curettage of, 105
    ulcers and, 250
  etiology of, 205–206
  malignant melanoma as, 212–213
  squamous cell carcinoma as, 207–211, 250
  sun exposure and, 76, 80, 206, 207, 212
  surgery for, 105
  tumors and, 202–205
    benign, 45–47, 202
    electrosurgery for, 106
    malignant, 202–203
    premalignant, 203–204
    (See also specific kinds of tumors)
  turnover time in, 73
  X-ray therapy and, 109
Skin debris, removal of, 278–279
Skin diseases, 52–65, 263–272
  definitions of terms dealing with, 52–65
  emotions and, 21, 263–271
  health care personnel's attitude toward, 260–262
  hypochondriacal, 264, 272

Skin diseases:
  patient's perception of, 259–260
  prejudice toward, 258–259
  of psychiatric patients, 274–275
  psychosomatic and psychiatric approach to, 262–263
  psychotic or phobic, 264, 271
  range of, 2
  related to sebaceous glands, 112–121
  (See also specific skin diseases, for example: Skin cancer; Urticaria)
Skin ecology, 147–150
Skin protection, 278
Skin reactions, 71–96
  to drugs, 89–91
  eczema as, 91–96
    (See also Eczema)
  healing of wounds as, 81–82
  immunity, allergy and hypersensitivity as, 83–85
  inflammation as, 73–75
  to insect bites, 86
  interplay of, 97
  primary irritant dermatitis as, 96–97
  repair, regeneration and hyperkeratosis as, 75
  sunburn as, 75–80
  to thermal injuries, 82–83
  turnover time as, 72–73
  vascular reaction patterns, 86–89
Skin tags (acrochordons, cutaneous tags, fibroepithelial polyps), 46, 49, 106
SLE (systemic lupus erythematosis), 21, 228, 229, 288
Smallpox (variola):
  cutaneous signs of, 216, 220–222
  primary cell damage in, 240
Soaks, 281–282
Solar keratoses (see Actinic keratoses)
Specific agents (therapeutic), 285–286
Spirochetal infections:
  alopecia and, 21
  responsible for BFP, 196
  (See also Syphilis)
Spirochetes (treponema pallidum), 188, 189, 191, 193, 194
Spitz juvenile melanoma (compound melanocytoma), 42
Spongiosis:
  defined, 92
  as first stage of blister formation, 239, 240
Squamous cell carcinoma (epidermoid carcinoma), 207–211, 250
Staphylococcal pyodermas, 280
Staphylococcal scalded skin syndrome (SSSS), 247
Staphylococcemia, cutaneous signs of, 216, 224
Staphylococcus:
  albus, 147, 154, 156
  aureus, 148, 152, 157
  epidermidis, 147

Stasis dermatitis, 50
  causes of, 93, 95
  ischemia and, 250, 252
Statsis ulcers, 251
Stevens-Johnson syndrome (*see* Erythema
  multiforme)
Stomatitis:
  angular, 161, 162
  aphthous, 186–187
Stratum corneum:
  of the aged, 49
  characteristics of, 11–12
  described, 9
  hair compared with, 17
  thickening of, 60–61, 75
Strawberry mark (capillary hemangioma,
  nevus vasculosus), 39, 40
Stress:
  acne and, 115
  alopecia and, 21
  alopecia areata and, 264, 267–268
  atopic dermatitis and, 266
  as cause of pruritus, 67
  physiologic responses to, 263–265
  psoriasis and, 122
  role of, in adolescent skin diseases, 44
  skin's reaction to, 71
Sturge-Weber syndrome, 39
Subacute bacterial endocarditis, cutaneous
  signs of, 216, 224–225
Subcutaneous tissue (adipose layer,
  panniculus adiposus), 6, 15
Suction, blister formation by, 240
Sudamina (miliaria crystallina), 137, 138
Sun exposure:
  melasma and, 140
  for pityriasis rosea, 142
  skin cancer and, 76, 80, 206, 207, 212
  for vitiligo, 142
Sun spectrum, biologic phenomena and, 79
Sunburn, 75–80, 287
Sunburn spectrum, 78
Superficial fungus infections, 95
Superficial spreading melanoma, 208
Surgery, 105–107
  for basal cell carcinoma, 207
  for Bowen's disease, 205
  for dermal melanocytosis, 42
  for dermato fibromas, lipomas, and cysts,
    47
  for hemangiomas, 40
  for hidradenitis suppurativa, 158
  for malignant melanomas, 212–213
  for rhinophyma, 118
  for squamous cell carcinoma, 209–210
  for warts, 173
  (*See also* Cryosurgery; Electrosurgery)
Sweat, composition of, 27
Syphilis, 189–196
  acquired by sexual contact, 188
  early, 189–193
  infectivity of, 280–281
  late, 193–194
  as major venereal disease, 187

Syphilis:
  secondary: cutaneous signs of, 216, 218–
    219
    effects of, 21, 191–192
    tests to detect, 194–195
Syphilophobia, 264, 272
Symptom relief as goal of therapy, 277–278
Systemic diseases:
  cutaneous signs of, 214–225
  etiology of, 215
Systemic lupus erythematosis (SLE), 228,
  229, 288
Systemic mastocytosis, cutaneous signs of,
  231
Systemic therapy, 286–288

Tabes dorsalis, described, 194
Tars, 286
Telangiectasia:
  in acne rosacea, 118
  in actinic keratosis, 204
  defined, 58–59
  hereditary hemorrhagic, 232
  paronychial, 236
Telangiectatic nevus (plane nevus, nevus
  flammeus, diffuse capillary
  hemangioma), 39, 40
Telogen effluvium, causes of, 19
Telogen phase of hair follicles, 18–19
TEN (toxic epidermal necrolysis, scalded
  skin syndrome), 216, 247
Terminal hairs:
  affected by androgens, 20
  described, 18
Therapy, 277–288
  for acne rosacea, 117–119
  for acne vulgaris, 107, 108, 115–117
  for actinic keratoses, 203–204
  for allergic contact dermatitis, 94–95
  for allergies, 286–287
  for alopecia areata, 287
  for aphthous stomatitis, 187
  for atopic dermatitis, 96, 132–133, 267,
    286, 287
  for bacterial infections, 280
  for burns, 82–83
  for candidiasis, 163
  for carbuncles, 157
  for chancroid, 198
  for collagen diseases, 288
  for contact dermatitis, 94–95, 287
  for dermatomyositis, 168, 288
  for diaper dermatitis, 37
  dressings as, 282–284
  for dry skin, 44–45, 277–278
  for ecthyma, 154
  for eczema, 96, 108, 287, 288
  for EM, 88, 247, 287
  emotional aspects of, 272–274
  for erythrasma, 152
  for exfoliative erythroderma, 287, 288
  for furunculosis, 156
  goals of, 3, 277–280
  for gonorrhea, 197–198
  for granuloma inguinale, 199

Therapy:
  for herpes simplex, 178–179
  for hyperhidrosis, 265
  for ichthyosis, 281
  for impetigo, 153–154
  for insect bites, 86
  for lichen planus, 144
  for lymphogranuloma venerium, 198
  for melasma, 139–140
  for miliaria, 137, 139
  for molluscum contagiosum, 174, 175
  for mycosis fungoides, 235
  for nummular eczema, 133
  for pediculosis, 181
  for pemphigus diseases, 243, 288
  for pityriasis rosea, 142
  precautions against infectivity in, 280–281
  for pruritus, 69, 277, 287
  for psoriasis, 107–108, 124–125, 286, 287
  for Rocky Mountain spotted fever, 222
  for scabies, 181
  for seborrheic dermatitis, 120–121, 286
  for seborrheic keratoses, 46
  soaks and baths as, 281–282
  to stimulate regrowth of hair, 21
  for syphilis, 195
  systemic, 286–288
  for TEN, 247
  for tinea versicolor, 169–170
  topical, 284–286
  for ulcers, 252–253
  ultraviolet light, 107–108
  for urticaria, 87, 286, 287
  for vitiligo, 142
  for warts, 105, 106, 108, 172–174
  (*See also* Cryosurgery; Curettage; Electro-
    surgery; Surgery; X-ray therapy)
Thermal injuries (burns):
  blisters in, 240
  as cause of alopecia, 21
  skin cancer and, 207
  skin reactions to, 82–83
Thickness of skin, variations in, 6, 8
Third-degree burns, 82, 83
Thrombosis, ulcers and, 250
Thrush, 161
Thyroid acropachy, 226
Thyroid disorders (*see* Endocrine disorders)
Timing of lesions, etiology of systemic
    disease and, 215
Tinea capitis (scalp ringworm), 109, 164,
    165, 281
Tinea corporis (body ringworm), 164, 165
Tinea cruris (groin ringworm, jock itch),
    164–167
Tinea manum (palm ringworm), 166
Tinea pedis (feet ringworm), 165, 166, 265
Tinea versicolor (TV), 168–170
Topical steroids, 285–286
Topical therapy, 284–286
Toxic epidermal necrolysis (TEN, scalded
    skin syndrome), 216, 247
Toxic erythema (erythema neonatorum,
    urticaria neonatorum, erythema
    neonatorum allergicum), 35

Trauma:
  alopecia and, 21, 22
  as cause of ulcers, 250
  ischemia and, 250, 252
Treatment (*see* Therapy)
Treponema pallidum (spirochetes), 188,
    189, 191, 193, 194
Treponemal tests, administration of, 194–195
Trichomonas vaginalis, 188
Trichomoniasis acquired by sexual contact,
    188
Trichotilomania:
  defined, 22
  psychological components of, 264, 270–271
Trypanosomiasis as cause of BFP, 196
Tuberculosis as cause of BFP, 196
Tuberous sclerosis:
  cutaneous signs of, 235
  under Wood's light, 103
Tumors, 202–205
  benign, 45–47, 202
  electrosurgery for, 106
  malignant, 202–203
  premalignant, 203–204
  (*See also specific kinds of tumors*)
Turnover, 72–73
  peeling from sunburn as, 76, 77
  in psoriasis, 123
TV (tinea versicolor), 168–170
Typhoid fever (enteric fever), 216, 218
Typhus as cause of BFP, 196
Tzanck tests, 103, 241

Ulcers, 62–64, 247–255
  arterial, 251
  bedsores as, 253–255
  causes of, 250
  dermatoses manifested by, 247–248
  erosion and, 248–249
  factitial, 253, 255, 264, 271
  incontinence and, 275
  ischemic, 250–253
  neurotrophic, 249, 251
  post-radiation, 251
  rodent (*see* Basal cell carcinoma)
  stasis, 251
Ultraviolet (UV) light therapy, 107–108
Undertucked cells, 28
Uremia as cause of pruritus, 67
Urethritis, 176
Urticaria (hives), 56
  as allergy, 87, 90, 91, 227
  atopy in, 128
  DH and, 248
  in EM, 246
  as manifestation of cancer, 233
  pruritus in, 57, 85
  serum sickness as, 219
  therapy for, 87, 286, 287
Urticaria neonatorum (toxic erythema,
    erythema neonatorum, erythema
    neonatorum allergicum), 35
Urticaria pigmentosa, cutaneous signs of,
    230–231

UV-A (*see* Long ultraviolet radiation)
UV-B (*see* Middle ultraviolet radiation)
UV-C (*see* Short ultraviolet radiation)

Vaginal thrush, 161
Vaginitis, 48
  monilial, 116
Varicella (*see* Chicken pox)
Variegated color of malignant lesions, 213
Variola (*see* Smallpox)
Vascular nevi (hemangiomas), 37–41
Vascular reaction patterns, 86–87
Vasculitis:
  allergic, 216
  palpable purpura and, 236
  purpura and, 89
  ulcers and, 250
V.D. (*see* Venereal disease)
Vehicles (medication bases) types of, 284
Vellus hairs (Panugo hairs), 18
Venereal disease (V.D.), 187–199
  acquired by sexual contact, 188
  adolescent fear of, 44
  chancroid as, 196, 198
    acquired by sexual contact, 188
    as minor venereal disease, 187
  gonorrhea as, 197–198
    acquired by sexual contact, 188
    as major venereal disease, 187
  granuloma inguinale as, 199
    acquired by sexual contact, 188
    as minor venereal disease, 187
    ulcers and, 250
  lymphogranuloma venerium as, 187, 188,
    198
  obtaining information on, 44
  syphilis as, 189–196
    acquired by sexual contact, 188
    early, 189–193
    effects of, 21, 191–192
    infectivity of, 280–281
    late, 193–194
    as major venereal disease, 187
    secondary, 216, 218–219
  tests to detect, 194–195
Venereal warts (condyloma accuminata),
  171, 172, 188
Venous insufficiency, 50
  ulcers and, 250, 252
Venous stasis dermatitis, pruritus and, 68
Vernix caseosa, composition of, 23
Verruca filiformis (filiform warts), 171, 172
Verruca plana (flat warts), 171, 172
Verruca plantaris (plantar warts), 171, 172
Verruca vulgaris (common warts), 171, 172
Vesicles, 58
  defined, 57
  systemic disease manifested by, 216, 220,
    223
Vesicular eczematous dermatitis, 96
Viral exanthems:
  cutaneous signs of, 216, 218
  in oral cavity, 186
  pruritus and, 67

Viral infections, 170–179
  alopecia and, 21
  herpes simplex as, 175–179
    disseminated, 216
    eczema and, 131
    infectivity of, 281
    multinucleate cells of, 102
    primary cell damage in, 240
  molluscum contagiosum as, 174, 175
    acquired by sexual contact, 188
    as benign neoplasms, 205
    scooping out of, 105–106
    primary cell damage in, 240
    responsible for BFP, 196
  warts as, 170–174
    as benign tumors, 205
    infectivity of, 281
    therapy for, 105, 106, 108, 172–174
    types of, 170–172
    venereal, 171, 172, 188
Viral tonsilitis, 176
Vitiligo:
  characteristics of, 140, 141
  described, 56
  hyperthyroidism and, 226
  psychological component of, 264
  treatment of, 142
  under Wood's light, 103
Von Recklinghausen's disease (neuro-
    fibromatosis), 235
Vulvitis, 48
Vulvovaginitis, herpes simplex and, 176

Warts, 170–174
  as benign tumors, 205
  infectivity of, 281
  therapy for, 105, 106, 108, 172–174
  types of, 170–172
  venereal, 171, 172, 188
Weil-Felix test, 222
Wens, 47
Wet dressings, 282
Wet-to-dry dressings, 283–284
Wheals, 56–58
Wickham's striae, described, 144
Wood's light examination, 101–103, 152, 166,
  169
Wound healing granulation tissue in, 81
Wright's stain, 103
Wrinkling:
  due to sun exposure, 76, 80
  in xeroderma pigmentosum, 206

Xeroderma pigmentosum, described, 206
X-ray:
  alopecia and, 21, 22
  primary cell damage from, 240
  skin cancer and, 207
  ulcers caused by, 250
X-ray therapy, 40, 108–109, 158

Yeast infections (*see* Fungus infections)

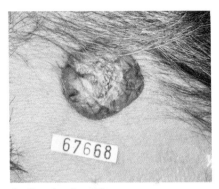

A Basal cell carcinoma

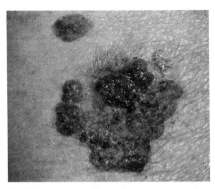

B Squamous cell carcinoma

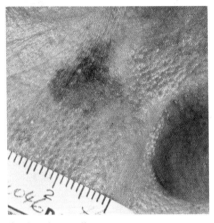

C Lentigo maligna

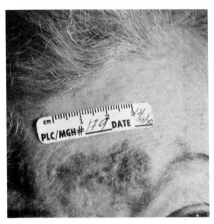

D Malignant melanoma type 1

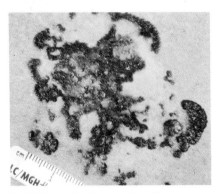

E Malignant melanoma type 2

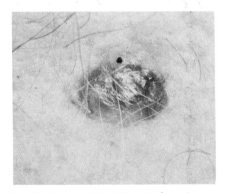

F Malignant melanoma type 3